Clinical Management of Renal Transplantation

DEVELOPMENTS IN NEPHROLOGY

Volume 32

The titles published in this series are listed at the end of this volume.

Clinical Management of Renal Transplantation

Editor

Mary G. McGeown

CBE, DSc (Hon), DMSc (Hon), MD, PhD,
FRCP (Lon., Edin. and Dublin)

Professorial Fellow of Medicine
Queen's University of Belfast
United Kingdom

Kluwer Academic Publishers

Dordrecht / Boston / London

Library of Congress Cataloging-in-Publication Data


```
Clinical management of renal transplantation / editor, Mary G. McGeown
      p.    cm. -- (Developments in nephrology ; v. 32)
    Includes index.
    ISBN 0-7923-1604-5 (hb : alk. paper)
    1. Kidneys--Transplantation.  2. Kidneys--Diseases--Patients-
  -Hospital care.    I. McGeown, Mary G.  II. Series: Developments in
  nephrology ; 32.
    [DNLM: 1. Kidney Transplantation.   WJ 368 C641]
  RD575.C558   1992
  617.4'610592--dc20
  DNLM/DLC
  for Library of Congress                                  91-46770
```


ISBN 0-7923-1604-5

Published by Kluwer Academic Publishers,
P.O. Box 17, 3300 AA Dordrecht, The Netherlands.

Kluwer Academic Publishers incorporates
the publishing programmes of
D. Reidel, Martinus Nijhoff, Dr W. Junk and MTP Press.

Sold and attributed in the U.S.A. and Canada
by Kluwer Academic Publishers,
101 Philip Drive, Norwell, MA 02061, U.S.A.

In all other countries, sold and distributed
by Kluwer Academic Publishers Group,
P.O. Box 322, 3300 AH Dordrecht, The Netherlands.

Printed on acid-free paper

Printed in the Netherlands

Dedicated to the staff of the Renal Unit who worked so loyally as a team with me over the years from 1968 to 1988, and to the patients for whom we were privileged to care.

"For mercy has a human heart;
Pity, a human face;
And Love, the human form divine;
and Peace, the human dress.
Then every man, of every clime,
That prays in his distress,
Prays to the human form divine:
Love, Mercy, Pity, Peace."

– William Blake.

Table of contents

About the editor

After graduating in medicine, the editor worked for three years in the Queen's University Department of Biochemistry obtaining the degree of PhD. Returning to medicine, she spent some five years on research on calcium metabolism and the causes of renal calculi. In 1959 she set up a service for the treatment of acute renal failure. During the next decade this service was expanded to include the management of nephrological problems in general, and the treatment of advanced chronic renal failure by haemodialysis. A renal transplant unit was established in 1968. The results of renal transplantation achieved in the Belfast Unit have been acknowledged as being amongst the best in the world. In 1983 she was made an honorary Doctor of Science by the New University of Ulster, and in 1991 an honorary Doctor of Medical Science by the Queen's University of Belfast. In 1985 she was appointed Commander of the British Empire by Her Majesty the Queen.

List of Contributors

John P. Alexander, MB, Bch, BAO, FRCPI, FFARCSI, DA, Consultant anaesthetist, Intensive Care Unit, Belfast City Hospital, Belfast.

J. Henry Brown, MD, MRCP, Senior registrar, The Mary G. McGeown Regional Department of Nephrology, Belfast City Hospital, Belfast.

Ciaran C. Doherty, MD, FRCP, Consultant nephrologist, The Mary G. McGeown Regional Department of Nephrology, Belfast City Hospital, Belfast.

Richard A. Donaldson, BSc, MB, BCh, BAO, FRCS, Consultant urologist and consultant transplant surgeon, Department of Urology, Belfast City Irospital, Belfast.

James F. Douglas, MB, BCh, BAO, FRCP, BCL, Consultant nephrologist and head of The Mary G. McGeown Regional Department of Nephrology, Belfast City Hospital, Belfast.

Claire M. Hill, MD, FRCPath, FRCPI, Senior lecturer and consultant pathologist, the Queen's University of Belfast, Institute of Pathology, Royal Victoria Hospital, Belfast.

S. Robin Johnston, FRCS, Consultant urologist, Department of Urology, Belfast City Hospital, Belfast.

Patrick F. Keane, MD, FRCS, Senior registrar, Department of Urology, Belfast City Hospital, Belfast

Joseph A. Kennedy, MCh, FRCS, Consultant urologist and head of the Department of Urology, Belfast City Hospital, Belfast.

Robert M. Kernohan, FRCS Ed, Consultant transplant surgeon and consultant urologist, Departments of Urology and Nephrology, Belfast City Hospital, Belfast.

Alan Larkin, MB, BCh, BAO, MRCP, Consultant radiologist, Department of Radiology, Belfast City Hospital, Belfast.

Gavin G. Lavery, MD, FFARCS, Consultant anaesthetist, Robert Gray Regional Intensive Care Unit, Royal Victoria Hospital, Belfast.

W. Gordon G. Loughridge, MA, MB, BCh Camb, MD, FRCS Ed, Consultant urologist, Department of Urology, Belfast City Hospital, Belfast.

A. Peter Maxwell, MD, MRCP, Senior registrar, The Mary G. McGeown Regional Department of Nephrology, Belfast City Hospital, Belfast.

Derek Middleton, BSc, MD, MRCPath,
Top scientific officer and head of
Department of Tissue Typing, Central
Laboratories, Belfast City Hospital,
Belfast.

**Mary G. McGeown, CBE, DSc (Hon),
DMSc (Hon), MD, PhD, FRCP, FRCPE,
FRCPI,** Professorial fellow, the Queen's
University of Belfast, Department of
Medicine, Belfast City Hospital, Belfast.

Peter T. McNamee, MD, MRCP,
Consultant nephrologist, The Mary G.
McGeown Regional Department of
Nephrology, Belfast City Hospital, Belfast.

William Nelson, MD, MRCP, Consultant
nephrologist, The Mary G. McGeown
Regional Department of Nephrology,
Belfast City Hospital, Belfast.

Brian G. Wilson, MCH, FRCP, Senior
registrar, Department of Urology, Belfast
City Hospital, Belfast.

Preface

Young doctors often come to work in a kidney transplant centre, as part of their training rotation, without previous knowledge of transplantation and indeed without the intention of staying there for any lengthy period. They may well be bewildered about where to begin reading on the subject, which takes in a number of specialties, including nephrology, transplant surgery, immunology, tissue typing, urology, general medicine and general surgery, not to mention laboratory sciences such as bacteriology, haematology and biochemistry, and presupposes some knowledge of them all. Publications at all levels abound on these subjects, but the doctor new to the field cannot read and digest them immediately on arrival. We have tried to provide a clear and concise picture of the care needed by patients who are being prepared for renal transplantation or who have recently received a kidney transplant. This account has been written in a form which we hope can be easily understood by senior medical students and nurses, as well as the medically qualified.

Renal transplantation commenced in the Renal Unit of the Belfast City Hospital in 1968, and over the 22 year period over 600 transplants have been carried out, using mainly cadaveric donors. During this period the team working in the Belfast Renal Transplant Unit has acquired considerable experience of all aspects of renal transplantation. We have together written this book in the hope that it will prove to be of use as an introduction to the subject.

Acknowledgements

All departments of the Belfast City Hospital have contributed in one way or another to our work of renal transplantation and without them it would not have been possible. We are very grateful for their help.

We wish to acknowledge the invaluable support of the Northern Ireland Kidney Research Fund and its devoted fund-raisers, and their Research Secretary, Mrs Pat Watters.

We wish to thank Mrs Pauline Patterson and Mrs Ruby Watson for typing the final text.

Emeritus Professor Gordon Dunstan, MA, FSA, DD (Hon), kindly read chapter 2 and gave much helpful advice.

CHAPTER 1

History of renal transplantation

MARY G. McGEOWN

1. History of renal transplantation

Fra Angelico's famous picture of the Saints Cosmas and Damian grafting a black leg onto a white patient is often shown as the first transplantation. Another picture of this mythical event, by an unknown artist, shows the patient with a black thigh, the remainder of the limb being apparently his own. A bystander is proudly showing his black thigh to the patient, no doubt reassured by seeing that a previous similar graft has succeeded. Modern transplantation has not yet caught up with the reputed skill of Cosmas and Damian.

Leaving the realms of speculation, transplantation could perhaps be considered to begin with the discovery about 1860 by Reverdin and others that slivers of skin could be transplanted from one part of the body to another, but failed if transferred from one individual to another. It was claimed that fragments of solid organs could also be transplanted.

At the beginning of this century methods of suturing blood vessels were developed and paved the way for attempts to transplant the kidney. In 1902 Ullmann demonstrated to the Vienna Medical Society a dog with the kidney transplanted from the normal site to the neck vessels, the ureter being left free through the skin producing urine. At the same year in another Viennese hospital Decastello carried out a dog-to-dog transplant and the kidney produced urine. A similar experiment by Ullmann also succeeded but neither of them seems to have carried the experiment further. About 1905 Carrel, working in Jaboulay's laboratory in Lyon, using improved methods of suturing, carried out kidney grafts between cats and dogs, then removed the animals' own kidneys, and found that they functioned well for a few days after which urine ceased. Carrel left to work in the United States, where he continued to develop methods of suturing blood vessels, for which he was given the Nobel Prize in 1912. He is still remembered and referred to in later chapters of this book.

Jaboulay, Carrel's teacher, is credited with the first transplantation of animal organs to man. During the first decade of this century he transplanted

Mary G. McGeown (ed.), Clinical Management of Renal Transplantation, 1–8.

a goat and a pig kidney into patients with chronic renal failure. In each case the kidney produced urine but ceased after about an hour. In 1910 in Berlin Unger also attempted transplantation of kidneys between animals and man, but urine was not produced in his experiments.

In 1923 Williamson in Boston repeated the dog to dog experiments and again the kidneys functioned for a short time. He examined the failed kidneys and used the word "rejection" in his description.

The first patient to patient kidney grafts were carried out in the Ukraine by Voronoy. He transplanted cadaver kidneys on six occasions between 1933 and 1949, but none of them achieved useful function. In 1946 in Boston a human kidney was transplanted to the vessels in the arm but it functioned only briefly.

Further attempts to transplant cadaver kidneys were made in the early 1950s by Küss and Dubois in Paris and by Murray, Holden and Hume in Boston. Small doses of ACTH or cortisone were given to some of the recipients in the hope of preventing the rejection which occurred in the animal experiments, and in a few the kidney survived for a short time. The early grafts were placed superficially in the thigh, but soon thereafter the pelvic vessels were used, placing the kidney within the iliac fossa.

Simultaneously with the clinical attempts at transplantation, in both Europe and America the nature of the rejection process was being studied, by the behaviour of skin grafts in mice and of kidney grafts on dogs. It was shown that skin could be successfully transplanted between litter mates, but not between different litters of the same parentage. This suggested that it should be possible to transplant kidneys between individuals whose genetic inheritance was sufficiently close without fear of rejection. The kidney is a duplicated organ. One can be spared.

The first, and successful kidney transplant between identical twins, was carried out in Boston by Murray and his colleagues in 1954. The kidney supported the patient for eight years, until recurrence of the original disease (nephritis) led to its failure. Over the next few years transplantation between identical twins was carried out in several centres in both Europe and America. Some of the grafts failed for technical reasons but in none was there evidence of rejection. The first transplant in Belfast in 1962, between identical twins, was a technical failure.

Although not directly related to the transplant operation, the invention of the first useful artificial kidney by Kolff in Holland during the Second World War was a very important development which facilitated the support of the patient with kidney failure. At first the artificial kidney could not be used to support the patient for more than a short time as superficial blood vessels were used up at each treatment. The invention of the semi-permanent arterio-venous shunt by Scribner in 1962 allowed the same pair of blood vessels to be used repeatedly for haemodialysis until transplantation could be arranged. Later technical advances in haemodialysis, and the invention of the subcutaneous arterio-venous fistula made it possible to support patients with terminal renal failure for many years if necessary.

Few patients reaching end stage renal failure are fortunate enough to have an identical twin who is willing to donate a kidney and can spare one. Attempts to graft kidneys between non-identical twins, between siblings, or from parent to child all failed. It was obvious that a way of preventing rejection had to be found if kidney transplantation was to become clinically useful.

The first attempts to prevent rejection used total body irradiation prior to transplantation. Between 1958 and 1960 this was used in Boston for 12 recipients, one, between non-identical twins, was successful. In Paris in that period one sibling graft succeeded. These attempts showed that rejection could be suppressed, but while irradiation prevented rejection most patients died from overwhelming infection and/or bone marrow toxicity. A less toxic method of immunosuppression was needed and the search began for a drug which was effective at suppressing rejection but was non-toxic or nearly so. The pursuit of the Holy Grail of a non-toxic and totally effective immuno-suppressive drug has continued over more than three decades but it must be admitted that it has not yet been found. The story of immunosuppression will be considered further in Chapter 15.

2. Development of renal transplantation in Northern Ireland

2.1. *1962–1965*

In 1962 when kidney transplantation began to move from the realm of pure experiment, there was already a renal unit established in Northern Ireland. The Renal Unit, like others at that time, had been set up in the Belfast City Hospital in 1959 for the treatment of acute renal failure, in patients whose kidney function was likely to recover if supported for a relatively short time. Inevitably some of the patients who received this treatment did not recover worthwhile renal function. There was as yet no method of longer term replacement of kidney function, and such patients died. While the Scribner arterio-venous shunt had just been invented it was not fully evaluated. These circumstances led to my early interest in renal transplantation.

There was much discussion about the possibility of keeping kidney patients alive indefinitely, and even at work, using the Scribner shunt for regular haemodialysis. Nevertheless it seemed to me that transplantation would eventually prove to be the best way to replace kidney function. However haemodialysis might play an important part, by being used to make these very ill patients fit for surgery and to maintain them until a kidney could be found. If the graft failed it was hoped that the patient would return to dialysis therapy and could have a second, or even a third or fourth graft.

This eventually came to pass and now thirty years later in Northern Ireland there are some patients who have functioning third transplants and two who have survived to have their fourth functioning graft.

The first patient to be transplanted here was a young woman who arrived in the Renal Unit in 1962 suffering from advanced renal failure and severe hypertension. She was almost blind from bilateral detachment of the retina. This patient differed from many others in that she had an identical twin who was willing to donate and could spare a kidney. The evidence of identity rather than ordinary sibship lay in their close resemblance, allowing for the difference due to illness and profound anaemia, the sharing of the same ABO group and minor red cell groups, and finally the non-rejection of transplants of skin between them. A kidney was removed from the healthy girl and transplanted into her sister, but the kidney never functioned.

About this time several other centres in Great Britain began to attempt renal transplantation, using live related donors. In Belfast over the next three years three patients with end stage renal failure were investigated with a view to finding a kidney donor from their family. Two patients, with the consenting relative (a parent in each case), were sent to other centres in Great Britain for a transplant but neither survived. It is interesting that the failures were due not to rejection but to technical complications of the transplant operation. The third patient, who did not have a suitable relative, received a transplant from a cadaver donor but died from bone marrow toxicity due to the immunosuppressive drug, cyclophosphamide.

2.2. *1965–1968*

In Belfast early in 1965 it became possible to attempt to maintain patients by regular artificial kidney treatment (haemodialysis), at first treating one patient at a time, later two patients. By this time the technique of insertion and care of the arterio-venous shunt had been mastered, though the only equipment available was the twin coil Kolff kidney needed for the treatment of patients with acute renal failure. For this reason the early patients with chronic renal failure received their treatment during the night.

Early in 1965 I was able to arrange for St. Mary's Hospital, London, then very actively engaged in the development of renal transplantation, to take a patient for a cadaver kidney graft. This graft survived and the patient returned to Northern Ireland for immunosuppression to be continued here. The kidney continued to function well for over eight years, but was lost after the patient developed deep venous thrombosis on the side of the graft following a plane journey. Following this success a continuing arrangement was developed with St. Mary's Hospital and later with Professor (now Sir) Roy Calne's Unit in Cambridge. The second patient, transplanted in August, 1965, also received a cadaver graft which continues to function well over 27 years later. When a patient was admitted to the Belfast Unit who seemed in every way suitable, he/she was presented to one or other of these units and, if found acceptable, the patient was maintained with regular haemodialysis until transferred for a place on their programme.

The waiting period sometimes lasted for several months or even a year or more, before there was a space for a patient of the appropriate blood group, as the transplant centres tried to have in readiness one recipient of each ABO group to receive any appropriate kidney which became available. Matching was on the basis of ABO group only. The lymphocyte cross match had not yet been discovered. After two months or more the patient returned to Northern Ireland and immunosupressive therapy was continued under my supervision at the Belfast City Hospital.

This system of transplant brokerage was continued until facilities for transplantation were provided in Belfast towards the end of 1968. A total of 14 patients, including the three above, received transplants in UK centres, those after 1965 being carried out in London or Cambridge. Nine returned with functioning grafts and three remain alive with good function of the graft now 27, 25 and 25 years later, while four other grafts functioned for 5 years or longer. It is remarkable that all of the successful grafts came from cadaver donors, and those from live related donors failed. This experience may partly explain my strong preference for cadaver donation.

Towards the end of 1965 there was a modest expansion of the facilities for haemodialysis and it became possible to provide treatment for four patients regularly twice weekly. Once four patients had commenced treatment, no further patients could be accepted until a space was created by either the provision of a transplant for, or the death of, an existing patient. The system of "transplant brokerage" which had grown up, while useful, was in no way sufficient to allow for the treatment of the new patients who continued to arrive. More facilities were badly needed.

3. Expansion of renal replacement therapy

In 1968 a small purpose-built unit was provided to accommodate a haemodialysis area and facilities for transplantation. By the time the unit was ready the demands for treatment had already outstripped the six places provided. Home haemodialysis was being used in other parts of the UK to allow the treatment of more patients but was not feasible here because of the serious civil disturbances which commenced about this time.

A 10-bed ward for haemodialysis was opened in May 1972, funded at first to treat 20 patients. During the first year of its existence there was a small outbreak of hepatitis B (four cases) which required the setting up of an isolation area for the infected patients. About this time many British units suffered outbreaks of hepatitis B which caused deaths among patients and staff. In the Belfast Unit no new patients were admitted for nine months (six months after the last infection was diagnosed – the recommended practice).

A rigorous routine for prevention of hospital borne cross-infection was instituted. While over the years the routine has lapsed in most units, it has been reintroduced recently in some areas where the patients may be carriers of HIV virus, and perhaps hepatitis also.

There have been increases in funding for haemodialysis several times over the years allowing increased numbers of patients to be treated. The existing ward was used more intensively, dialysis sessions increased to six days weekly, night dialysis was reintroduced in 1980, more efficient dialysis equipment made it possible to shorten each session while still giving adequate treatment. By 1991, 92 patients are receiving regular treatment in the same area.

Haemodialysis treatment has been provided closer to home for some patients living in the western part of Northern Ireland in a 6 bed satellite unit in the Tyrone County Hospital in Omagh. This is used for patients already stable on treatment, when constant attendance of trained nephrologists is not necessary.

3.1. *Continuous ambulatory peritoneal dialysis*

The introduction of continuous ambulatory peritoneal dialysis (CAPD) by Nolph in 1976, developed by Oreopoulos into a practical tool which patients could quickly learn to use at home, allowed a world wide expansion of treatment of patients with end-stage renal failure. We recall that Oreopoulos spent three years training in nephrology in the Belfast Unit before he emigrated to Canada in 1970.

CAPD was first used in Belfast in 1978 for an elderly patient who quickly learned the simple techniques involved and continued his own treatment even when in hospital for a femoral bypass. CAPD has been used for the treatment of children and for elderly patients who are medically unsuitable for transplantation, and for patients for whom it is difficult to find a graft because they have high titre antibodies or rare tissue type. Unfortunately, although only very simple equipment is needed and no staff are involved, CAPD is almost as expensive as haemodialysis because of the cost of the sterile fluids and disposables. However it has been used as extensively as funding allows, and the number of patients on renal replacement therapy has thereby been increased to about 182.

4. Renal transplantation in Belfast after 1968

The experience gained from the management of the patients who were sent to have their renal transplants in other centres was invaluable and was used

Table 1. Belfast recipe for renal transplantation

1. Special unit designed to minimize infection
2. Organization of team – each member assigned own duties
3. Cadaver donors (usually)
4. Preparation of recipient
5. Tissue matching
6. Transplant operation – duties planned
7. Immunosuppression – precribed by nephrologist
8. Long term follow-up very important

in planning. The plan later came to be known as the "Belfast Recipe for Transplantation" (Table 1).

During the 1960s a major cause of graft loss was the death of the patient from infection. This lesson was made clear by the fact that three of the five patients who did not return to Belfast after transplantation had died from infection. The heavily immunosuppressed patient with a new wound was clearly very susceptible to infection, and we decided to take special measures to protect against hospital cross-infection.

The new renal unit was designed with "clean" and "dirty" corridors, between which the single patient wards were situated, with graded positive pressure ventilation (Figure 1). On the opposite side of the "clean" corridor from the wards was the operating theatre, the dialysis room, and the sterile goods store. All used items from the patient's wards were disposed of through double-door hatches to "dirty" corridor. Staff changed into sterile theatre clothing before entering the "clean" area. Visitors were limited in numbers and wore clean gowns, masks and over-shoes.

The function of each member of the staff was carefully considered and each member of the team had a list of his/her specified duties and knew exactly what was to be done when a transplant was to take place. From the beginning, we expected that most donor kidneys would come from cadavers, and planned for this rather than for live related donors which was then the usual procedure.

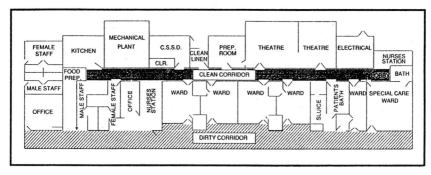

Figure 1. Plan of the Renal Unit.

The investigation and preparation of the recipient, the arrangements for tissue matching, the details of anaesthesia, the transplant operation, and immunosuppression were all discussed and agreed by the team. These arrangements, and the modifications introduced as our experience increased, will be described in later chapters.

CHAPTER 2

Ethical considerations

MARY G. McGEOWN

The Reverend Professor Gordon Dunstan, Emeritus Professor of Moral and Social Theology, King's College, London, has defined ethics in a medical context as "the obligations of a moral nature which govern the practice of medicine". He expresses these obligations as the duty to serve and protect the interests of the patient in ways consistent with the ethics of the profession and the moral values held in common by society. Ethics play an important role in the practice of nephrologists. Once treatment of a patient has been initiated ethics must be considered in every aspect of management. The acceptance of the patient for treatment in the first place is fraught with decisions of an ethical nature. Once accepted ethical considerations may be involved in what treatment should be given and how it should be managed within the context of the patient's family. The decision that a renal transplant should be arranged produces a new crop of ethical dilemmas, particularly if a live donor, related or unrelated, is considered. Termination of treatment, either at the request of the patient, or by others is not very uncommon – how and when (if ever) can it be contemplated? Finally ethics are involved in the global decision as to how medical resources should be managed – does our duty to our own patients outweigh our duties to the provision of treatment for other sick people?

1. Dialysis

In former times once renal function had ceased permanently life ended within a short time as there was no effective treatment. The prospect was changed dramatically by the introduction of the arterio-venous fistula by Quinton and Scribner in 1960. This permitted the repeated regular use of artificial kidney treatment and opened up the possibility of prolonging the life of patients with terminal renal failure almost indefinitely. It also introduced a series of ethical problems which have increased in number and complexity with the passage of time.

When first introduced in 1962 regular dialysis therapy (RDT) was available

Mary G. McGeown (ed.), Clinical Management of Renal Transplantation, 9–26.
© 1992 *Kluwer Academic Publishers, Dordrecht. Printed in the Netherlands.*

only in Seattle and only for very few patients. Over the next few years it was developed elsewhere, by enthusiastic young doctors usually working in academic centres. They were able to cater for only a handful of patients. In this respect its development did not differ from that of new advances in other specialties. However it did differ in that its availability or non-availability meant the difference between life and death for individual patients. Everywhere the treatment facilities were capable of accepting only a few patients, the number being far below those in need of it. Thus from the very earliest days nephrologists were brought face to face with the ethical dilemmas surrounding the decisions of which patient should receive treatment and which left to die.

Scribner and others set up committees to help spread the responsibility for the decisions which had to be made. There was no way by which all those in need could be treated. Once the life-boat was full taking in more people merely reduced the chances of survival of those already in the boat, unless a space was created by the removal of an existing patient either by death or by transplantation. I faced similar awesome decisions in Belfast. I remember with sorrow many young and in every way worthy people for whom, at their time, there was no room in the boat. The stark reality at the beginning was that we could treat two people and two only.

So we had to face the first of our ethical dilemmas – shortage of facilities, more patients than could be treated, with the corollary of the need to decide who should have treatment and who left to die. Many more patients can now be treated, but this dilemma still remains in underdeveloped countries where large numbers of patients still die from renal failure. The decision and the dilemma may still be present even where they seem to have disappeared.

At this stage transplantation lagged well behind regular dialysis therapy and was associated with a much higher mortality. Most renal physicians considered that dialysis was safer. Expansion of facilities for regular haemodialysis seemed the way forward. In 1964 Shaldon, at the Royal Free Hospital in London, began to train patients to undertake haemodialysis in their own homes, thus effectively creating more facilities outside the hospital. Home haemodialysis was shown to be possible and it was developed mainly in the United Kingdom. It never took off in Europe and had limited application in America. At its peak it catered for a few hundred people, and was eventually ousted by what had been regarded as the Cinderella of RDT – peritoneal dialysis.

During the early 1960s peritoneal dialysis was still in its infancy – catheters were improvised from urethral rubber catheters, peritoneal dialysis fluid was prepared from mixtures of the intravenous electrolyte solutions then available. Peritoneal dialysis usually failed because of peritonitis and it was regarded as a very inferior form of treatment.

Continuous ambulatory peritoneal dialysis (CAPD) was more than a decade away. However when Nolph recognised that the efficiency of peritoneal dialysis could be greatly increased by leaving the dialysis fluid in continuing contact with the peritoneal membrane, and the technique was simplified and developed by Oreopoulos, CAPD was born, in 1976. The treatment could be mastered rapidly even by patients of modest intelligence and was soon being offered to many who would otherwise have been excluded. At first it was used mainly for older and otherwise disadvantaged patients, and for the very young where it meant that children could be treated at home and spared the trauma of needling. Soon its advantages to the patient of freedom from the need to fit into hospital timetables and the possibility of undertaking the treatment at work or when travelling made younger, fitter patients request it. It was not however cheaper than home haemodialysis because of the high cost of the bags of dialysis fluid and other disposable items.

1.1. *Availability of dialysis*

In the Western World during the past two decades, particularly since the introduction of CAPD, the numbers of patients receiving RDT have increased rapidly. In the Third World provision for sufferers of end-stage renal failure has not improved and most still die.

Although the pioneers of home haemodialysis, and amongst the first to introduce RDT on a wide scale, the United Kingdom (U.K.) has lagged far behind other European countries and the United States (U.S.) in its provision of dialysis facilities, particularly for older patients and those with diabetes and other disabilities. U.K. centres are able to accept up to 65 new patients per million population per annum, compared with 88.6 in Austria and 83.6 in Western Germany (1989 figures).

Aware of the shortfall, the Renal Association of Great Britain carried out recent epidemiological studies in England and Northern Ireland (1990). These have shown that there are 75–80 new adult patients per million population per annum, suffering from terminal renal failure, well above the 55 per million currently being accepted in many centres. The considerable shortfall must represent patients at present excluded from treatment, for largely unknown reasons. One reason appears to be that some patients, particularly the older and the diabetic, are never referred to a renal unit by their doctor, who perhaps expects that they will not be treated because of lack of resources.

The cost of RDT has always been high. More sophisticated equipment, improved dialysis membranes and better dialysis fluid have made shorter periods of treatment adequate and removed many of the discomforts that some patients experienced. Improvement in equipment has been a factor in making treatment more expensive. A 1978 report by the Office of Health Economics estimated the cost of haemodialysis in hospital at £10,800. In 1991 the cost had escalated to £18,000 per annum.

At the 1988 rate of acceptance of 55 per million population the reservoir of patients on RDT is about 8,000. The accumulation of new patients is well above the rate of removal of existing patients by transplantation and death so that the stock of patients will continue to increase for a number of years before a steady state is reached. The patients supported by a renal transplant will also increase and continue to consume resources (for immunosuppressive drugs, hospital outpatient attendances, etc., are estimated to cost £3,000 per annum).

There will come a point even in the richest countries when the needs for renal replacement therapy will come into conflict with those of other medical services. The treatment of renal patients consumes resources directly, and also laboratory, radiological and other services already under pressure by other specialties. More renal units are needed in U.K. – it has 1.3 dialysis centres per million population compared with 4.4 in France and 7.1 in Italy. More doctors with training in nephrology will be needed to staff the new units.

1.2. *Termination of dialysis*

The wider acceptance of patients for RDT has brought a new problem to light. The earlier more formal assessment of patients before dialysis favoured young patients who in general were more fit and had a stronger motivation to live. Now elderly chronic renal failure patients with significant other disease, especially of the cardiovascular system, receive treatment. These patients are unlikely to be "rescued" by a renal transplant: they are sicker and spend more time in hospital for treatment of their other problems. With this trend has come an increase in withdrawal from dialysis (when dialysis is still technically feasible). Recent data from both Canada and the European Dialysis and Transplant Association suggest that voluntary withdrawal from dialysis treatment is becoming common and in some studies accounts for up to 25% of deaths in dialysis programmes. Before 1980 this accounted for only 5% of deaths. Termination of treatment may be even more common than this suggests as such a death may be recorded under the disease being treated rather than withdrawal of treatment. Half the patients in one study were mentally competent when the decision to cease treatment was made and 39% of the mentally competent patients had no new medical complications. It was suggested that the patients' own perception of their condition was the crucial factor in the decision to discontinue dialysis. Amongst the incompetent patients (who had recent medical complications) the decision to withdraw treatment was initiated by the physician in 73% of cases. It could be argued that patients and their families would have been spared misery and unhappiness if treatment had not been offered in the first place. Another view, and one that I would subscribe to, is that families are likely to be happier if they feel that every possible effort has been made to save their relative's life. From the viewpoint of the doctor it is much easier to accept than to exclude a patient from treatment.

It is beyond doubt that treatment should be provided for all patients who could be expected to benefit. Provision of treatment ought to be on the generous side to allow for patients, such as those discussed above who later withdrew voluntarily from treatment, who might have benefited. But doctors are not providers of treatment, they dispense it. Are they then responsible when there is not enough treatment to go round? Nephrologists have been accused of being acquiescent in accepting the situation, thus condoning the death of patients. Renal physicians feel that they have spent themselves tirelessly hammering at Government to provide more money. They have obtained much support in the public as well as in the medical press, but the large increase in spending needed at the "coal face" of patient care has not been forthcoming. The high cost of renal replacement therapy is brought into sharper focus in the U.K. where it has to be provided from the global sum allocated to the health services, rather than being paid for per item of treatment as elsewhere. Nevertheless the Government has at last accepted the profession's estimate of the need and admitted the magnitude of the problem. There may be grounds for hope that future provision for end-stage renal failure will be on a much more generous scale.

If our problems can be solved, what then of those of the Third World?

1.3. *Informed consent*

At this point informed consent needs to be considered. The patient who is to undergo renal replacement therapy must be given a clear explanation of the nature of his illness, and its prognosis should treatment not be given. The methods of treatment available must be described. After the patient has had opportunity to consider the information and to ask questions, he may wish to know which method the doctor considers to be the best option available and why. He has a right to ask this question. The doctor who answers it honestly and clearly is not being paternalistic but is fulfilling his duty to his patient. The patient must be made aware that whatever option is chosen, it may require to be changed at some time.

In most cases the patient will first require some form of dialysis but sooner or later the question of renal transplantation will arise. The implications of a renal transplant must be described in detail, and the patient given a realistic estimate of the chances of having a functioning graft, not only immediately, but after one year, three years and five years. The source of a kidney will be mentioned and the patient may suggest that a relative may wish to donate a kidney. The patient should be told that if a relative wishes he (or she) can contact the doctor for further information. The patient should not be made an intermediary for arrangements for possible live donation. Whether or not the possibility of a relative becoming a donor is mentioned, it should be

14

clearly stated that most kidneys come from recently dead individuals. The patient should not be made to feel responsible for finding the donor, or the donor feel pressurized to donate. If a relative wishes to donate or simply to have information the doctor can be contacted directly. The question of a live donor coming forward should not be explored further with the patient.

2. Transplantation

2.1. *The living related donor*

The earliest transplants were between identical twins. Doctors did not seem to be concerned that they might not be ethical. Transplants were then attempted between non-identical twins, and other less close relatives. It seems to have been generally assumed that a related donor is acceptable. This ignores the fact that there may be hidden pressures and attempts to exploit within the family. The bond between parent and child is almost always strong and consent for donation of kidneys is usually freely and voluntarily given although even when the prospective donor is a parent there may be pressures unknown to the doctor.

One such "volunteer" donor was the father of a 28-year-old man. Both parents were alive and the patient had one brother, a priest. At interview, both parents and the brother expressed willingness to give a kidney, if suitable. The mother and the brother were of a different blood group from the patient, the father matched. While the father was being investigated he confided that when undergoing appendicectomy in youth he had nearly died during the anaesthetic, and he had been told that he would not survive another anaesthetic. The situation was complicated by the fact that his wife was a Roman Catholic, while he was a Protestant and the children had been brought up in the Catholic faith. He felt that the family, especially his wife, would never forgive him if he refused to donate a kidney to his son. He preferred to risk what he regarded as certain death to refusal to donate. The father was led to believe that his kidneys were unsuitable on the pyelogram. This seemed the only humane solution. The patient later had a cadaveric kidney graft, which continues to function well more than 26 years later.

In other cases a sibling had emigrated many years previously from Ireland to Australia or the United States and there developed renal failure. The doctors responsible for treating the faraway patient, on discovering that there were siblings in Ireland, contacted the family and asked that they should have blood group and tissue type done to see if they could provide a kidney. In several cases the recipient had not seen the family or even kept in contact by frequent letters for as long as 20 years. There were the wives and children (who were young) of the prospective donors and in one case the sister's fiancé, to be considered. In the latter case I had lengthy discussions with the sister (and sometimes the fiancé) on at least five occasions, after which, in spite of the man's objections, the sister decided to go to America to see her brother. I was never told whether she did donate a kidney in the end!

Another conflict arises when an unmarried sibling or other unmarried less close relative is elected by the family to be the donor. The elected one may be too timid to refuse to "donate". It takes courage to say that you don't want to give a kidney to save Uncle Tom.

2.1.1. *Informed consent*: *the donor*

When a live donor is contemplated, the initial contact will usually be with the recipient's doctor, who will try to ensure that the offer is voluntary, that there is no benefit of any sort for the donor and that coercion has not been used. The motive for the offer should be sought, which ought to be altruism and love of the recipient. Once this is established investigation of the individual for suitability as a donor can proceed.

From the genuine case histories above it is obvious that every prospective donor must be interviewed without the recipient or other family members present. Should it be necessary to use an interpreter, this should not be a member of the family or the recipient's doctor. In the past one surgeon usually looked after both recipient and donor. Present thinking is that a different doctor should have responsibility for the donor and look after the donor's interest. When the donor is not genetically related to the recipient, or the relationship is more distant than permitted under the Human Organ Transplant Act 1989, in the U.K. the case must be referred to the Unrelated Live Transplant Regulatory Authority (Chapter 2.3).

The duties of the donor's doctor are to ensure that the donor:
1. is a volunteer;
2. has had no financial or other inducement to give a kidney, and has not been subjected to coercion;
3. understands the nature of the act for which he/she is volunteering, its consequences and risks.

The donor should be informed that despite all care, no operation is free from risk. The operation will be undertaken solely for the benefit of the recipient, and will entail more extensive surgery than would be required for the removal of a diseased kidney. It should be put bluntly "You may die". The risk of death is currently assessed as 1 in 1600 donor operations. The donor should also be informed that if he so wishes he can change his mind right up to the moment of commencement of surgery.

The view of other religions and races may need to be considered. Islam regards the donation of organs as an act of charity, benevolence, altruism and love of mankind. Donation of organs is not regarded as an act of transgression against the body.

The Chief Rabbinate of Jerusalem has stated (1990) that declaration of brain death is acceptable as establishment of death, provided that three physicians are present (elsewhere two are sufficient). One objective test of brain death is required, usually the auditory test. Jews are not only permitted but are obligated to donate: it is now a *mizveh*, a commandment to do so. Israeli law does not require consent from the family, but the doctors are required to inform the family about the intention to remove organs.

In Japan, brain death is not accepted as death, despite extensive discussion by the public, and a series of committees to examine the question, including a Japanese conference on the subject held in Copenhagen (1991). Great concern was aroused by a heart transplant carried out in Japan soon after Professor Barnard's first heart transplant. The Japanese transplant failed and the public seem to have been left with deep suspicion of the diagnosis of death in this case, and of the suitability of the recipient for surgery.

2.2. *Unrelated living donor*

When there is no related donor available the spouse may be considered. The spouse is often very willing to become a donor – for one thing life restricted by the partner's illness and treatment will be improved if the transplantation is successful. The situation is not always thus, and special care needs to be taken that the spouse is a true volunteer, especially if the pair come from overseas. Evidence is needed that the marriage is of such duration that it could not have been entered into for the purpose of procuring a donor. This information is readily available when the pair are members of the doctor's community, but in other circumstances marriage certificates, photographs of children (which may show family likenesses), affidavits etc. may be needed. Partners in stable relationships outside marriage may ask to be considered. The situation may then be more difficult to assess. The "Guidelines in Renal Transplantation and Dialysis" of the Australian Kidney Foundation has put the true meaning well – "The reason for donating should unmistakably be a charitable act arising from a special relationship between the donor and recipient. All motives other than those associated with an unfettered gift should be excluded." Donations proposed from more distant genetically related individuals should be regarded in the same way.

Particular care is needed where an offer of donation comes from a follower of the same religion who did not previously know the patient personally. The offer may stem from a truly altruistic desire to serve a much respected church member, but the emotion of the moment may out-weigh proper appreciation of what is involved.

In the early 1960s in America very occasionally a convicted criminal became a donor. It was said that the felon was being given a chance to expiate his crime, but not explicitly stated that there would be amelioration of sentence. This was regarded as wrong later. There has been a recent report that patients from Hong Kong are going to mainland China where a transplant operation can be purchased, the kidneys, in some cases at any rate, coming from executed felons.

In India kidneys bought from poor individuals are marketed for transplantation, often without appropriate medical preparation and protection for recipient and donor. The whole question of commercialism in kidney transplantation will be discussed later in relation to the Human Transplant Act.

2.3. *Cadaveric transplantation*

At first kidneys to be used for transplantation were taken after heart-beat had ceased and life was extinct. In the U.K. kidneys were removed for transplantation having regard to the Human Tissue Act of 1961. This Act addressed the responsibility for the body of the deceased. It stated that the person lawfully in possession of the body could give permission for the removal of its parts for therapeutic purposes, medical education or research, when the deceased had requested this, and there was no reason to believe that the request had been withdrawn. It further stated that where such a request had not been made such permission could be given by the person lawfully in possession of the body provided, there was no reason to believe that the deceased had any objection to this, "and that the surviving spouse or any surviving relative do not object". The interpretation of the wording "any surviving relative" produced difficulty until the Department of Health issued a circular stating that it was sufficient to make such enquiries from surviving relatives as were reasonable within the time available. Doctors seeking permission to remove organs, even when the decreased is known to have given consent, are wise not to press for donation if the relatives are strongly opposed to it, and most do not do so. Consideration for the feelings of relatives is important in the long-term strategy for increasing the supply of cadaveric organs.

During the 1970s it began to be recognised by many, not only those concerned with the supply of organs for transplantation, that brain stem death is equivalent to total brain death and therefore somatic death (Chapters 3 and 10). Early in 1978 the Transplant Advisory Panel advised the Departments of Health of Great Brain and Northern Ireland that a code of practice was needed for procedures relating to the removal of organs for transplantation. A Working Party under the chairmanship of Lord Smith of Marlow was set up to draft a code for the use of medical, nursing and administrative staff. I was privileged to be a member of the Working Party. The Code of Practice was issued in October, 1979. It included a transplantation check-list and the criteria for diagnosis of brain-death. The tests were to be carried out separately by two doctors, one of whom should be the consultant in charge of the case, or his deputy, who should have been registered for at least five years and who should have had adequate previous experience in such cases. The booklet contained the relevant sections of the Human Tissue Act, 1961.

However a small but vociferous group of doctors refused to accept that brain stem death can be regarded as "real" death. There followed a programme on television dealing with kidney transplantation, in which it was alleged that kidneys had been removed from patients diagnosed as brain dead who had still been alive by ordinary standards. The allegations were refuted and in one set of cases withdrawn. Nevertheless the number of kidney transplants was greatly reduced over many months and dialysis units were overwhelmed with new patients for whom there were no facilities.

The Code of Practice was revised by the same Working Party and reissued in February, 1983. It included more details on the diagnosis of brain death.

The doctor attending a dying patient has a duty to care for that patient as long as he lives. Professor Dunstan says that duty does not oblige the doctor "to prolong the patient's life, or his dying, by all possible means; at some point the medical management must be changed from serving the patient's interests in recovery or longer life into serving his interests in a peaceful dying. Once his patient is dead he has a presumptive duty, if asked, to help his colleagues in transplant surgery to serve patients of theirs."

A few doctors continue to question the validity of accepting brain stem death as total brain death. Professor Dunstan points out that it is essential that the criteria of brain stem death are always applied strictly. This excludes by definition patients in a persistent vegetative state where severe damage has been largely confined to the cerebral hemispheres, and the brain stem is capable of sustaining respiration and circulation spontaneously. This condition of coma or semi-coma may persist for years if fluids and nutrients are given. Lamb says a "a 'hopeless' condition does not justify either death *by* organ removal or death *for* organ removal." In an anencephalic infant the tests for brain stem death cannot be applied, and there can be no certain diagnosis of death until circulation and respiration have ceased.

3. Human Organ Transplant Act

Quite apart from the fact that the new Code did not satisfy the few objecting doctors, the profession itself became worried that living donors were being used without adequate protection for the donor. Living donation was not addressed by the Human Tissue Act and the members of the British Transplantation Society were concerned that rumours of commercialism in live donation within private practice might have some foundation in fact. They wanted a Register of all transplants to be set up. The Department of Health was unwilling to request further legislation which they regarded as not necessary, and which would erode the professional freedom of doctors.

The British Transplantation Society issued their own "Recommendations on the use of living donors in the United Kingdom", in the British Medical Journal in July, 1986 (Appendix 1, Chapter 2). The Transplantation Society at about the same time stated its views, which were very similar. The General Medical Council gave its approval of this effort by the profession to regulate its own affairs.

Negotiations with the Department of Health were still continuing when, in January, 1989, the press and other media published details of kidneys which were purchased from Turkish donors and transplanted in the Humana Hospital in London. This was followed by the passage of the Human Organ Transplant Act in July, 1989.

The Act is given in Appendix 2 of this Chapter and is discussed further in Chapter 3. It is given effect by a series of detailed Regulations. Under the Act it becomes an offence to make or receive payment for the supply of, or offer of supply of, an organ which has been or is to be removed from a dead or living person and is intended to be transplanted into another person whether in Great Britain or elsewhere. Advertisements relating to the supply of organs for transplantation are prohibited. It permits donations of organs from persons within defined degrees of genetic relationship, and specifies the ways by which the fact of the relationship is to be established. Donations from donors more distantly related than those permitted under the Act, and those from living unrelated donors may be permitted under certain restrictions. Proposals for such donations must be referred to a new statutory body, the Unrelated Live Transplant Regulatory Authority (ULTRA) for approval. The Authority may have 11 or 12 members, and is chaired by a medically qualified person who is not engaged in transplantation. A Register of all organ transplants (corneal grafts are excepted at present) was set up.

The Authority undertakes to consider quickly proposals referred to it. It has issued advice to clinicians wishing to refer proposals to it. Apart from matters directly referred to in the Act, it is charged with the duty of looking after the donor's interest. Donors must understand the nature of the medical procedure and the risks involved in donating a kidney. They must be told "You may die". A leaflet has been prepared which can be given to intending donors.

The prospective donor must be interviewed in private. The recipient or other family members must not be present. If the donor is unrelated the regulations require a report from an independent third party who has interviewed both the donor and recipient and who is acceptable to ULTRA for this purpose. In general, to be acceptable to ULTRA the person making the report should be a physician, surgeon or psychiatrist of NHS consultant or equivalent professional status who is not otherwise party to the transplant proceedings, nor a close associate of one who is. He or she should not be practising in the fields of renal medicine or renal transplantation. It is important that the third party understands that he or she is helping the Authority to satisfy the requirements of the law and is acting in an altruistic capacity.

4. The Islamic view

The view of Islam is of concern to many people. Although Islam teaches that the sanctity of the human body is not lessened by departure of the soul and death, it has permitted transplantation from early times – arab surgeons were experts at tooth transplantation over 1000 years ago. The use of porcine bone grafts which take much better than other xenografts, was recommended despite the fact that Muslims consider the pig and its products untouchable. In 1959 a Fatwa (decree) sanctioned blood transfusion, and corneal grafts from cadavers. A series of fatwas from that time onwards have all stated that donation of organs should not be regarded as transgression against the body. At the Third International Conference of Islamic Jurists held in Amman in 1986 a resolution was passed by a majority of votes, which equated brain death with cardiac and respiratory death. The Fourth International Conference in Jeddah in 1988 endorsed all previous fatwas on organ transplantation, and clearly rejected trading or trafficking in organs.

There are still some doctors who advocate the view that individuals have a right to sell parts of their body if they so wish. The view of the majority is expressed in "Guiding principles on human organ transplantation", recently issued by the World Health Organisation. The Guiding principles for the first time specifically prohibit the removal of an organ from the body of a living minor for the purpose of transplantation, though an exception may be made under national law in the case of regenerative tissues. It is stated firmly "The human body and its parts cannot be the subject of commercial transactions".

5. Conclusion

The ethical problems associated with the use of cadaveric donors are much less than those with living donors, whether related or not. There is a strong argument for avoiding the use of living donors altogether. The removal of organs from a cadaver with the consent of the family harms no one, often gives some measure of comfort to the bereaved, can restore normal health to the fortunate recipient, and in the case of kidneys allows new needy patients to be accepted for dialysis. If the cadaveric kidney transplant fails, there is no need to agonize about the fate of the kidney or the disappointment of the donor, no need to push immunosuppressive drugs at increased risk to the recipient.

Unfortunately the number of patients on all transplant waiting lists continues to grow as more older and diabetic patients are accepted, and grafts fail in some already transplanted. Some patients have to wait years before an acceptably matched cadaveric kidney is found. It will still be necessary to continue to use kidneys from live related donors, even very occasionally unrelated donors, for some time to come.

The solution for the future may lie in xenografts. Grafts may come from closely related (concordant) or widely divergent (discordant) species. Grafts from covergent species are acutely rejected by mainly cellular mechanisms similar to allograft rejection. Graft survival can be prolonged by appropriate antilymphocyte sera or subtotal irradiation: chemotherapy is less effective. Grafts from divergent species are rejected hyperacutely by largely humoral mechanisms and immunosuppression is not effective. The concordant species for man, the primates, are slow and expensive to breed, and the most suitable for size, the chimpanzee, orangutan and gorilla, are endangered and protected species which can hardly be used. ABO blood group compatibility is necessary for transplantation and blood group O, which constitutes the majority of patients of graft waiting lists, is uncommon in the baboon and other smaller primates. However it is already possible to produce discordant transgenic animals in which the human MHC genes are transferred into, for example, the pig genome. The organs of these genetically engineered animals would be less aggressively rejected and immunosuppression would be more effective. Discordant combinations could be chosen to be easy to breed, suitable for size, and perhaps favouring blood group O individuals.

Appendix 1

Recommendations on the use of living kidney donors in the United Kingdom. British Transplantation Society.

Report compiled on behalf of the British Transplantation Society by Robert A. Sells, R. W. G. Johnson and I. Hutchinson, *Br. Med. J.* 1986; 293: 257–258.

Recommendations on the use of living kidney donors in the United Kingdom

BRITISH TRANSPLANTATION SOCIETY

Cadaveric donor transplantation remains the preferred form of treatment for end stage renal disease, and the British Transplantation Society will continue to encourage an increase in the availability of cadaveric organs. The society believes that the only justification for the use of living donors in renal transplantation is the continuing shortage of cadaveric donors.

When living donors have been used by transplant units in the United Kingdom it has been traditional to accept only blood relatives as they offer a very good chance of success. In other countries where there is a severe shortage of cadaveric donors and resources living unrelated donors have been used. With improved results of kidney transplantation from unrelated cadavers, doctors are being asked to consider a broader choice of donor. The society believes that such donors should be used only exceptionally, when a cadaver or living related donor cannot be found. We consider that it would be wrong to exclude totally living unrelated donors in the United Kingdom, but their use will require extremely rigorous safeguards to avoid the exploitation of donors and the manipulation of recipients and to afford adequate protection for doctors. Safeguards are also required to minimise the chance of a surgeon

This report was compiled on behalf of the British Transplantation Society by Robert A Sells, R W G Johnson, and I Hutchinson.

Correspondence to: Mr R A Sells, Royal Liverpool Hospital, Liverpool L7 8XP.

using a donor organ from a living non-relative when he has been led to believe that the donor and recipient were blood relatives.

The society, therefore, has adopted the following guidelines. Before accepting a living donor the transplant surgeon must be satisfied that all of the following conditions have been fulfilled.

Related donors

(1) Blood relatives willing to donate organs must provide evidence of their relationship with the recipient. A family group often provides witnesses to the consanguinity of donor and recipient, and the facts must be checked by the surgeon with the family practitioner. A surgeon must not proceed to transplant a kidney from an alleged living related donor until he is convinced that the evidence is overwhelmingly in favour of the fact of consanguinity. When doubt exists about the truth of verbal evidence or (in the case of a foreign donor) written evidence about consanguinity the surgeon should insist on additional evidence being obtained to confirm or refute consanguinity. Studies on the patient and relevant family members should be performed using some or all of the following techniques: HLA A, B, and DR typing; erythrocyte antigen subtyping; globulin allotyping; and deoxyribonucleic acid (DNA) "fingerprinting."

Tests with DNA hybridisation can establish with a high degree of certainty a first degree relationship. When the patient and the proposed donor claim a more distant relationship the availability of blood from a common first degree relative would be valuable. When the surgeon's final opinion is that the evidence indicates an unacceptably high risk of non-consanguinity he should refuse to perform the operation.

The normal practices which have applied to organ donation from living relatives in the United Kingdom should be applied in all instances.

Unrelated donors

(2) When no suitable living consanguineous donor has come forward and in cases where cadaveric transplantation is not practical or possible a surgeon may, exceptionally, consider the transplantation of an organ from a living unrelated donor, provided that the following conditions apply.

(*a*) The donor is either the spouse of the recipient or a blood relative of the spouse (in law relative) or a friend who has a close and enduring relationship with the recipient.

(*b*) The donor has achieved the age of legal majority in the United Kingdom.

(*c*) The relationship claimed by the donor with the recipient must have been established beyond reasonable doubt.

(*d*) It may be necessary to seek documentary or collateral proof of the duration of the relationship.

(*e*) Any aspects of the relationship between the recipient and the donor or within the family that might indicate that the donor was the subject of pressure of whatever kind from the recipient, his family, or anyone else must have been completely investigated. If there is evidence of improper pressure the surgeon must refuse to perform the operation.

(*f*) The psychiatric and emotional suitability of the donor must have been established: he must understand the procedure and its attendant risks and be a suitably mature person for the act of donation. Due regard must have been paid to the social and family obligations of the prospective donor.

(*g*) Consent must have been freely given by the donor. He must have been given sufficient information to allow him to make his decision, and there must be clear evidence that he has understood it.

(*h*) There must be clear evidence that the motivation of the donor is both altruistic and charitable and that neither blackmail nor extortion is a motive for the donation; that the donor is receiving no money over and above his reasonable expenses and reimbursement of earnings lost through the act of organ donation; and that the donor does not seek publicity.

(*i*) The rules of confidentiality will apply to the treatment of both donor and recipient.

(*j*) There must not have been any advertising by the potential donor, the potential recipient, or any agency acting on behalf of donor or recipient.

(*k*) The diagnostic and operative procedures performed on the donor and the recipient must carry no undue risks, and there must not be any factors

BRITISH MEDICAL JOURNAL   VOLUME 293   26 JULY 1986

which are likely to decrease the chances of success of the transplant. All surgical and medical procedures are to be performed only in recognised institutions whose staff are experienced in transplanting kidneys from living related donors and cadavers.

Register and review panel for transplantations

The principle of acceptance of living, unrelated kidney donors, even rarely and in the exceptional circumstances described above, intensifies the need for a register of all organ donations and transplant operations in the United Kingdom; the society wishes all such activity to be monitored so that it may report developments to its members. To this end we urge the government to establish a compulsory register of all imports of transplantable tissues and organs into the United Kingdom, all exports of tissues and organs from the United Kingdom, and all transplant operations taking place within the United Kingdom. A record card should be completed at each such event to include not only relevant medical details but also a signed declaration by the responsible surgeon that the British Transplantation Society guidelines have been followed. A copy of each card will be filed with the Department of Health and Social Security.

A review panel will be elected by the society, the chief function of which will be to monitor this register, seek additional information from transplant teams as necessary, and report to the members of the society. In addition, the panel will advise any surgeon intending to transplant a kidney from a living unrelated donor or from a living donor whose blood relationship with the recipient is not clearly established. Donors and recipients should be informed that material identifying them may have to be made available on occasions to the panel.

The panel will consist of three members of the British Transplantation Society, but lay or professional members may be coopted in an advisory role. Transplant teams must be prepared to divulge relevant medical and personal information to the panel on request, but the panel will have no powers of enforcement.

The case of any person not acting in conformity with these guidelines will be reported to the appropriate authorities; if the person is a member he or she will be expelled from the society.

Appendix 2

Human Organ Transplant Act 1989.

A

BILL

INTITULED

An Act to prohibit commercial dealings in human organs intended
for transplanting; to restrict the transplanting of such organs
between persons who are not genetically related; and for
supplementary purposes connected with those matters.

A.D. 1989.

B E IT ENACTED by the Queen's most Excellent Majesty, by and
with the advice and consent of the Lords Spiritual and Temporal,
and Commons, in this present Parliament assembled, and by the
authority of the same, as follows: —

5   1.—(1) A person is guilty of an offence if in Great Britain he—

    (a) makes or receives any payment for the supply of, or for an offer
to supply, an organ which has been or is to be removed from a
dead or living person and is intended to be transplanted into
another person whether in Great Britain or elsewhere;

10   (b) seeks to find a person willing to supply for payment such an
organ as is mentioned in paragraph (a) above or offers to supply
such an organ for payment;

    (c) initiates or negotiates any arrangement involving the making of
any payment for the supply of, or for an offer to supply, such an
15   organ; or

    (d) takes part in the management or control of a body of persons
corporate or unincorporate whose activities consist of or
include the initiation or negotiation of such arrangements.

    (2) Without prejudice to paragraph (b) of subsection (1) above, a
20 person is guilty of an offence if he causes to be published or distributed, or
knowingly publishes or distributes, in Great Britain an advertisement—

    (a) inviting persons to supply for payment any such organs as are
mentioned in paragraph (a) of that subsection or offering to
supply any such organs for payment; or

25   (b) indicating that the advertiser is willing to initiate or negotiate
any such arrangement as is mentioned in paragraph (c) of that
subsection.

Prohibition of
commercial
dealings in
human organs.

HL Bill 77   50/2

(3) In this section "payment" means payment in money or money's worth but does not include any payment for defraying or reimbursing—

    (a) the cost of removing, transporting or preserving the organ to be supplied; or

    (b) any expenses or loss of earnings incurred by a person so far as reasonably and directly attributable to his supplying an organ from his body.

(4) In this section "advertisement" includes any form of advertising whether to the public generally, to any section of the public or individually to selected persons.

(5) A person guilty of an offence under subsection (1) above is liable on summary conviction to imprisonment for a term not exceeding three months or a fine not exceeding level 5 on the standard scale or both; and a person guilty of an offence under subsection (2) above is liable on summary conviction to a fine not exceeding level 5 on that scale.

Restriction on transplants between persons not genetically related.

2.—(1) Subject to subsection (3) below, a person is guilty of an offence if in Great Britain he—

    (a) removes from a living person an organ intended to be transplanted into another person; or

    (b) transplants an organ removed from a living person into another person,

unless the person into whom the organ is to be or, as the case may be, is transplanted is genetically related to the person from whom the organ is removed.

(2) For the purposes of this section a person is genetically related to—

    (a) his natural parents and children;

    (b) his brothers and sisters of the whole or half blood;

    (c) the brothers and sisters of the whole or half blood of either of his natural parents; and

    (d) the natural children of his brothers and sisters of the whole or half blood or of the brothers and sisters of the whole or half blood of either of his natural parents;

but persons shall not in any particular case be treated as related in any of those ways unless the fact of the relationship has been established by such means as are specified by regulations made by the Secretary of State.

(3) The Secretary of State may by regulations provide that the prohibition in subsection (1) above shall not apply in cases where—

    (a) such authority as is specified in or constituted by the regulations is satisfied—

        (i) that no payment has been or is to be made in contravention of section 1 above; and

        (ii) that such other conditions as are specified in the regulations are satisfied; and

    (b) such other requirements as may be specified in the regulations are complied with.

(4) The expenses of any such authority shall be defrayed by the Secretary of State out of money provided by Parliament.

(5) A person guilty of an offence under this section is liable on summary conviction to imprisonment for a term not exceeding three months or a fine not exceeding level 5 on the standard scale or both.

(6) The power to make regulations under this section shall be exercisable by statutory instrument.

(7) Regulations under subsection (2) above shall be subject to annulment in pursuance of a resolution of either House of Parliament; and no regulations shall be made under subsection (3) above unless a draft of them has been laid before and approved by a resolution of each House of Parliament.

3.—(1) The Secretary of State may make regulations requiring such persons as are specified in the regulations to supply to such authority as is so specified such information as may be so specified with respect to transplants that have been or are proposed to be carried out in Great Britain using organs removed from dead or living persons.

Information about transplant operations.

(2) Any such authority shall keep a record of information supplied to it in pursuance of the regulations made under this section.

(3) Any person who without reasonable excuse fails to comply with those regulations is guilty of an offence and liable on summary conviction to a fine not exceeding level 3 on the standard scale; and any person who, in purported compliance with those regulations, knowingly or recklessly supplies information which is false or misleading in a material respect is guilty of an offence and liable on summary conviction to a fine not exceeding level 5 on the standard scale.

(4) The power to make regulations under this section shall be exercisable by statutory instrument subject to annulment in pursuance of a resolution of either House of Parliament.

4.—(1) Where an offence under this Act committed by a body corporate is proved to have been committed with the consent or connivance of, or to be attributable to any neglect on the part of, any director, manager, secretary or other similar officer of the body corporate or any person who was purporting to act in any such capacity, he as well as the body corporate is guilty of the offence and is liable to be proceeded against and punished accordingly.

Offences by bodies corporate.

(2) Where the affairs of a body corporate are managed by its members, subsection (1) above shall apply to the acts and defaults of a member in connection with his functions of management as if he were a director of the body corporate.

5. No proceedings for an offence under section 1 or 2 above shall be instituted in England and Wales except by or with the consent of the Director of Public Prosecutions.

Prosecutions.

6. An Order in Council under paragraph 1(1)(b) of Schedule 1 to the Northern Ireland Act 1974 (legislation for Northern Ireland in the interim period) which contains a statement that it is made only for purposes corresponding to the purposes of this Act—

Northern Ireland. 1974 c. 28.

(a) shall not be subject to paragraph 1(4) and (5) of that Schedule (affirmative resolution of both Houses of Parliament); but

26

Further reading

Albar, M. A. Organ transplantation – an Islamic perspective. *Saudi Med. J.* 1991; 12: 280–284.

Donnelly, P. K., Clayton, D. G., Simpson, A. R. Transplants from living donors in the United Kingdom and Ireland: a centre study. *Br. Med. J.* 1989; 298: 490–493.

Donohoe, J. Kidney transplants from living donors. *J. Irish Coll. Phys. Surg.* 1990; 19: 12–13.

Dunstan, G. R. Ethics in kidney transplantation. *Irish J. Coll. Surg. Phys.* 1992; 21: 189–192.

Hirsch, D. J. Death from dialysis termination. *Nephrol. Dial. Transplant.* 1989; 4: 41–44.

Land, W., Dossetor, J. B., eds. *Organ replacement Therapy: Ethics, Justice, Commerce.* 1991; Berlin; Springer-Verlag.

Neu, S. Kjellstrand, C. M. Stopping long-term dialysis. An empirical study of withdrawal of life supporting treatment. *New Engl. J. Med.* 1986; 314: 14–19.

The Transplantation Society, Council of. Commercialisation in transplantation: the problems and some guidelines for practice. *Lancet* 1985; 2: 715–716.

CHAPTER 3

Legal aspects of renal transplantation

J. F. DOUGLAS

The kidney to be used for renal transplantation may be taken from a living donor or from a cadaver.

1. General principles

The Common Law (i.e. the general non-statutory law of the land, derived mainly from case precedents) regards organ transplantation as it does all other forms of medical practice: the process is governed by the general laws of crime, tort (civil wrong) and contract.

Living donation, whether or not related, is governed by the rules of Common Law and is certainly not illegal. Provided the donor gives adequate informed consent and a reasonable level of care and skill is used during the operation and the follow-up afterwards, a doctor is not at risk of any special liability.

The status of postmortem donation is somewhat uncertain. The Common Law depends very heavily on the principles of decided cases (*rationes decidendi*). Very little material is available for decision as, until the transplant era, the fate of dead bodies was rarely a matter of controversy. It is clear that no proprietary rights are recognised in a dead body. Provided that certain rights of "possession for disposal" and certain statutory powers (e.g. of the Coroner) are recognised, cadaver organ retrieval does not seem to be illegal under the Common Law. Medical practice in this area may, however, be constrained by the general principles mentioned above. It is also subject to the control of the General Medical Council (GMC), a statutory body, as regards ethical issues, although the GMC's ultimate sanctions are professional rather than personal.

2. Statutory control of cadaver organ retrieval

The near-vacuum of Common Law rulings, together with public and parliamentary concern regarding the harvesting of post mortem tissue, led to

Mary G. McGeown (ed.), Clinical Management of Renal Transplantation, 27–34.
© 1992 *Kluwer Academic Publishers, Dordrecht. Printed in the Netherlands.*

statutory intervention, culminating in the Human Tissues Act 1961 (HTA). This important Act, which replaced the earlier Corneal Grafting Act 1952, set out to clarify the law on cadaver organ retrieval and the post mortem removal of human tissue in general. It does not apply to living donor transplantation.

Lawful removal of organs is covered by Section 1 of the Act. Section 1 (1) deals with *prior consent*. If a person has expressed an intention to donate, either in writing at any time or orally in the presence of at least two witnesses during his (or her) last illness, then the person lawfully in possession of the body after death (usually a hospital) may legally authorise removal of tissue in accordance with the request. A properly completed "Donor Card" (of which many are in circulation in the community) satisfies this condition, although it is made clear by the Section that evidence of later withdrawal of consent by an individual nullifies the effect of the document. Section 1 (2) deals with the situation (much the most common) in which there has been *no prior consent*. In this case, the person lawfully in possession may authorise the removal of tissue as above, provided that, after "such reasonable enquiry as may be practicable" there is no evidence of any objection on the part of either the deceased, the surviving spouse or any surviving relative. To satisfy the Act, all removals must be effected by a fully registered medical practitioner "who must have satisfied himself by personal examination of the body that life is extinct" (Section 1 (4)). In cases in which the Coroner is involved (the large majority), the Act invariably requires his consent (Section 1 (5)).

The HTA produces few problems in practice. There is a theoretical risk of conflict if a donor has expressed an intention to donate, in writing, which is opposed by his (or her) next-of-kin. The HTA permits retrieval, but this could in some circumstances be frustrated through insistence by the next-of-kin on their Common Law right to immediate possession of the body for the purpose of disposal. It is thus wise not to ignore the wishes of the next-of-kin, except in extreme circumstances.

In site of a surprisingly large number of "loose ends", the HTA has provided an effective legal framework for organ retrieval for more than 30 years. There are a number of reasons for this. First, the majority of cases *do* require consent, both of Coroner and/or spouse or relatives. Second, the Act is essentially a clarifying statute, which does not attempt to break new ground, but merely sets out conditions under which organ donation is undoubtedly lawful. Since it expressly retains the effect of Common Law (Section 1 (8)) it is by no means clear that organ retrieval other than under its conditions is necessarily *unlawful*. Third, breach of its conditions carries no sanction and appears unlikely to be the basis for any civil claim for compensation or restitution. The Act is really no more than an enacted "Code of Practice". Its main beneficial effect is to reassure the practitioner who has complied with its terms that he (or she) does not run the risk of any liability.

Because it is squarely based on consent, few accuse the HTA of going too far. A strong body of opinion, however, believes that it does not go far enough. Supporters of this point of view claim that many organs are "wasted" due to absence of consent or failure to request it. Some advocate the introduction of "opting-out" legislation, under which organ retrieval may be allowed without reference to the donor's relatives, unless an active objection is made. Some others also support "required request" legislation, which imposes penalties on practitioners who fail to ask for organ donation in appropriate circumstances. There is evidence from some European countries and American states that such measures can be associated with an increased donation rate. However these effects are not uniform and, where effective, are also often accompanied by other donation-enhancing measures. Attempts to introduce legislation along these lines have been resisted by the United Kingdom Parliament, while a recent survey of deaths in intensive care units (ICUs) suggested that fewer potential organ donors had been overlooked than previously thought. There is evidence that potential donors in non-ICU centres (e.g., victims of cerebro- and cardiovascular events) exist in considerable numbers. New legislation might increase donation from such centres. However, past experience suggests that greatly increased donor support and transplant co-ordination would be necessary for effective and ethically acceptable results in this sector. An overall impression is that "opting-out" and "required request" legislation is unlikely to come into effect in the United Kingdom or Eire within the foreseeable future.

3. The legal concept of death

The HTA authorises the removal of organs from a donor's body "after his death". However, the clarity of this authorisation has been obscured by the intervention of modern technology, which has led to a re-appraisal of the meaning and time of "death".

It has long been known that different body structures and tissues die at different rates following irreversible cardiac arrest and the onset of "traditional death". The diagnosis of such "traditional death" has always given rise to certain difficulties (e.g., those of profound bradycardia and "suspended animation") but in general has been reliably linked to the persistent presence of asystole. Because of this linkage, the Common Law has never evolved a precise definition of death, but has merely required medical evidence that it exists. Nevertheless, with increased scientific investigation of the "death process" and the development of techniques to support "partial life" in certain types of patient, it has become increasingly clear, first, that cardiac asystole cannot be identified with death if the other vital organs can be kept alive by medical means, and, second, that the presence of a cardiac output does not guarantee the existence of a state which can be equated with life. The development of cardiac resuscitation, heart-lung bypass and cardiac transplantation are ample evidence for the first proposition, while the second is supported, not only by the long-recognised, though macabre, effects of decapitation, but by the "physiological decapitation" noted in many patients maintained in ICUs on ventilation and other life support systems. The concept of "brain death" (permanent loss of cognitive functions) has been extended to that of "brain stem death". This means the permanent loss of cognitive function associated with permanent loss of brain stem function. Since permanent loss of brain stem function, which can be diagnosed by straightforward clinical means, is incompatible with the survival of any other part of the body without artificial support and is also associated with permanent absence of cognition, it has gradually been accepted, in medical and legal thinking, that "brain stem death" should be accepted as, and equated with, "traditional death" – i.e. the end of the life process. A widespread practice has grown up, based on this concept, of declaring a patient dead, despite maintenance by artificial life support systems, as soon as brain stem death has been clearly diagnosed. Ventilation is then discontinued because, since the patient is now dead, further support of the cadaver is valueless except in so far as it may aid in the procurement of organs for transplantation.

The above concept of death has much to recommend it, not only because it gives primacy to the brain, the centre of self awareness, as the essential seat of "life", but also because it recognises that, in the absence of a living brain stem, the rest of the body cannot survive unaided. Brain stem death has been accepted as *de facto* medical evidence of death in numerous countries, while in others there has been explicit statutory recognition of its validity. In some countries, however, while brain stem death and its consequences are accepted, it is not equated with the state of "overall death". There remain, in addition, many countries in which brain stem death has neither medical nor legal recognition.

In the United Kingdom, medical practice has generally followed guidelines laid down in a Code of Practice drawn up by a Working Party of the Health Department of Great Britain and Northern Ireland in 1983. This states (Section 28) "There is no legal definition of death". Death has traditionally been diagnosed by the irreversible cessation of respiration and heart beat. This Working Party accepts the view held by the Conference of Royal Colleges that death can also be diagnosed by the irreversible cessation of brain stem function – 'brain death'. In diagnosing brain death the criteria laid down by the Colleges should be followed."

The British Code of Practice is widely followed in the United Kingdom. It appears to have the sanction of the Courts in that cases in which it has been applied have not been judicially criticised. However, it is important to realise that it does not have the force of the law and that the Courts, up to this time, have not specifically stated that brain stem death in artificially ventilated patients can be equated for all purposes with "traditional death". Since the Common Law practice has been to follow medical evidence in the diagnosis of death, it seems probable that the British Courts will accept irreversible death of the brain stem, however caused, as the one true test of death. A "double standard" of death would be extremely difficult to apply to the British legal system, for which the concept of death at one particular instant has enormous importance. The law of succession to property provides an obvious example. If property is left by Will to a person on artificial life support, such a bequest is invalid if the beneficiary is irreversibly "dead" at the time of the testator's death, but takes effect, and becomes part of the beneficiary's disposable property, if he is not regarded as "irreversibly dead" until the life support is withdrawn and circulatory arrest has occurred. The situation would become even more complicated if the testator were also to be on artificial life support, which is not wholly improbable (as in the case of two close relatives involved in the same accident). British law thus really "demands" a single definition of death, which is probably satisfied by that of brain stem death. However, without a confirmatory case decision at the highest level, the legal validity of brain stem death cannot be regarded as absolute.

Experience, biological science, logic and philosophy, as well as religious thought, morality and expediency all tend to confirm the "rightness" of "brain stem death" as the true test of irreversible dying. Nevertheless public, and even some medical, opinion remains perturbed by the divergence produced by modern technology between "personal" life and physical survival of the body in the presence of a defunct personality. British lawyers are proud of the case-led Common Law, arguing that it permits evolution of the law to cope satisfactorily with changing circumstances. However, it is not well suited to resolving the complicated issues raised by modern science and medicine. There is a strong case for the introduction of a statutory definition of death which stresses the primacy of the death of the brain stem but integrates this concept with that of "circulatory" or "traditional" death in such a way as to avoid a double definition of death. A number of models for this already exist.

Brain death is usually taken as meaning "whole brain death" (i.e. death of the cerebral hemispheres and brain stem). It should not be equated with a persistent "vegetative" or decerebrate state in the absence of evidence of death of the brain stem. Some have argued that such decerebrate patients should be regarded as "dead" because of the total absence of cognition. Such patients can breathe spontaneously, swallow, and show a response to painful stimuli. Their eyes are open and their hearts can beat normally for long periods of time. Despite some protests, present medical and legal thinking do not regard such patients as "dead". In spite of the hopeless state of such persons, it is best to regard them as still alive until the emergence of evidence of irreversible brain stem death.

4. The Human Organ Transplant Act 1989

Although the HTA 1961 confirms the lawful nature of organ retrieval under certain circumstances, there is no real evidence that, under the Common

Law, organ donation and transplantation, whether living or cadaver, are illegal in themselves. General principles of criminal law, tort and contract apply, as elsewhere. In addition, markedly unethical activities may fall foul of the powers of the GMC. Organ donation for profit might in some circumstances be regarded as contractually illegal and therefore unenforceable. However, legal attitudes towards blood donation and kindred procedures make this unlikely. Nevertheless, with the growing effectiveness of kidney transplantation and a continued world-wide shortage of organ donors, it was inevitable that the situation would be exploited for commercial purposes. During the 1980s, a "kidney trade" emerged in the British private medical sector and elsewhere. Certain living donors, from poor countries, were induced to donate kidneys, for profit (often modest) to wealthy, unrelated but adequately matched recipients in operations carried out at a private British clinic. Widely, though not universally, condemned, these operations were, at least in part, open to the control of Common Law remedies and the discipline of the GMC. An increasingly large body of opinion, however, regarded all organ donation for profit as unethical. The Human Organ Transplant Act 1989 (HOTA) was brought into force in order to curb such practices and regulate solid organ transplantation in general. The Act (with its subordinate regulations) does three main things. First, it prohibits commercial dealings in organs for transplantation, both generally and in specific ways. Second, it prohibits living donor transplantation except where (i) a close genetic relationship is proven or (ii) a specifically constituted body, the Unrelated Live Transplant Regulatory Authority (ULTRA), is satisfied that the donation has no commercial basis and is made freely, after adequate information and explanation. Third, it requires notification of all transplant operations to various Authorities, both central and local, together with sufficient information to allow these Authorities to monitor transplant practice and compliance with the Act. Any breach of the rules becomes a criminal offence, punishable on summary conviction.

The HOTA sets out clear rules for the majority of organ donation situations encountered by doctors in the United Kingdom, but, like the HTA, poses a number of difficulties. First, it applies only to transplants carried out in the territory of Great Britain (although Northern Ireland is covered by similar separate legislation) and is thus open to evasion. Second, it may be capable of being flouted by determined donors and recipients who would regard the penalties of the Act as a small price to pay for the benefit of transplantation. Third, the regulations governing proof of the genetic relationship raise several problems related to the extent of testing and the standard of proof required to establish criminal liability. Fourth, the setting up of ULTRA represents an unprecedented intrusion into the doctor/patient relationship, whose strength should be an essential part of long-term management in chronic renal failure.

Many of the difficulties of the HOTA relate to the position of the unrelated living donor. There is considerable support in British transplantation circles for a further statutory ban on all such donations (excepting spouses and certain others) although this move would not solve all the problems of the Act. A contrary view is that the Act goes too far and should have been limited to a ban on commercial dealing and the compulsory registration of transplants.

5. The future: international agreement on organ donation?

It should be remembered that the "ethical viewpoint" varies throughout the world. Different countries, cultures and religious beliefs influence public and medical attitudes. The availability of organs for donation and of renal replacement services in general (including dialysis) are also important factors. Steadily increasing transplant waiting lists do not make the issues easier to resolve. It appears probable that further statutory regulation of the whole field of organ donation will be attempted in the future. In this context, a recent "statement of guiding principles" issued by the World Health Organisation is of considerable interest. The following main principles are proposed:

1. Organs may be removed from the bodies of the deceased persons for the purpose of transplantation if: (a) any consents required by law are obtained; (b) there is no reason to believe that the deceased person objected to such removal, in the absence of any formal consent given during the person's lifetime.
2. Physicians determining that the death of a potential donor has occurred should not be directly involved in organ removal from the donor and subsequent transplantation procedures, or be responsible for the care of potential recipients of such organs.
3. Organs for transplantation should be removed preferably from the bodies of deceased persons. However, adult living persons may donate organs but in general such donors should be genetically related to the recipients. Exceptions may be made in the case of transplantation of bone marrow and other acceptable regenerative tissues. An organ may be removed from the body of an adult living donor for the purpose of transplantation if the donor gives free consent. The donor should be free of any undue influence and pressure and sufficiently informed to be able to understand and weigh the risks, benefits and consequences of consent.
4. No organ should be removed from the body of a living minor for the purpose of transplantation. Exceptions may be made under a national law in the case of regenerative tissues.
5. The human body and its parts cannot be the subject of commercial transactions. Accordingly, giving or receiving payment (including any other compensation or award) for organs should be prohibited.
6. Advertising the need for or availability of organs, with a view to offering or seeking payment, should be prohibited.
7. It should be prohibited for physicians and other health professionals to

engage in organ transplantation procedures if they have reason to believe that the organs concerned have been the subject of commercial transactions.

8. It should be prohibited for any person or facility involved in organ transplantation procedures to receive any payment that exceeds a justifiable fee for the services rendered.

9. In the light of the principles of distributive justice and equity, donated organs should be made available to patients on the basis of medical need and not on the basis of financial or other considerations.

Further reading

Skegg, P. D. G. *Law, Ethics and Medicine*. Oxford; Oxford University Press, 1984.

Working Party on behalf of the Health Departments of Great Britain and Northern Ireland. Cadaveric organs for transplantation: a code of practice including the diagnosis of brain death. London, H.M.S.O., 1983.

World Health Organisation. Guiding principles on human organ transplantation. *Lancet* 1991; 337:1470–71.

CHAPTER 4

Assessment of the patient before renal transplantation

J. F. DOUGLAS

An illness has healed when it has vanished without significant trace or consequence. It is cured when medical (or other) intervention has had the same
effect. Renal replacement therapy for end-stage renal failure cannot be
described in these terms. Despite their remarkable ability to extend life and
well-being, dialysis and transplantation remain flawed techniques. Nevertheless, progressive improvements in both allow us to hope that they might in
future lead to a "quasi-cure" for end-stage renal failure. This may be defined
as a situation in which the life and health of the sufferer has been restored
as completely as if a cure had truly been effected. The closest possible
approximation to such a "quasi-cure" should be the goal of all contemporary
management of renal failure. It follows that dialysis and transplantation
should be applied in any individual case, not as competing ends in themselves
but as a means of achieving the above objective.

In assessing the suitability of a patient for transplantation it is useful
to keep this principle in mind. Three important questions require to be
answered:

1. is transplantation a reasonable way of achieving a good result for the
   patient?
2. does transplantation offer a better way than dialysis in any given set
   of circumstances?
3. if transplantation is the better way, what preparation is necessary in
   order to improve the benefits and minimize the problems that it will
   involve for the patient?

The first two questions are considered below, while the third will be examined
in succeeding chapters.

1. Selection of patients

Who can have a kidney transplant? Selection criteria have changed considerably during the short history of transplantation. In the early days, both

Mary G. McGeown (ed.), Clinical Management of Renal Transplantation, 35–60.
© 1992 *Kluwer Academic Publishers, Dordrecht. Printed in the Netherlands.*

dialysis and transplantation were new techniques, largely untried clinically. Very few patients would have access to them and their long-term benefit was uncertain.

In the case of dialysis it was at once clear that the potential demand for treatment far outstripped the supply. Scribner in Seattle who was the first in 1962 to attempt long-term maintenance haemodialysis, reacted to the problem of selection by devising a rigid double committee selection process through which patients were screened before being accepted for treatment. They were first interviewed by a panel of physicians knowledgeable in renal disease, who decided on their medical suitability. Standards were strict: few under 15, over 45, or with ancillary disease were deemed acceptable. The next stage was a mixed lay and medical committee who decided on the patients' social and economic suitability. Many early units followed Scribner's pattern and set up selection committees, which usually included some lay members and senior nurses. Gradually the selection process became less formal, although still very thorough. Detailed guidelines were necessary in order to alleviate the agonizing nature of judgments that committee members were called on to make. Selection for dialysis largely controlled selection for transplantation. The first cadaver transplants had poor results, and haemodialysis was usually necessary until a suitable living related donor could be found. Transplantation was a relatively rare event. Since the kidney usually came from a living relation, who was put at risk by a major operation, it was very important that the recipient should both survive and prosper, in order to justify the procedure. The ideal candidate was a young adult, free from disease other than renal failure itself. The criteria for acceptance onto haemodialysis were also useful in selection for transplantation – indeed they had often been already applied to the patient. Where transplantation succeeded, its beneficial effects were markedly greater than those of dialysis. This was the main stimulus to the search for improved methods of matching and immunosuppression, leading to decreased mortality from infection and gradually improving graft survival.

Today both dialysis and transplantation (cadaver or living related) are widely practiced in developed countries and their availability to the community has greatly increased. Although expense and the inadequate supply of donors restrict both therapies and lead to increasingly long waiting lists for transplantation, it is now usually possible to assess suitability for treatment on medical grounds only without recourse to the non-medical criteria forced on Scribner and his contemporaries, as well as on ourselves in Belfast for many years. Selection and assessment effectively become the same thing, since the only issue to decide is how dialysis and transplantation can be integrated to provide the longest survival and associated higher quality of living to any given patient.

2. Assessment for transplantation

It is not always easy to decide between dialysis and transplantation, since each has its own benefits and drawbacks; nor is the decision immutable once made. Both are developing technologies and the balance between them has swayed with the decades. In the nineteen-sixties and early seventies the high mortality of post-transplant infections led many units to opt for dialysis as their primary treatment. Units which followed the Belfast low steroid regime, however, were able to combine excellent graft survival with low mortality and thus offer most patients the improved quality of life obtained by successful transplantation. From 1978 the introduction of cyclosporin began a trend of improved graft survival and reduced mortality which, by the late nineteen eighties, had led transplantation to be widely regarded as the preferred treatment, not only for uncomplicated cases, but also for patients at increased risk due to age or other factors. As the nineteen nineties begin, however, some aspects of dialysis again seem increasingly attractive. Improved quality of dialysis, the advent of high-flux biocompatible membranes, the elimination of such problems as acetate toxicity and dialysis dementia and the ability, through recombinant erythropoietin, to reverse the anaemia of end-stage renal failure, are important contributing factors to this change. The continued scarcity of transplants, the steady rise in the mean age of patients on renal replacement therapy and the greater general availability of dialysis are also relevant. While there is a tendency to try to "place" transplants where they will do most good in terms of survival and well-being, there is also an increased ability to discuss treatment openly with patients, who no longer have to feel that treatment will be denied for non-medical reasons. Such discussion, however, can lead to problems. Few people like dialysis. Even the most strict and apparently well-adapted patient tends to see a successful transplant as a liberative event – "like stepping into the light from darkness". Doctors underestimate the mental imprisonment of dialysis and are in danger of interpreting the patient's relief at its end as evidence of improved well-being. Steroid-induced euphoria can also be misinterpreted. The advantages of transplantation are thus sometimes described in an over-optimistic way to patients whose only real choice is to follow medical advice. Some of the disheartening problems of transplantation – weight gain, steroid effects, infection and neoplasia are frequently glossed over before the operation. It is true that cyclosporin has helped to reduce the full impact of steroid toxicity. Nevertheless, many other drug effects remain, including those of cyclosporin itself. Thus, while it is right to take account of the benefits of transplantation, it is a mistake to attempt, uncritically, to achieve them in every patient who might conceivably benefit. The wisest course is to aim for the "transplant miracle" in those patients for whom it is most likely to occur and to be increasingly cautious in seeking it when multiplying clinical problems make it less easy to foresee.

Table 2. Factors in assessment for renal transplantation

1. Personal
2. Primary renal disease
3. Urinary tract
4. Cardiovascular system
5. Other pre-existing diseases
6. Infections
7. Immunological status
8. Information and constant
9. Cost-effectiveness

Factors which are useful in the assessment of possible transplant recipients are shown in Table 2.

3. Personal

3.1. *Age*

In the past, transplantation was considered to be most successful in recipients aged from 15 to 40 years. Young children tended to develop serious steroid-induced side effects, such as obesity and stunting of growth. Elderly patients were at increased risk of cardiac, cerebrovascular, pulmonary, gastric, intestinal and skeletal disease; and, in addition to a naturally lower survival rate, there were higher rates of drug-related disease.

Modern steroid-sparing regimes have improved the position. In children from 5–15 years, patient and graft survival are comparable to those for young adults. There is increasing evidence that transplantation in younger children (down to as young as six months) can provide satisfactory results. Cyclosporin regimes (with minimal or no steroid) allow more normal development, notably of pre-pubertal growth. Freedom from dialysis is also basically beneficial. However, for small children, a few years on CAPD may allow a period of growth, without excessive hardship, which could make for easier transplantation in the end.

For older patients, too, steroid-sparing regimes can produce excellent results. There is no definite upper age limit for transplantation. However, both patient and graft survival decline with increasing age, making transplantation a less desirable alternative to dialysis. In face of a continued shortage of donors, younger recipients, with better long-term survival, must be given priority. In practice, therefore, it seems likely that few patients over 70 will receive transplantation in the foreseeable future.

3.2. *Sex*

There is no discernible sex difference in the survival of patients or of grafts. However, sex may be important in determining the acceptability of transplantation. Weight gain and cyclosporin-induced hirsutism can provoke a crisis of "body-image" particularly in young or middle-aged women, sometimes involving suicidal urges. Where an acceptable dialysis alternative exists transplantation for such women should not be considered until possible side-effects have been fully discussed, and accepted.

3.3. *Race*

In the United States, black recipients of cadaver donors show a lower rate of graft survival than white recipients, although their survival on dialysis is slightly better than that of whites. There is also evidence that rejection rates among Arabs in Israel are lower than among Israeli recipients. The reason is unclear. It has been suggested that transplantation between individuals in regions of racial homogeneity will show better results than in regions with heterogeneity. Such assertions are difficult to prove. In any event homogeneity may be better described in terms of HLA antigen compatibility than in terms of racial likeness. The gradual spread of transplantation throughout the world can be expected to produce better understanding of this subject.

3.4. *Social and mental factors*

These have been extensively considered in the past. In the early days of renal replacement therapy, social deviance and mental subnormality led to the exclusion of such patients from dialysis for non-medical reasons. This is no longer an appropriate stance. Renal replacement by dialysis should be freely available, subject only to the physical practicality of applying it. Transplantation, which remains a scarce therapy, is in a slightly different position. It should be offered where it promises a better quality of survival than dialysis. In some cases of social deviance (e.g. drug abuse) or severe subnormality this might not be true. In extreme situations the issue of whether any treatment can be beneficial may arise. In typical cases, however, (e.g. inadequacy, criminality or low IQ) the only proper course is to ignore the abnormality and treat these patients in the same way as their more fortunate fellow-sufferers. Whatever the form of dialysis, some sort of family support is usually essential. Although the need for dialysis can precipitate a crisis in the home, the patient living and coping alone is often at a serious disadvantage. Intelligent social work can be very valuable, not only in defining the initial situation, but also in monitoring its evolution as the patient continues to bear the strain of continued renal replacement therapy.

3.5. *Psychological factors*

It is essential that the patient be capable of following the strict discipline of regular dialysis and adhering to the rules of dietary and fluid restriction. After transplantation the immunosuppressive drugs must be taken regularly and appointments for regular reviews kept. It is helpful if the patient is seen some time before the need for renal replacement and attends the renal clinic, giving opportunity for assessment of personality and ability to follow discipline. The patient who is already very ill with seriously deranged blood chemistry at the first visit may be much more difficult to assess. The family doctor, school teachers or the employer may be able to attest that the patient is reliable and co-operative, but on the other hand may present an over-optimistic view hoping to help the patient.

Motivation is very important for without it the patient can become discouraged when the going is rough. Married patients, especially when they have children, are usually strongly motivated to get well. Adolescents pose difficult problems. Their schooling is often seriously interrupted already and plans for future training may have to be postponed, apparently indefinitely. They feel that they are different from others in their age group and often bitterly resent the restrictions imposed by their ill-health. These problems seem particularly to afflict young males, who may be very difficult with both their families and the renal unit staff. Late adolescent girls seem to manage better, especially if they already have a steady emotional relationship. Younger children may be sensitive about their appearance, especially their small size for their age, and about skeletal deformities such as knock knees, bow legs or scissors gait.

The mental stability and motivation of the patient are much more important than his intelligence. Indeed the highly intelligent patient who constantly demands information, who introduces modifications to his treatment according to what he has heard or read, can be very difficult to treat. Less intelligent patients often fare better, follow instructions carefully and with common sense, and are more tolerant of restriction and discomfort. Mentally deficient patients may be accepted as dearly loved members of their family even though problems as to future support can be foreseen.

4. Primary renal disease

Table 3 shows a list of conditions for which transplantation may be indicated. Glomerulonephritis remains the commonest cause, as shown by Table 4. There is a steady increase in the number of cases of diabetic nephropathy, non-diabetic multisystem disease and renal vascular disease; this reflects the widening scope of transplantation rather than an increasing incidence of these conditions. The nature of the primary diagnosis can have considerable bearing on the question of whether or when to transplant.

Table 3. Causes of renal failure for which transplantation may be indicated

Main causes	Example
Chronic glomerulonephritis	Most forms
Chronic pyelonephritis	Reflux nephropathy
Hypertensive disease	Hypertensive nephrosclerosis
Hereditary disease	Polycystic Kidneys Medullary cystic disease Hereditary nephritis (including Alport's syndrome) Cystinuria
Systemic disease	Systemic lupus Vasculitis Scleroderma Haemolytic uraemic syndrome
Metabolic disorder	Diabetic nephropathy Amyloid disease Cystinosis Oxalosis Fabry's disease Gout
Urological disease	Renal stones Chronic obstruction Megacystis
Drugs and toxins	Analgesic nephropathy
Irreversible acute renal failure	Cortical necrosis
Trauma	
Tumours	Renal cell carcinoma Wilm's tumour Myeloma Other

Table 4. Causes of renal disease in age range 16–64

Disease	% of total
Glomerulonephritis	28.3
Pyelonephritis/interstitial nephritis	17.1
Diabetes mellitus	10.2
Cystic kidney disease	9.4
Renal vascular disease	8.3
Non-diabetic multisystem disease	4.6
Drug nephropathy	3.3
Hereditary	2.3
Miscellaneous	3.3
Aetiology uncertain	12.8

4.1. *Glomerulonephritis*

This is the commonest cause of renal failure in patients being assessed for transplantation. Recurrence in the graft is the main potential problem (Table 5). The following points should be noted:

Table 5. Recurrent glomerulonephritis in transplanted kidneys

Original disease	Recurrences	
	% Incidence	% Graft Loss
Membranoproliferative gomerulonephritis (type 1)	15	5
Membranoproliferative glomerulonephritis (type 11)	90	10
Focal glomerulosclerosis	25	12
IgA nephropathy	50	5
Crescentic glomerulonephritis (postinfectious/idiopathic)	30	10
Anti-glomerular basement membrane (AGBM) nephritis	5	1
Idiopathic membranous glomerulonephritis	20	0
Lupus nephritis	<1	0
Henoch–Schonlein purpura	25	8

4.1.1. In the case of many proliferative lesions graft recurrence declines with time from an acute nephritogenic episode. Transplantation should not be considered until such episodes have fully subsided. For example, in the case of anti-GBM nephritis it should not be considered until anti-GBM antibodies fall to near-zero levels.

4.1.2. The rate of graft loss is lower than that of recurrence and is more important in assessing the appropriateness of transplantation.

4.1.3. Diagnosis of recurrence may be difficult. Immunosuppression may alter its histopathological pattern. In addition the rejection process may itself mimic various forms of glomerulonephritis.

Although in conditions with higher graft loss rate it may be unwise to consider living-related donor grafts, recurrence is not in general a bar to transplantation.

4.2. *Chronic pyelonephritis (reflux nephropathy)*

This condition is apparently caused by a combination of urinary infection and vesico-ureteric reflux (VUR), leading to intra-renal reflux into the compound papillae of infants and young children. The forcing of infected urine into the renal tubules triggers a process of inflammation and interstitial fibrosis which leads to scarring and distorted growth, usually with severe hypertension. Gross congenital abnormalities (e.g. megacystis-megaureter), as well as various acquired infective or inflammatory lesions of the bladder, may cause reflux. However, it most commonly results from deficiency or immaturity of the musculature of the trigone region and of the ureterotrigonal insertion, so that the normal pinch-valve action of bladder contraction fails to operate. New scarring rarely occurs in adult life, when reflux has usually been ended by bladder growth and the kidney itself is less vulnerable to intra-renal reflux. Most cases of renal failure follow childhood scarring. Infection without reflux rarely, if ever, causes pyelonephritic scarring. Thus, while end-stage reflux nephropathy may be associated with an increased rate of post-graft urinary infection, this is not a contra-indication to transplantation, which can be carried out with a high success rate. Bilateral nephro-ureterectomy has been widely practised for ureteric reflux, both before and after transplantation. Its relative merits will be discussed later.

4.3. *Hereditary renal diseases*

Where these are limited to renal lesions, as in the cases of medullary cystic disease and hereditary nephritis or polycystic disease, in which cysts in other organs, such as liver and pancreas very rarely give rise to symptoms, there is no evidence that the outcome of transplantation, as regards patient or graft survival, differs from that of other types of primary renal disease.

4.4. *Metabolic diseases*

4.4.1. *Diabetes mellitus.* Diabetes is now the third commonest cause of end-stage renal failure in many series (see Table 3). Treatment involves many difficult problems and the approach, both to dialysis and to transplantation, has varied widely in different countries and centres. Although survival rates are lower than for other diseases, it is clear that transplantation can be the best option for certain patients. Blindness appears to be largely irrelevant in spite of some reports that it is stabilized after transplantation. Much more important are age and the extent of secondary vascular lesions. Where marked coronary artery and iliofemoral artery disease are already present at the time of transplantation, there is an unacceptably high incidence of early myocardial infarction and peripheral gangrene, although these are not necessarily accelerated by the procedure. The worst vascular disease is seen in older, non insulin-dependent patients, although length of disease, degree of hypertension and other factors, such as the habit of smoking, strongly influence the situation. The older and higher risk patients are often better maintained on dialysis. Nevertheless, younger insulin-dependent patients without severe vascular disease usually merit transplantation. Although recurrent diabetic nephropathy has been increasingly reported and probably limits the long-term survival of many grafts, it is in practice not a contra-indication to transplantation in well selected patients. Concurrent pancreatic transplantation offers the hope of a simultaneous "quasi-cure" of the underlying disease. Early results were disappointing, but the development of islet cell implantation (whether or not contemporaneously) by various techniques allows some hope for the future.

4.4.2. *Amyloidosis*. Due to its multisystem involvement, primary amyloidosis carries an increased mortality, whatever form of renal replacement is chosen, particularly in the older patient. This raises the question of whether transplantation is justified in these circumstances. However, although it will eventually recur, graft (as opposed to patient) survival is not significantly worse than in glomerulonephritis. Transplantation may be acceptable, therefore, when a reasonable quality of life cannot be attained by dialysis. Secondary amyloidosis may also recur in grafts if the primary cause has not been removed. The outcome for the patient is affected largely by this cause. In rheumatoid arthritis and familial mediterranean fever it does not differ significantly from that for glomerulonephritis. In bronchiectasis, however, the risk of fatal respiratory infection may be a reason to avoid transplantation.

4.4.3. *Gouty nephropathy*. This in general responds well to transplantation. Alluprinol and azathioprine have combined to produce severe marrow depression in some cases, while cyclosporin has been known to precipitate gouty attacks by contributing to a rise in serum uric acid.

4.4.4. *Cystinosis*. This autosomal recessive disorder causes widespread cystine deposition in young children, with multi-organ involvement, including renal failure. Although cystine continues to be deposited following transplantation, the results are good. An early graft should be sought in order to minimize the stunting of growth produced by the combination of the primary disease and renal failure.

4.4.5. *Cystinuria*. (easily confused with the preceding disorder) is an autosomal recessive condition characterised by a urinary leakage of the amino-acids cystine, ornithine, arginine and lysine. The disease is due to a specific defect of proximal tubular amino-acid transport. Cystine, which is rather insoluble in acid media, tends to form multiple, progressive and often massive calculi which can lead to end-stage renal failure. Despite the genetically-mediated nature of the lesion, transplantation is entirely appropriate, since the donor kidney, "programmed" by different genes, cannot develop the tubular defect.

4.4.6. *Oxalosis.* This rare genetically determined disease results in widespread tissue deposition of oxalate, usually causing renal failure in late childhood or early adult life. Transplantation is feasible, but since oxalate deposits continue in the recipient, the graft is immediately exposed to them. Aggressive measures to prevent early oxalate deposition, including intensive preoperative dialysis, maintenance of post-operative diuresis and magnesium, phosphate and pyridoxine administration have produced reasonable results in at least one series of living-related donations. In general transplantation should be avoided unless early function can be assured.

4.4.7. *Fabry's disease.* Fabry's disease, an X-linked recessive condition, is caused by deficiency of a specific alpha-galactosidase enzyme. This leads to widespread accumulation of trihexoside in numerous tissues, including the glomeruli and tubules. Patients develop multiple features, including limb pain, cutaneous papules, vascular disease and renal failure. Despite hopes that a donor kidney would both reverse renal failure and supply the missing enzyme, there has been a high post-graft mortality, with only a few long term survivals. Transplantation should therefore be approached with caution, if at all.

4.4.8. *Multisystem disorders.* The outlook for systemic lupus erythematosis (SLE) has improved considerably in recent decades, even when it results in end-stage renal failure. Many cases appear to have "burned out" by this stage and, in these, the results of transplantation are satisfactory. However, where the disease is still active at the time of grafting, high rates of recurrence have been reported. It is advisable to delay transplantation until evidence of disease activity has disappeared.

The vasculitides form a related group of diseases with an autoimmune basis and a high mortality if untreated, to which the risks of therapeutic immunosuppression must be added. Polyarteritis nodosa (rarely), microvascular vasculitis and Wegener's granulomatosis are the forms most likely to lead to renal failure. As in the case of SLE, if the disease process has become inactive without undue cost to the patient, transplantation can lead to good results. During the active phase, recurrence is likely. For microvascular vasculitis and Wegener's granulomatosis the anti-neutrophil cytoplasmic antibody level (ANCA) is a reliable measure, both in diagnosis and in assessing activity. Transplantation should be deferred until overactivity, however judged, has subsided.

Systemic sclerosis is associated with multiple organ improvement, much disability and a sclerosing glomerulopathy, frequently leading to renal failure with severe hypertension. Angiotension conversion enzyme (ACE) inhibitors may delay progression and control hypertension. Limb involvement often causes difficulty with both haemo- and peritoneal dialysis. Satisfactory results have been reported after transplantation, which is thus probably the treatment of choice where the disease is inactive and the patient is judged fit enough to benefit.

Haemolytic uraemic syndrome may cause reversible acute renal failure, but many cases progress to a chronic state. Fairly good graft survival has been achieved in adults, but in children a high rate of recurrence, often with graft loss, has been reported. In view of the variable outcome it is probably best not to use living-related donor grafts in these patients.

4.4.9. *Tumours*

4.4.9.1. *Primary renal tumours.* Occasionally benign renal tumours (e.g. vascular multiple hamartomata) have led to the need for bilateral nephrectomy and renal replacement therapy. Early transplantation has plainly been desirable in such cases. The main malignant tumours which may lead to the same result are bilateral or recurrent renal cell carcinoma (by far the commonest), Wilm's tumour and tumours of the urinary tract. The question of transplantation in such cases depends on the pathology of the tumour, its natural history, degree of differentiation, the likelihood of metastases and the length of "tumour-free" survival. No such patient can be guaranteed safe from secondary recurrence, even in the absence of transplantation and post-graft immunosuppression greatly increases the risks. Nevertheless, in selected cases, excellent graft and patient survival has been achieved. Treatment of the tumour may affect preparation for transplantation, e.g. in extreme cases of urothelial tumours (which may recur throughout the tract) removal of *all* urothelial tissue, from the pelvis to the urethra, may be necessary. Cystic degeneration in end-stage renal failure is associated with an increased incidence of renal tumours. Thus, patients who have waited many years for transplantation (e.g. due to sensitization) should be screened for this development and if necessary considered for pre-graft bilateral nephrectomy.

4.4.9.2. *Secondary renal tumours.* Renal failure following secondary deposits in the kidneys never merits transplantation. Infiltrative lesions may occasionally be different. Good results have been reported in cases of multiple myeloma. After remission had been achieved with chemotherapy a few patients remained well for up to nine years after the graft procedure.

5. Urinary tract

5.1. *Stone disease*

Urinary calculi cause end-stage renal failure by a combination of back pressure, infection and renal cortical atrophy. Progression of the disease is slow, with well-maintained urinary output. Hypertension is relatively rare, probably due to the presence of a sodium-losing tubular dysfunction in many patients. Potentially reversible factors (e.g. infection, continuing obstruction and electrolyte or water imbalance) should be excluded before committing patients to dialysis and transplantation. Bilateral nephrectomy should not be considered until it is clear that all useful residual renal function has been lost.

5.2. *Obstructive disease*

The previous arguments also apply to this condition. However, since indolent renal infection is less likely, the issue of bilateral nephrectomy does not usually arise. All evidence of obstruction should be fully investigated for reversibility which in some cases may lead to near-total return of renal function.

Case history

A 42 year old man presented with severe uraemia, accompanied by normochromic normocytic anaemia. Renal imaging suggested kidneys of low-normal size. The patient was given dialysis therapy and prepared for transplantation. Bilateral nephrectomy was planned, but before this could be done the patient developed unexpected fluctuations in serum creatinine, urea and urinary output. Full urological assessment revealed retroperitoneal fibrosis which was relieved by surgery. The patient achieved near-normal renal function and was eventually discharged from follow-up.

5.3. *Lower urinary tract*

Disease of the lower urinary tract is not in itself a bar to transplantation, because, where necessary, urinary diversion can produce a satisfactory drainage system. However all lesions must be fully assessed. In some cases, the nature of the disease (e.g. malignant tumour or active infection) may preclude transplantation. In others, the extent of preparatory surgery may justify a decision to reject it as too dangerous for the patient.

6. Cardiovascular system

Cardiovascular disease causes over 50 per cent of deaths in patients on renal replacement therapy. In the 38–54 age group "myocardial ischaemia" deaths are twenty times and cerebrovascular deaths fifty times more common than in the general population. For those over 55 the factors are ten and twenty times respectively. Peripheral vascular disease is increased in a similar ratio.

The risks are already high for dialysis patients and there is no evidence that they are reduced by transplantation. Hypertension usually improves after grafting, as do triglyceride and lipoprotein abnormalities, but both often persist. Steroid therapy itself may induce hypercholesterolaemia. It is often said that patients at high risk of cardiovascular, cerebrovascular or peripheral vascular disease ought not to be offered transplantation. Unfortunately this is a meaningless statement unless that risk can be defined. In view of the figures just quoted it could mean that nobody should be offered transplantation! Against such a background, "extra" high risk is particularly hard to determine. Much of the hoped-for future improvement in transplantation depends on better identification and reduction of these risks.

6.1. *Hypertension*

About 80 per cent of renal failure patients are hypertensive when they start dialysis. Good blood pressure control on dialysis is possible, and important, although not always easy to achieve. However, the state of blood pressure control is rarely a reason for deciding against transplantation. If it is good the patient should benefit while if it is poor transplantation will probably improve control. The most important comparison is between those who are hypertensive when starting dialysis and those who are not. The latter group has better survival on all forms of renal replacement therapy. Improved survival for the hypertensive group probably depends upon good blood pressure control from the first development of hypertension, which may precede dialysis by years or decades.

6.2. *Cardiovascular disease*

Some degree of premature vascular disease is present in most cases of chronic renal failure. Non-renal factors such as age, heredity, diet and smoking exacerbate the renal factors, which include hypertension, hyperlipidaemia, hyperparathyroidism, hyperphosphataemia, insulin resistance and (when present) diabetes. Prevention and elimination of these risk factors are important for the reduction of mortality. The major clinical question remains: what is the point beyond which vascular disease prohibits transplantation? There are two possible extreme positions. The first is that mortality is increased in any event so that every patient deserves the improved quality of life offered by transplantation. The second is that the scarcity of grafts requires them to be given to those who have the best overall prognosis. Common sense demands an intermediate approach, but there is no easy solution and disappointing early deaths will occur. To reduce these experience teaches a number of points. Hypertension is no bar to transplantation for the reasons already given. Cardiomegaly due to left ventricular hypertrophy, can also usually be ignored. Many patients enjoy excellent survival and health in spite of it – indeed left ventricular function has been shown to improve significantly after successful grafting. The same applies to heart failure which is not accompanied by other evidence of cardiac dysfunction. However, heart failure combined with hypotension or dysrhythmias, particularly when provoked by haemodialysis, is less innocent. Supraventricular arrhythmias are not particularly alarming, especially where there is an extra-cardiac cause (e.g., hyperparathyroidism in the case of atrial fibrillation). The presence of any degree of heartblock is disturbing, especially since, if intermittent, it may be missed.

Case history

A 62 year old man with a history of aortic aneurysm and generalised vascular disease had made good progress on CAPD and after full assessment was put "on call" for transplantation. After a year a suitable kidney became available. At pre-operative assessment the patient reported recent "fainting attacks" but ECG showed sinus rhythm with some ischaemic changes. Shortly after anaesthetic induction he developed complete heartblock with profound bradycardia requiring cardio-pulmonary resuscitation. The transplant was abandoned. Two years later, after insertion of a ventricular pacemaker, he remains on CAPD, with the issue of transplantation unresolved.

Coronary artery atherosclerosis is so common that it cannot be regarded as contra-indication. Nor can angina, particularly if associated with anaemia and correctable by transfusion or erythropoietin. Indeed in several cases transplantation has successfully cured the angina for periods in excess of ten years. One, or even two, episodes of myocardial infarction need not prevent grafting if there are no persistent cardiac sequelae and risk factors are vigorously corrected. Persistent severe angina or repeated infarction should be investigated by coronary artery angiography and selection of patients for angioplasty or by-pass surgery, after which many successful transplants have been carried out with prolonged patient survival.

However, widespread inoperable coronary atheroma is often unacceptable. Unfortunately it is sometimes silent and therefore undetected.

Case history

A 42 year old woman with a family history of ischaemic heart disease and a heavy smoking habit developed renal failure due to chronic pyelonephritis. Pre-transplant assessment showed mild hypertension with normal heart size and ECG. Nevertheless, fatal cardiac arrest occurred at the end of operation. Autopsy revealed massive generalised coronary artery atheroma with near-total occlusion of all vessels.

The prognosis of ischaemic heart disease depends upon multiplication of risk factors. Where the risks are many, with evidence of advanced myocardial disease, it may be wise to decide against transplantation, particularly since steroid-induced hypercholesterolaemia may exacerbate them.

Valvular and *congenital* heart disease should usually be regarded as contra-indications to transplantation. Early results are often good, but the five year mortality from bacterial endocarditis has been high. Although such risks also exist without renal replacement therapy, it appears ethically unacceptable to increase them by the deliberate addition of immunosuppressive drugs.

6.3. *Cerebrovascular disease*

Similar arguments apply in this case but with a slightly different emphasis. The argument against grafting in cases of severe disablement is that the patient cannot experience complete rehabilitation (although it may be claimed that management will become easier). Certain points may be learned from experience. Stable stroke patients in whom the cause (e.g., hypertension, embolus or subarachnoid haemorrhage) has been corrected, can often be transplanted with little risk. Victims of massive stroke are unlikely to be well rehabilitated following transplantation. However, youth counts in the patient's favour.

Case history

A 35 year old man with a strong family history of vascular disease developed renal failure due to hypertensive nephrosclerosis. Shortly after starting haemodialysis he developed a dense left hemiplegia and required admission to a geriatric unit. In order to "ease terminal care" it was decided to opt for transplantation and a poor quality, poorly matched cadaver was successfully implanted. Thereafter the patient's condition gradually improved. Sixteen years later he remains well, having outlived his parents and siblings and with only marginal neurological defect.

6.4. *Peripheral vascular disease*

It is possible to achieve good results despite severe peripheral vascular disease but a high risk of amputation must be accepted – the feet are at much greater risk than the hands. Where severe ischaemia exists before transplantation, eventual necrosis and amputation are almost inevitable. The limb on the transplant side is more often affected. Secondary infection is common and the mortality is high, particularly for diabetics. Occasional high risk patients are found to be untransplantable due to near-total occlusion of the iliofemoral arteries. In all cases of suspected disease preliminary arterial assessment, including arteriography, is desirable. Peripheral vascular disease can also produce damage in the other end organs, although this is comparatively rare relative to the limbs. Retinal lesions, however, are common and are usually underdiagnosed.

6.5. *Lipoprotein abnormalities*

Hyperlipidaemia greatly increases the risk of ischaemic heart disease in the general population. Thus its increased incidence in uraemia and dialysis patients is significant. Total cholesterol is normal or low, but there is marked hypertriglyceridaemia. High density lipoprotein (HDL) cholesterol is reduced. There is increased size and triglyceride content of low density lipoprotein (LDL) with increased concentration and cholesterol enrichment of very low density lipoprotein (VLDL). This combination of abnormalities with triglyceride-rich lipoprotein remnants is highly atherogenic in dialysis patients. After transplantation HDL cholesterol usually returns to normal, but triglycerides, LDL cholesterol and VLDL cholesterol remain elevated, and aggravated by steroid maintenance doses greater than 12.5 mg/day. The trend to lower steroid doses reduces hyperlipidaemia, but cyclosporin, even in monotherapy, is also associated with significant increases in total and LDL cholesterol. There is thus no evidence that transplantation reduces the atherogenic risk of hyperlipidaemia.

6.6. *Overall atherogenic risk of transplantation*

It has often been suggested (i) that dialysis increases the rate of atherogenesis and (ii) that transplantation further accelerates the process. This is understandable in view of the very high incidence and mortality rates noted above, but there is in fact no firm evidence of such acceleration in either group. Coronary and other vascular events do show a relationship to known risk factors which are similar to those of age-matched non-uraemic patients with similar risk factors. These include hypertension, age, diabetes, hyperlipidaemia and smoking. Conversely, uraemic patients with a background of low risk show a low relative rate of late atherogenesis. It thus appears that while some features of uraemia and dialysis (e.g., hyperparathyroidism and hyperphosphataemia) as well as some effects of transplantation (e.g., steroid- and/or cyclosporin-induced hyperlipidaemia) do have an atherogenic potential, these are outweighed by the major risk factors which exist before the start of renal replacement therapy and which largely date from the onset of renal disease. Elimination of these risks is in theory possible and will be necessary in practice if the goal of "quasi-cure" with normal longevity is to be realised. At present the decision on whether to transplant patients with severe atheromatous vascular disease must continue to depend on clinical judgment in individual cases of the prospect for overall survival and benefit.

7. Other pre-existing diseases

Disease in other body systems is commonly found, and indeed is often responsible for, the patient's renal failure. Such conditions not only increase the risk of transplantation but also contribute to mortality and decreased rehabilitation.

7.1. *Respiratory system*

Chronic bronchitis and emphysema are not major risk factors unless they are associated with respiratory failure and *cor pulmonale*.Bronchiectasis is often found as a cause of end-stage renal failure due to secondary amyloidosis. Good post-graft survival has been obtained, but there is a risk of fatal chest infection. The key factors in deciding on transplantation in these cases are the severity of the disease, the number of other risk factors and the quality of life obtained by dialysis.

7.2. *Gastro-intestinal system*

7.2.1. *Hiatus hernia* is usually acceptable in a transplant recipient as long as it is not gross and is under medical control. An increased incidence of post-graft reflux oesophagitis can usually be managed by H_2 blockers.

7.2.2. *Peptic ulceration* is much increased in renal failure. Nearly one quarter of transplanted patients have a previous history of ulcer disease. Nearly 30 per cent of transplant patients show evidence of upper GI inflammation or ulceration on endoscopy, with a high gastric acid secretion. A high mortality from complications was formerly experienced both before and after transplantation. Surgical intervention, on an emergency or prophylactic basis, was common. Early use of H_2 blockers and a reduction in post-transplant steroid doses has greatly improved the situation. All potential recipients should be screened for evidence of disease which should be treated if active. Transplantation should not be considered until the ulcer has healed on endoscopy. H_2 blockers should be continued after grafting. Patients who are symptomatic for the first time post-transplant should undergo prompt endoscopy, followed by treatment with H_2 blockers. In all patients who require high dose steroid for rejection, H_2 blockers should be used prophylactically. Surgery, which is now rarely necessary, should be reserved for complications.

7.2.3. *Gallstones and chronic cholecystitis* are commonly encountered in dialysis patients. They usually have no association with renal failure. Transplantation is not contra-indicated but preliminary cholecystectomy may be advisable. The main post-transplant dangers are of ascending infection and carcinomatous change. In addition jaundice of uncertain cause and impaired liver function tests, possibly related to opportunist infection, often complicate immunosuppressive therapy, increasing the difficulty of diagnosing biliary tree disorders. Some centres have performed pre-transplant cholecystectomy in all patients with gallstones or non-functioning gallbladder. This has not been the Belfast policy, which is to treat symptomatic cases surgically and retain a high "index of suspicion" in the presence of clinically silent disease.

7.2.4. *Liver disease* may be present incidentally or as part of a multisystem disorder. When mild or moderate, we have not found it a serious bar to transplantation. However, jaundice of uncertain cause, usually drug-induced or related to opportunistic infection, often follows post-transplantation immunosuppression and this exacerbates any pre-existing liver damage. In cases of liver dysfunction following hepatitis B infection there is evidence of marked deterioration post-transplant with a significantly increased mortality.

7.2.5. *Appendicitis* is an occasional hazard after transplantation but is usually dealt with successfully, even if the graft is in the right iliac fossa. Nevertheless, in the event of pre-transplant abdominal surgery, the removal of the appendix is desirable. In the days of routine abdominal bilateral nephrectomy, appendicectomy was performed in many cases, but with changing practice opportunities are less.

7.2.6. *Diverticular disease*, mainly of the sigmoid colon, is common in older patients. Despite a few cases of diverticular rupture following immunosuppression, prophylactic surgical intervention has not been our practice and serious complications have been rare. All patients over 45 should be screened for evidence of disease and fully investigated where appropriate. Since the symptoms of acute diverticulitis can mimic those of graft rejection, some centres electively place the transplanted kidney in the right iliac fossa when diverticular disease is present.

7.2.7. *Unexplained gastro-intestinal bleeding* occurs in some patients before transplantation, raising concern about underlying lesions. This is an indication for full intestinal investigation. If, as often happens, extensive tests reveal no underlying cause, it is usually safe to put the patient "on call". In some older patients intestinal angiodysplasia may be present: this lesion tends to run a relapsing but benign course.

7.3. *Neurological system*

Minor, non-progressive or treated conditions are compatible with good post-transplant survival. Epilepsy, stable peripheral neuropathy, neuromyopathy and successfully-treated brain tumour fall into this category. Major conditions which produce effects amounting to organ failure, carry unacceptable risks of infection, or promise unacceptably low prospects for rehabilitation are usually not suitable for transplantation. Irreversible dementia, advanced multiple sclerosis and total respiratory paralysis are examples. Stroke disease has been considered under vascular disorders but can be classified as major or minor for this purpose according to its severity. Conditions of intermediate severity are the most difficult to resolve. Moderate stroke and disabling multiple sclerosis have been successfully transplanted. There have also been good reports of grafts in paraplegics, but experience in Belfast has been disappointing, several patients succumbing to infection before a kidney became available.

7.4. *Mental subnormality and severe psychiatric disorder*

Most patients are physically suited for transplantation. Cooperation, compliance and control are the key factors and vary with the degree of subnormality or disturbance. Excellent results have been obtained in selected cases. A period of observation on dialysis is helpful, since if the patient can cope with this procedure he (or she) can usually cope better with transplantation.

7.5. *Skeletal system*

7.5.1. *Renal osteodystrophy* is almost always present in end-stage renal failure, although clinical evidence may be slight. It is a major indication for transplantation.

7.5.2. *Osteoporosis*, masked by osteodystrophy, may be present, particularly in the older (over 60) woman of slight build. Devastating steroid-induced deterioration can occur in such patients after transplantation and there is a strong case for cyclosporin monotherapy if possible.

7.5.3. *Osteo- and rheumatoid arthritis* are often exacerbated by transplantation, usually by a combination of weight gain and increased activity. The pain can be debilitating and is not always controlled. In general, however, patients are ready to accept it as the "price" of successful grafting.

7.6. *Eyes, ears, nose and throat*

7.6.1. *Uraemia.* Uraemic visual defects are not cured by transplantation, although it has been claimed that diabetic retinopathy progresses less rapidly.

7.6.2. *Cataract* is liable to be exacerbated by posterior polar opacities but is eventually amenable to surgery. Sudden nerve deafness has occurred in both dialysis and transplant patients – there is often already a history of partial deafness. In the past some cases of oto- and vestibulo-toxicity have been caused by aminoglycoside therapy for secondary infection. Hearing should be tested in all patients, but rather to assess defects than to discover objections to renal transplantation.

7.7. Endocrine, metabolic, congenital and genetically-mediated conditions

Few, if any, of these conditions preclude successful transplantation. The practical requirements are: (i) the disorder should have a reasonable prognosis in its own right, and (ii) it should be under optimal medical control at the time of grafting. Thus, in the case of thyroid disorders, there should be no evidence of serious secondary development such as malignancy or cardiac arrhythmias. The patient should have been rendered euthyroid before going "on call" for transplantation.

Certain metabolic diseases, such as diabetes and hyperparathyroidism fall into a special category: they are either the cause or the consequence of renal disease and must be managed as such.

7.8. Malignancy

Transplantation should never be attempted in the presence of known or recently treated malignant disease. It is unacceptable to risk a fatal recurrence of metastatic spread due to suppressing the patient's immunological defences. Arguments, from whatever source, in favour of grafting should be resisted. The incidence of primary malignancy following transplant immunosuppression is already distressingly high. It is a doctor's duty to minimize such fearsome iatrogenic disease, even at the expense of "quality of life". However, in some cases of malignancy, transplantation several years after apparently successful treatment has been performed with good long-term survival. In deciding to transplant the nature and extent of the original lesion, its natural history, type of treatment and the length of time without recurrence are all important. The amount of immunosuppression may also be significant – there is evidence that the incidence of post-graft malignancy increases with the number of agents used.

8. Infection

8.1. Bacterial infections

Patients who have serious unresolved infection of major organs should not be put forward for transplantation.

8.1.1. Examples are suppurative bronchiectasis, subacute endocarditis, infected renal stones and active osteomyelitis. Once such infections have been fully eradicated, transplantation may be considered but should probably not be attempted if the potential for re-infection remains. Immunisation against certain organisms (e.g. pneumococcus) is available and safe, but is not at present a practical way of reducing overall risk. Minor infections (e.g. urinary or upper respiratory) are sometimes present when donor kidneys become available. In general, with proper management, they do not affect the outcome. Particular attention should be paid to treatment of dental caries, to prevent the development of dental abscesses after transplantation. Infections related to dialysis access (e.g. CAPD catheter tracts, A-V fistulae and indwelling venous catheters) should be aggressively treated but usually subside rapidly after transplantation as the need for dialysis disappears and access devices are removed.

8.1.2. *Tuberculosis* (TB) needs careful assessment. Active lesions obviously preclude transplantation. Treated cases may be transplanted after an appropriate time (several years) when prophylactic anti-tuberculous therapy should be given. In regions with a high incidence of TB infection there may be a case for routine antibiotic cover, both before and after transplantation. In the United Kingdom (and Northern Ireland) the possibility of active TB must still be remembered, particularly in the old, in those with a history of infection and in patients with radiologically or otherwise suggestive features. False negative tuberculin tests and cultures may occur in uraemic patients, making a clinical diagnosis necessary. Wherever possible biopsy of suspicious lesions should be performed.

8.2. *Viral infections*

8.2.1. *Hepatitis.* Hepatitis B virus (HBV) infection reached its highest level in dialysis populations in the early 1980s, when nearly 1800 new cases per year (over 10 per cent of all patients) were recorded in Europe, while a similar number were known to be chronic hepatitis B surface antigen (HBsAg) carriers. With increased vaccination and other preventive measures there has since been a pronounced fall in both incidence and prevalence of HBV and the carrier state.

New cases have become very rare in the United Kingdom where the disease is rare in the community and preventive measures (including routine testing of all blood products) have been available since the early 1970s. Nevertheless, it is probably wise to offer vaccination to all patients and staff of dialysis units, since this should lead to the eventual eradication of HBV. Transplantation should not be considered during the active phase of infection and probably not during the continuation of the carrier state. If biopsy and/or biochemical evidence of marked liver dysfunction persists, it is unwise to opt for transplantation. The long-term mortality in this situation is significantly above average. Hepatitis A infection is rarer and has fewer consequences for patients and staff – transplantation is safe, provided the active state has subsided. Hepatitis C is now recognised as a separate entity. It has increased both relatively and absolutely over recent years although its incidence in Northern Ireland remains very low. Transplantation should not be considered when the condition is active and offered with caution in cases where long-term hepatic dysfunction persists.

Hepatitis C antibody testing is now carried out routinely on all organ donors and all potential kidney transplant recipients in the Belfast Unit. This test, when positive, indicates past exposure to the virus, not its present activity, and should be interpreted with this in mind. Testing for the presence of hepatitis C antigen may also soon be freely available.

8.2.2. *Cytomegalovirus.* (CMV) infection is one of the commonest opportunistic infections in transplant recipients. Transmission rarely occurs through staff or other patients. Whole blood (especially if fresh) or leucocyte infusions may be responsible, but the main source of primary infection in previously uninfected patients is the transplanted organ from a seropositive donor. Secondary infection may occur either through the donor kidney or by reactivation of the patient's own virus. It is thus important to establish the CMV status of all potential recipients in order to prevent CMV positive donation to CMV negative recipients. Where this is not possible, immunisation and/or prophylactic use of acyclovir are likely to reduce morbidity and mortality.

8.2.3. *Varicella zoster virus.* (VZV) occurs annually in three per cent of transplant patients (10 times the normal rate). Fatal pneumonitis, encephalopathy and meningitis can occur, while zoster produces painful and sometimes disabling lesions, particularly of the eyes.

Immune status should be determined pre-transplantation where possible. Susceptible patients should receive immunisation and be considered for prophylactic treatment in the event of post-transplantation exposure.

8.2.4. *Human immunodeficiency virus.* (HIV) status should be checked in all potential recipients. Present knowledge suggests that HIV positive patients should not be transplanted, not only because of their overall poor prognosis, but also because immunosuppression is likely to accelerate and exacerbate progression to the AIDS syndrome.

8.2.5. *Epstein–Barr virus.* (EBV) and *human polyoma viruses* are known to carry potentially serious consequences following post-graft infection in previously sero-negative patients. Some other viruses may be in the same position. In all these situations, seroconversion may be possible now or in future. Adenoviruses, influenza A virus and other RNA viruses do not appear to pose excessive risks following transplantation, but some centres support pre-graft immunisation against these infections where feasible. Patients sometimes present for transplantation with clinical evidence of self-limiting infection by these and similar organisms. This should not automatically rule out the operation.

8.3. *Infestations*

These should be considered in all pre-transplant assessments, as fatal proliferation has been recorded in immunosuppressed patients. This is particularly important if the patient has a history of residence in certain regions.

Case history

A 48 year old Chinese woman from Hong Kong was treated in Belfast for chronic renal failure. While on dialysis she complained of occasional abdominal pain, but investigations were negative. Two years after successful transplantation she developed an acute abdominal and pulmonary state, to which she succumbed. Later histological examination revealed widespread hyper-infestation by *Strongyloides stercoralis*, with marked involvement of lungs and abdominal organs. In retrospect, pre- and post-graft thiabendazole might have proved life-saving.

Numerous other cases of pre-graft infection, or infestation with unusual or tropical organisms may be cited. Painstaking and thorough pre-graft exclusion of such diseases is mandatory, together with prophylactic therapy (on clinical suspicion if necessary) and all other appropriate measures. It is easy to "park" a patient on dialysis and cease active investigation pending transplantation. Continuous constructive thinking aimed at the reduction of post-graft infection risks is the best way of reducing their impact.

9. Immunological status

The need to monitor immunological activity in diseases which may recur in the graft has already been discussed. In addition, blood group and tissue type information is required on all patients. This knowledge is necessary in order to arrange the desired degree of tissue matching between donor and recipient. It will be discussed in detail in Chapter 9. Knowledge of unacceptable antigens (e.g., from marital partners or previous graft donors) is usually necessary. The determination of HLA antigens of blood relations often helps to resolve uncertainties in the patient's personal tissue type. In the case of potential living related donors they help to confirm the relationship to the patient and the closeness of tissue matching. Regular screening for cytotoxic antibodies is mandatory. These are often present in multiparous women or after loss of a previous graft. Antibodies may appear transiently after transfusion so that early sampling is necessary. It is usually unwise to put a graft into a patient who has demonstrated incompatible antibodies, even if these appear to be absent in the latest sample examined before transplantation. These issues are discussed in more detail elsewhere.

10. Information and consent

No assessment is complete without an interview in which the benefits of transplantation are fully outlined to the patient and in which he (or she) is given a chance to discuss the negative side of the "transplant miracle". As renal replacement therapy has become more generally available it approximates more closely to other treatments than in its early days, when survival could be offered only to the selected few. Due to scarcity of donors it is not at present possible to offer transplantation on request. Medical assessment of suitability must continue to have precedence. However, it is often appropriate to leave the decision to the patient. In all cases adequate explanation is necessary in order to fulfil the legal obligation to allow informed consent. In any interview the following points should be covered as a minimum: (i) the need for replacement therapy; (ii) the comparative benefits in terms of length and quality of survival of dialysis and transplantation; (iii) the disadvantages of transplantation, particularly as regards immunosuppressive drug effects and other serious complications; (iv) in cases where transplantation is not offered, a reasoned explanation of this decision.

11. Cost effectiveness

The total requirement for renal replacement therapy is not yet clear. It is certainly greater than the 40 to 50 cases per million/year that assessments in the 1970s suggested, but may be less than the 140 per million/year suggested by recent figures from the USA and Japan. Spectra of disease seem to differ from country to country and acceptance policies certainly do. On present assessments, a reasonable upper limit for new cases of treatable renal failure in the UK may be between 80 and 100 per million/year. Provision of treatment on such a scale involves an enormous financial outlay from Government health funds which even the wealthiest states find difficult, although total outlay remains moderate in comparison to that for heart or lung diseases, because of the relative rarity of renal failure. Dialysis, in all its forms, is expensive and rendered more so by recent innovations which improve its quality and acceptability. Successful transplantation, in addition to providing a higher quality of life than dialysis in most cases, is also significantly cheaper, reducing costs to less than 20% those of dialysis in the second and subsequent years of treatment, even when the use of cyclosporin is taken into account.

For this reason it appears ethical to encourage its use in most cases which are suitable, since not only does it combine cost-effectiveness with high duration and quality of survival, but also it releases expensive centre spaces and equipment for the support of new patients, thus reducing the expense of expanding these facilities.

Further reading

Chapman, J. R., Allen, R. D. Dialysis and transplantation. In *Kidney Transplantation*, Morris, P. J., ed. 3rd ed. Philadelphia, Saunders, 1988; 37–69.

Strom, T. B., Tilney, N. L. Renal transplantation: clinical aspects. In *The Kidney*, Brenner, B. M., Rector, F. C. eds. 3rd ed. Philadelphia, Saunders, 1986; 1941–1976.

CHAPTER 5

Preparation for transplantation 1

J. F. DOUGLAS

The object of preparation for transplantation is to ensure that the donor kidney is accepted with the minimum risk of rejection or complications. In addition, however, pre-transplant survival and quality of life must be considered. The patient may spend many years, first with conservative therapy and later on dialysis, before a successful transplant is eventually achieved. All phases of survival are important and nothing should be done which benefits one at the expense of another. For example, bilateral nephrectomy brings some advantage for the transplanted patient but may affect the quality of life on dialysis. Multiple blood transfusions improve uraemic anaemia but may compromise transplantation by encouraging the formation of cytotoxic antibodies. At all times the overall welfare of the patient must take priority over the specific benefits expected from individual treatments.

1. Dialysis

The need for dialysis has been variously estimated in different times, countries and age-groups. In the United States, current estimates suggest that 100–140 new patients with treatable end-stage renal failure per million population (pmp) can be expected to present for treatment annually. In the United Kingdom studies in the early 1970s found 40–50 new cases pmp yearly in the under 60 age-group. More recent surveys involving all ages show an increase to at least 80 pmp. Countries differ with respect to both the causes and management of end-stage renal failure. In the US and Scandinavia, for example, 25 per cent of the dialysis population is diabetic; in the UK the figure is 10–15 per cent. This could represent differences either in the nephropathic potential or in management strategy between the countries. Australia and Switzerland have in the past reported much higher rates of analgesic nephropathy than elsewhere. In Japan, the average age of dialysis patients is younger than in Europe which could indicate a different spectrum of pathology or (more probably) a greater readiness to give dialysis early. There is thus still uncertainty as to the true need for dialysis. However, given the

Mary G. McGeown (ed.), Clinical Management of Renal Transplantation, 61–76.
© 1992 *Kluwer Academic Publishers, Dordrecht. Printed in the Netherlands.*

increasing incidence of renal failure with age and the rising life expectancy of Western populations, a minimum yearly figure of 80–100 pmp seems likely.

Provision of dialysis in the UK has risen from acceptance rates of under 40 pmp in 1985 to over 60 pmp in 1991. Further development will place an enormous, and costly, burden upon dialysis services. Most of the increase is in the over 60 age-group, in keeping with previous experience in the US. Many of these patients are unsuited to transplantation. However, it remains important to maximize the role of transplantation wherever appropriate in order to lessen the impact of dialysis need and integrate the two treatments as fully as possible.

1.1. *Principles of dialysis*

A full account of dialysis will be found elsewhere. The following account outlines the general nature of the treatment, particularly as it applies to the potential transplant recipient.

1.2. *Haemodialysis*

The chemical principle of dialysis through a semi-permeable membrane was discovered by Graham (1861). Abel (1913) performed the first experimental haemodialysis and the first human trial was made by Haas (1924). Wilhelm Kolff (1944) carried out the first successful reversal of acute renal failure using haemodialysis. Maintenance haemodialysis, pioneered by Scribner and others for the treatment of chronic end-stage renal failure, dates from 1960.

The principles of haemodialysis are depicted in Figure 2. It involves the diffusion of small and medium-sized molecules, including uraemic toxins, into a pre-prepared dialyate across an intervening semi-permeable membrane. Ultrafiltration of water and its solutes of suitable size can also be achieved, and controlled, by maintaining and regulating a trans-membrane hydrostatic pressure. Clinical haemodialysis involves both principles. Electrolyte loss is controlled by providing appropriate concentrations of different ions in the dialysis fluid. A typical "mixture" is shown in Figure 3. Potassium is low in order to prevent, or treat, hyperkalaemia. Sodium and chloride are normal, to preserve plasma tonicity. If they are lower, increased sodium loss, with hypotension, may result. Acetate (which metabolizes in the liver to equivalent amounts of bicarbonate) and divalent calcium ion are both relatively high: they thus pass into the body by reverse dialysis and tend to correct the metabolic acidosis and hypocalcaemia usually found in uraemic patients. High levels (>100 µmol/l) of dialysate glucose were at one time necessary in order to ensure adequate water extraction. This often induced secondary hyperglycaemia and hyponatraemia. Modern volumetrically controlled machines make such levels unnecessary. Glucose-free dialysis is sometimes

HAEMODIALYSIS

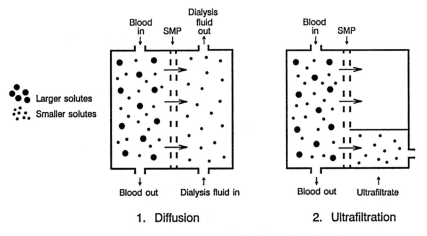

Haemodialysis combines (1) Diffusion of smaller solutes across a
semi-permeable membrane (SMP) down concentration gradient
(requires dialysis fluid) and (2) Ultrafiltration of H₂O and smaller
solutes across similar membrane by hydrostatic pressure (no
dialysis fluid required)

Figure 2. Basic principles of haemodialysis.

advocated to avoid exacerbation of raised lipid levels and discourage bacterial
growth. This can also produce hypoglycaemia, however. On balance a
"physiological" glucose level similar to that of fasting plasma (i.e. 5 μmol/l)
is desirable. The fluid is prepared by diluting concentrates, which are usually
"standard", with purified water in a proportioning system before delivery to
the dialysis membrane. At delivery, the fluid should be effectively sterile and
warmed to body temperature. The potential toxicity of dialysis fluid has been
increasingly recognised. High aluminium levels have caused many cases of
fatal encephalopathy as well as exacerbating bone disease and anaemia.
Acetate, when used as a convenient concentrate buffer, has caused numerous
toxic symptoms following its accumulation in the body during dialysis. These,
and other problems can now be overcome by better methods of water purification and dialysis fluid production.

Dialysis membranes were at first largely cellophane- and cellulose-based.
Although quite efficient, these are often poorly biocompatible and have
given rise to many complications related to unwanted complement activation,
including the long-term development of dialysis-related amyloidosis. Research has improved existing membranes and introduced new, more biocompatible substances, such as poly-acrylo-nitrile (PAN). Membrane performance has also been improved, allowing greater permeability to larger
molecules.

Increasing membrane permeability leads to greater fluid loss by ultrafiltration and convection. Sophisticated volume control mechanisms in modern

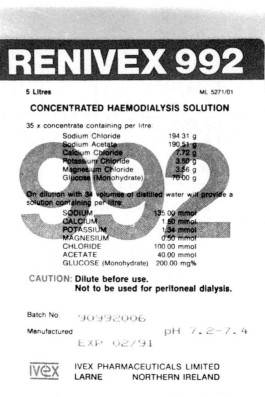

RENIVEX 992

5 Litres   ML 5271/01

CONCENTRATED HAEMODIALYSIS SOLUTION

35 x concentrate containing per litre:

Sodium Chloride	194.31 g
Sodium Acetate	190.51 g
Calcium Chloride	7.72 g
Potassium Chloride	3.50 g
Magnesium Chloride	3.56 g
Glucose (Monohydrate)	70.00 g

On dilution with 34 volumes of distilled water will provide a solution containing per litre:

SODIUM	135.00 mmol
CALCIUM	1.50 mmol
POTASSIUM	1.34 mmol
MAGNESIUM	0.50 mmol
CHLORIDE	100.00 mmol
ACETATE	40.00 mmol
GLUCOSE (Monohydrate)	200.00 mg%

CAUTION: **Dilute before use.**
Not to be used for peritoneal dialysis.

Batch No. 90992006

Manufactured   pH 7.2–7.4

EXP 02/91

ivex   IVEX PHARMACEUTICALS LIMITED
         LARNE   NORTHERN IRELAND

Figure 3. A container of concentrated dialysis fluid. On dilution it yields the solute concentrations listed on the outside label.

dialysis machines allow this to operate to the benefit of the patient so that excellent solute clearance is combined with sufficient fluid loss in a reasonably short treatment time. Haemofiltration is a form of high permeability treatment in which fluid and solutes, up to high molecular weights, are removed by convection alone, without the need for any dialysis fluid. A drawback of the technique is that considerable amounts of infused replacement fluid must be given to the patient to compensate for trans-membrane losses. This greatly increases its cost. Haemofiltration has been widely practised in Europe, notably in Germany. Its main advantages (apart from removal of large molecular weight toxins) are improved haemodynamic stability on treatment and better "general well-being". A further extension of the filtration principle is plasmapheresis. In this technique, plasma and its contents are completely separated from blood cells by filtration, followed by replacement infusion of fresh plasma or albumin. The patient's own plasma can be returned, if desired, minus any unwanted components. Plasmapheresis has a role in the treatment of acute immunologically-mediated glomerular disease (e.g.

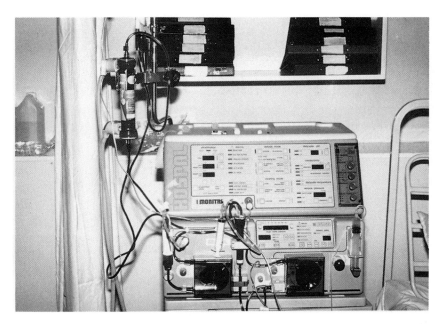

Figure 4. Dialyser and dialysis machine in use.

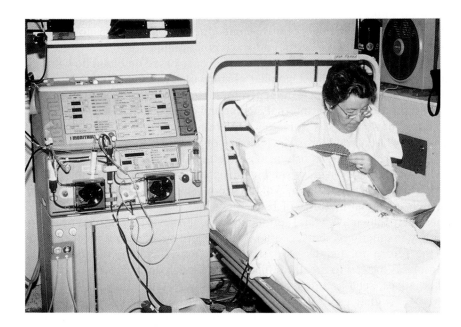

Figure 5. A chronic haemodialysis session.

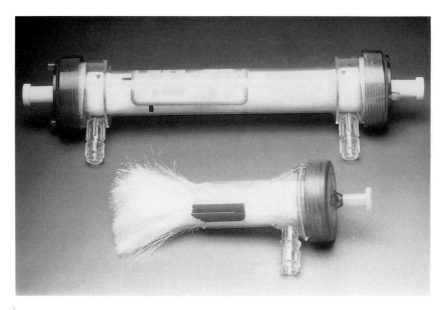

Figure 6. Capillary hollow fibre dialysers (a) intact (above) and (b) cut transversely to show fibre arrangement (below).

antiglomerular basement membrane nephritis) and in the removal of harmful cytotoxic antibodies, both before and after transplantation. However, although it does incidentally remove some uraemic toxins, it has no advantage in the routine management of end-stage renal failure.

A wide variety of dialysers is available. Those based on blood flow through hollow fibres are the most popular (Figure 6). Access to the circulation is made *via* double or single lumen routes, according to circumstances. For short-term use, femoral, internal jugular and in particular, subclavian venous catheters have almost completely replaced the arterio-venous shunt, first devised by Quinton (1958). The mainstay of access for long-term haemodialysis is the arterio-venous fistula, described by Brescia and Cimino in 1966. The preferred site is the wrist but many others have been used. Gradual hypertrophy ("arterialization") of the venous smooth muscle wall is necessary for full functional maturity of fistulae and this may require several months. Thereafter they may endure for many years. However, the spread of dialysis therapy to elderly patients, or those with severe circulatory disorder, as well as the return to dialysis of patients with long-standing, but now failed, transplants has led to greater difficulties of fistula construction in such cases. Alternatives, such as autogenous venous and prosthetic interposition grafts, have been widely used, with some success. Nevertheless, problems of access may persist. Occasionally, implantation of long-term central venous catheters has been necessary. Such patients tend to be unsuitable for transplantation.

Duration of dialysis, as well as frequency and site of treatment, vary considerably. Four hours three times a week or six to eight hours twice a week are commonly used. Logistic constraints are a major problem in Belfast, where the Northern Ireland Regional Dialysis Service has not yet achieved full decentralisation to provide a true "local" service for all parts of the province. Home dialysis, self-care, minimal-care and limited-care decentralised units lessen inconvenience and contribute to improved quality of life for most patients. However, some people, often elderly with or without ancillary disease, can only "manage" with the support of full hospital dialysis.

1.3. *Peritoneal dialysis* (*PD*)

It has been known for over 40 years that the peritoneal visceral membrane is capable of behaving as a dialysis membrane if the peritoneum is intermittently filled with an appropriate sterile dialysis solution. Acute uraemic crises have for many years responded well to this procedure. The development of the indwelling peritoneal catheter by Tenkhoff (1968) made possible the use of PD to treat end-stage renal failure. The most effective form has proved to be continuous ambulatory peritoneal dialysis (CAPD), developed in the late 1970s by Moncrief, Popovich, Oreopoulos and others. Three to five exchanges of up to two litres of suitable dialysis fluid are used per day. Dwell times of several hours are well tolerated, as are overnight dwells. The technique allows excellent control of uraemia and its symptoms. Various forms of intermittent PD, using automated delivery and monitoring systems, have been developed. Control of fluid and electrolyte loss is achieved by manipulating the tonicity and ionic composition of the dialysate bags of fluid.

PD (especially CAPD) has proved popular in a number of countries, notably the UK, often because it is a relatively cheap option in circumstances of haemodialysis under-provision. However, for younger patients it can produce a welcome sense of freedom and well-being, while for older patients it can appear haemodynamically more acceptable than haemodialysis. PD is an invaluable standby if vascular access fails repeatedly. It also spares valuable peripheral vessels which may prove life-saving in the future. The chief drawback of PD is peritonitis. The infection is usually mild to moderate in severity, not associated with fatal circulatory collapse and readily responsive to local and/or systemic antibiotics. The most common infections are due to skin organisms, such as staphylococcus epidermis and staphylococcus aureus. CAPD patients average one episode per 12–14 patient months. Errors of technique and infected catheter tracks are the main causative factors. Improving technology may be expected to reduce infection rates, which are falling in most centres. Recurrent infection may lead to sclerosing peritonitis, which precludes further PD and is a common reason for failure of PD. In some cases of recurrent infection the five year duration of treatment is under 40

PERITONEAL DIALYSIS

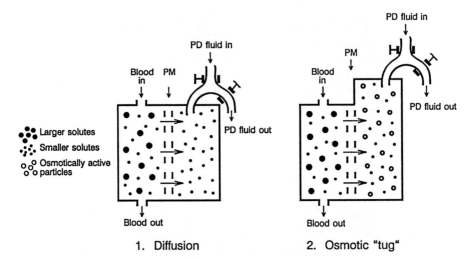

1. Diffusion   2. Osmotic "tug"

Peritoneal Dialysis (PD) combines (1) Diffusion of smaller solutes across peritoneal membrane (PM) down concentration gradient and (2) Osmotic "tug" of H_2O and smaller solutes across PM into PD fluid containing osmotically active particles, usually glucose.

Figure 7. Basic principles of peritoneal dialysis.

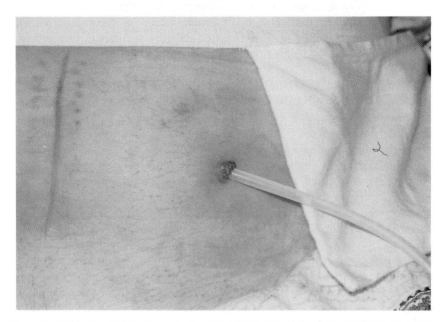

Figure 8. Access for CAPD. The use of a subcutaneous tunnel is important both to stabilize the catheter and to reduce the rate of peritoneal infection.

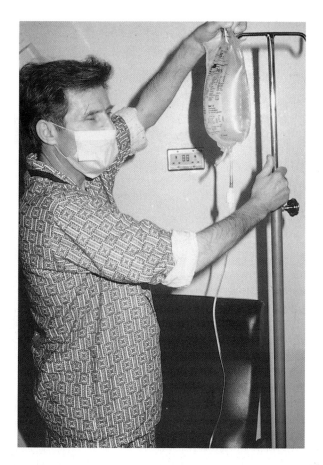

Figure 9. Setting-up for CAPD infusion. Training is relatively straightforward. An understanding of sterile technique is vital.

per cent. Patients with low infection rates may "clock-up" much longer times on treatment.

Apart from peritonitis, there is some doubt as to the long-term durability of the visceral peritoneum as a successful dialysis membrane. In some cases, the capacity to dialyse and/or ultrafilter has diminished or disappeared with time. A connection with the repeated use of hypertonic PD solutions to encourage fluid loss has been suggested. Nevertheless, there are a number of cases of proven survival on effective PD for periods of up to 10 years.

2. Choice of dialysis

For the potential transplant recipient, the "ideal" policy would be to map out a strategy which allows for survival and an adequate quality of life

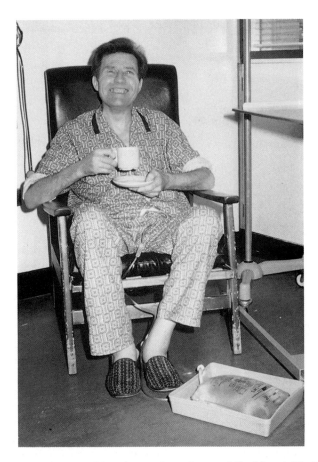

Figure 10. CAPD draining out. This patient performed successfully although blind from diabetic retinopathy.

pending successful transplantation but which does not reduce the options for dialysis at any time in the future, should it be required. Practical contingencies often intrude on this planning process and the future development of renal replacement therapy cannot be clearly seen. Nevertheless, the approach is in keeping with the already-stated philosophy of overall survival and welfare. For the younger, otherwise fit patient, CAPD is often a sensible first choice. In the absence of a serious bar to transplantation stemming from tissue type or cytotoxic antibody status, successful transplantation may be expected within two to three years at most, so that failure of the PD technique is unlikely. In the event of long-term graft failure, both haemo- and peritoneal dialysis remain fully available. There is a tendency for this to happen in Belfast. For some people, work or family commitments may dictate the method, while for others problems of access may leave no choice. Young children almost always do best on CAPD, which allows home care, does not involve unpleasant needling experiences and is compatible with on-going educational and social development.

3. Starting dialysis

It can be surprisingly difficult to fix the optimum time for starting dialysis. The clinical picture, or presentation, the underlying diagnosis, the general prognosis and the current biochemical findings are all important. Many patients still present in uraemic crisis and clearly need dialysis. If symptomatic and biochemical deterioration steadily recurs following treatment or if oliguria persists (especially in glomerular disease) the uraemia is probably terminal and regular dialysis is mandatory. The possibility of an acute, partly reversible, acute uraemic exacerbation should be remembered. Causes of this include hypertensive crisis, intercurrent disease inducing fluid and/or electrolyte imbalance, acute infective, obstructive or cardiovascular events and drug-mediated disturbances. The underlying disease tends to be tubulo-interstitial or urological rather than glomerular. Urinary volume is often well preserved. Following dialysis, the patient's condition remains stable with "viable" biochemical findings. Patients have been known to survive free of dialysis for up to 10 years after recovery from acute uraemic exacerbations requiring urgent dialysis. Progressive uraemic symptoms are a reliable sign of the need to treat, since, if they are ignored, the patient usually proceeds to a terminal state within a few months. Some patients (e.g. diabetics or sufferers from severe associated cardiovascular disease) develop symptoms "early", when creatinine levels are less than 700 micromol per litre, dialysis should usually be tried, and continued if it proves beneficial. Alarming biochemistry (creatinine over 1500 micromol/l, urea over 60 mmol/l, or potassium over 7 mmol/l) also demands dialysis. Asymptomatic uraemic patients can pose problems. They often decline dialysis and remain resolutely "well" for months, even years, despite creatinine levels persistently in excess of 1000 micromol/l. There is evidence, however, that 10-year survival is better (88 per cent) in those starting dialysis early (at a GFR of 10 ml/min) than in those (survival 55 per cent) who commence dialysis at a GFR of 2–4 ml/min. While this difference is to some extent obvious, it is true that late starters are also more prone to complications such as pericarditis and peripheral neuropathy. As a compromise, it seems reasonable to offer dialysis to asymptomatic patients when creatinine is consistently over 1000 micromol/l and GFR has fallen to five ml/min or less.

In the preferred situation, dialysis can be planned months or years in advance, following full assessment and with timely construction of access. Unfortunately, over 30 per cent of cases present as acute uraemic crises and require emergency management. Short-term vascular access with haemodialysis is the best response, allowing more time for assessment and choice of longer-term management.

4. Regular dialysis

Life on dialysis therapy should quickly become a well-understood and trouble-free, though tedious, routine, provided that access is satisfactory and that the procedure itself is tolerated without discomfort. Some aspects of treatment are shown in Figures 4–10.

While the likelihood of transplantation should be clear from an early stage of treatment, dialysis must be approached as if the patient could expect to live with it for many years. Apart from specific measures designed to benefit the transplanted state, dialysis is the same for all patients. Two common errors should be consciously avoided. The first is neglect by the doctor of the patient's medical state while on dialysis because he expects it to be "cured" by transplant. The second is "self burial" by the patient until all his ills are set right by the "miracle" of transplantation. Both these attitudes are a denial of the basic philosophy of treatment, which is to aim for as high a quality of survival as possible for as long as possible. This means that all medical problems of dialysis must be actively investigated and treated with as much consideration as an acute rejection episode. The patient must also be encouraged to recognise the current benefits produced by dialysis and be given a realistic, though optimistic, view of the likely effect of transplantation.

Patients returning to dialysis following graft failure fall into two categories, early and late. Early returners (under one year) have usually suffered acute graft rejection. It is important that return to dialysis occurs before the patient has developed undue side-effects of anti-rejection therapy and also that acute uraemic states are avoided. Confidence is severely shaken by abrupt emergency measures undertaken too late for an individual who has been exposed to the worst effects both of anti-rejection and of acute renal failure. Late return (over one year) may be necessary up to 10 or 20 years after transplantation following slow, mainly immunologically-mediated, graft failure. The decision to go back to dialysis should be clear, communicated in good time to the patient, and never deferred in the unreasonable hope of a slight extension of graft function. A full re-assessment is necessary, particularly of access problems and cardiovascular status. The patient should be made aware that further transplantation will not invariably be appropriate. Above all, he (or she) must be given the reassurance that all necessary support will be forthcoming throughout the duration of the renal disease. Integration of dialysis and transplantation in a smooth and effective way is a vital part of patient care. It requires (1) adequate dialysis facilities at all times and (2) control by a single consultant of all essential decisions related to the two modes of treatment for each individual.

Table 6. Factors influencing vulnerability of the kidney to nephrotoxins

High blood flow
High oxygen consumption
Large epithelial surface area
High enzyme activity
Medullary counter-current concentration gradients

5. Drugs and dialysis

The average dialysis patient takes a number of different drugs, not all of which are necessary and some of which are contraindicated. Among necessary drugs may usually be included anti-hypertensives, vitamin D analogues, phosphate-binding agents and erythropoietin. Sedatives, anti-pruritics, anti-emetics, diuretics and analgesics are frequently less valuable, though often used.

Pharmacological actions in renal failure may be divided into (1) nephrotoxic effects and (2) altered pharmacokinetics. Nephrotoxicity is common in patients with renal impairment. The kidney is vulnerable for a number of reasons (Table 6). Nephrotoxins may hasten the need for dialysis or diminish residual renal function in patients already on dialysis. Nephrotoxicity results from a number of different mechanisms (Table 7). In addition, indirect toxic mechanisms (related to drug-induced hypotension, dehydration, electrolyte imbalance and vasoconstriction) are an important cause of sudden dialysis-demanding emergencies. All uraemic crises should be screened for the possibility of reversible drug-related factors.

Pharmacological changes in renal failure are diverse, complex and still often poorly understood. The many variables include the extent of renal impairment, the drug-handling mechanisms affected and the effects on drug-handling of the different dialysis procedures. Pharmacokinetic mechanisms (e.g. bioavailability, distribution space, protein binding, end-organ responsiveness, biotransformation and elimination) are often affected differently by

Table 7. Mechanisms of nephrotoxicity

Mechanism	Example
Tubular damage	Heavy metals, Aminoglycosides
Hypersensitivity reactions	Drug induced angiitis Glomerulonephritis, Tubulo-interstitial nephritis
Papillary necrosis	Analgesic nephropathy (e.g. phenacetin)
Mixed vascular and tubulo-interstitial effects	Hypercalcaemia Cyclosporin

Table 8. Drugs usually requiring post-dialysis "top-up"

Aminoglycosides	Methyldopa
Cephalosporins	Atenolol
Penicillins	Procainamide
Chloramphenicol	Quinidine
Sulphonamides	Theophylline
Trimethoprim	Azathioprine
Flucytosine	Cyclophosphamide
Isoniazid	Methylprednisolone
Ethambutol	5-fluorouracil
Cycloserin	Salicylates
Fosfomycin	Water-soluble vitamins
Lithium	Barbital
Phenobarbital	

a single drug, so that the overall potential for toxicity may be unpredictable. In practical terms, therefore, prescribing should be cautious. It must be realised that the risk of drug toxicity is at least doubled in renal failure and also that drug-induced symptoms are frequently erroneously regarded as uraemic. An excellent maxim is:- if in doubt STOP ALL MEDICATIONS. When it is necessary to use a drug, it is usually best to stick to tried clinical practice. Normal loading doses are often acceptable, but thereafter increased spacing, decreased amounts, or both, may be appropriate.

Nomograms and tables relating drug dose to GFR and computer programmes outlining pharmacokinetic "modelling" for various drugs have been tried without conspicuous success. For some drugs (e.g. cyclosporin, aminoglycosides etc.) blood levels are valuable in predicting and preventing toxicity. In all cases, clinical judgment should have priority.

Dialysis induces a depletion of drugs analogous to, but by no means mirroring, renal elimination. Thus some post-dialysis "topping-up" may be desirable (Table 8). Haemo- and peritoneal dialysis are not identical in their effect. Where possible, tables of drug dialysis data should be consulted. Again, clinical considerations dominate. For example, methyldopa is quite well removed by dialysis of all types. However, since dialysis also improves blood pressure, extra doses of methyldopa are often not required.

6. Treatment of anaemia

Normochromic, normocytic anaemia is possibly the chief single cause of symptoms in end-stage renal failure. Tiredness and lack of energy are the main effects, but there are many others, including skeletal pain, dyspnoea and tachycardia, angina and heart failure. Poor concentration, loss of sexual desire and depression are also common. Deficiency of iron, vitamin B12 or folate may contribute, as may marrow toxins such as aluminium. Haemoglobin levels tend to be lower in haemodialysis than in CAPD patients, probably due to greater opportunity for blood loss related to needling, sampling or anticoagulation. In some younger women, the improved well-being produced by regular dialysis leads to a resumption of menstruation, severe menorrhagia and a profound exacerbation of anaemia. Hysterectomy may be necessary. Bilateral nephrectomy also significantly exacerbates anaemia.

Although some other factors operate, the chief cause of uraemic anaemia is clearly relative erythropoietin deficiency. Until the late 1980s, this was difficult to reverse. Blood transfusions provided temporary relief but carried a risk of cytotoxic antibody formation. Transfusion might also introduce diseases such as hepatitis B, HIV infection and CMV virus, although these can usually be excluded by routine screening. Recombinant erythropoietin, available through genetic engineering techniques for several years, promises to have a major impact on renal anaemia and thus on the quality of life on dialysis. In many cases it is able to restore haemoglobin levels to normal, although levels of 10–11 gms per cent may be preferable. Most cases of poor response are due to relative iron deficiency, which responds well to iron replacement. The greatest advantage of erythropoietin for the potential transplant recipient is that it avoids the need for possibly sensitising blood transfusions. Side-effects are few, but an exacerbation of hypertension is common. Some patients develop worrying episodes of hypertensive encephalopathy, while in others an increase of thromboembolic events has been noted. There is as yet no evidence that erythropoietin adversely affects transplantation, although one of our patients previously on effective erythropoietin therapy (as well as oral contraceptives) developed extensive post-graft arterio-venous thrombosis shortly following transplantation. In general, side-effects are more common at higher haemoglobin levels. It thus seems reasonable to aim for levels of 10–11 gms per cent in transplant candidates. Prophylactic post-transplant anticoagulation may also be advisable.

In general, the drug management of the potential transplant recipient does not differ significantly from the overall pattern. However, those drugs which interfere with cyclosporin metabolism (Table 9) should be avoided. Similarly, drugs which induce leucopenia (e.g., sulphonamides) or exacerbate gastro-intestinal disease (e.g. non-steroidal anti-inflammatory agents) are unsuitable since they may exacerbate the effects of azathioprine and steroids respectively.

An increasing number of patients return to dialysis following late graft failure. Removal of the transplant may be deferred or contraindicated for various reasons. The use and type of continued immunosuppression in such patients is not agreed. Gradual reduction to minimal doses is the best policy. Some patients seem able to manage without immunosuppression, although, in these, the possibility of late rejections episodes involving the failed graft should be remembered.

The secret of successful drug management on dialysis is undoubtedly regular patient AND drug chart review. Renal replacement therapy may be prolonged, with many switches and vicissitudes, for decades. The unwanted

Table 9. Important cyclosporin interactions

Cyclosporin level increased:	Corticosteroids
	Diltiazem
	Erythromycin
	Ketoconazole
Cyclosporin level decreased:	Isoniazid
	Phenobarbitone
	Phenytoin
	Rifampicin
Cyclosporin nephrotoxicity enhanced:	Aminoglycosides
	Amphotericin B
	Melphalan
	Sulphonamides
	Trimethoprim

accumulation of pharmacological "fellow-travellers" is best held in check by this salutary, and essential, process.

Further reading

Lazarus, J. M., Hakim, R. M. Medical aspects of hemodialysis. Ch. 49. In *The Kidney*, 4th ed., Brenner, B. M., Rector, F. C., eds. Philadelphia, Saunders, 1991; vol. 2: 2223–2298.

Maher, J. F. *Replacement of Renal Function by Dialysis*. 3d ed. Dordrecht, Kluwer Acad. Publishers, 1988: *passim*.

Nolph, K. D. Peritoneal dialysis. Ch. 50. In *The Kidney*, 4th ed., Brenner, B. M., Rector, F. C., eds. Philadelphia, Saunders, 1991; vol. 2: 2299–2335.

CHAPTER 6

Preparation for transplantation 2

J. F. DOUGLAS

1. Hypertension in end-stage renal failure

About 80 per cent of patients starting dialysis are hypertensive. In glomerulonephritis, diabetic nephropathy and primary vascular disease, the incidence of hypertension rises to over 90 per cent. Tubulo-interstitial and pelvi-ureteric disease carry a lower hypertensive risk. Atherogenesis in renal failure is closely related to blood pressure control. It is therefore disturbing to find that over 60 per cent of dialysis patients (and over 90 per cent of diabetics) have been shown to be under poor control. In the under 40 age-group, atherosclerosis is almost confined to patients with a history of hypertension. Long-term survival, both on dialysis and after transplantation, relates more closely to serial blood pressure levels than to any other single factor. Hypertension and its control are thus literally of vital importance to the patient. Unfortunately, it is probable that this is also the least effectively managed aspect of renal medical care.

The pathogenesis of renal hypertension is multi-factorial, but the contribution of the factors is not constant in all cases or even within the evolution of a single case.

Haemodynamic studies show a confusing picture, with some consistent features. Hypertensive uraemic patients display a persistently raised total peripheral resistance (TPR). Cardiac output and stroke volume are usually normal, although heart rate is usually increased. Anaemia decreases TPR, apparently through a mechanism of hypoxic vasodilatation. Correction of anaemia, by transfusion or erythropoietin (EPO), leads to a rise of TPR, although these two therapeutic measures are not haemodynamically identical. Viscosity effects of changing red cell mass may also play a part in TPR regulation. In addition, anaemia, together with coronary artery disease exacerbated by hypertension, alters cardiac function, adding the pathophysiology of heart failure to that of renal vasopressor effects. Hypoalbuminaemia, which may be present, due to proteinuria, peritoneal loss on PD, or malnutrition, alters plasma volume and its relationship to interstitial fluid volume.

Mary G. McGeown (ed.), Clinical Management of Renal Transplantation, 77–89.
© 1992 *Kluwer Academic Publishers, Dordrecht. Printed in the Netherlands.*

1.1. *Factors leading to hypertension in dialysis patients*

Among the many factors contributing to hypertension in dialysis patients the following appear to be the most important:-

1.1.1. *Sodium and water retention*

In end-stage renal failure an increase in plasma volume, ECF volume, total exchangeable sodium (NaE) and total body water is typically found. It was proposed by Starling, Borst and others that failure to excrete sodium and water produces an initial increase in ECF and blood volume with increased cardiac output, leading to hypertension. Following autoregulation, cardiac output falls to normal but hypertension is maintained by increased peripheral resistance. This sequence, though common, is not in fact always observed in clinical or experimental studies. It has been suggested, therefore, that sodium load may be the primary event. An increase in NaE may be followed by secondary volume expansion, but hypertension is produced by different and non-volume-related mechanisms. These contribute to raised TPR in various ways:- changes in blood vessel wall structure, tone and reactivity, stimulation of the renin-angiotensin-aldosterone axis, reflex regulation, reduction of sodium-potassium pump activity or altered transcellular sodium exchange, leading to increased intracellular calcium and heightened smooth muscle tone. The ability of dialysis to control blood pressure by fluid and solute removal demonstrates the importance of the overload theory but does not indicate which version is closer to reality.

1.1.2. *The renin-angiotensin system*

This system is not destroyed in end-stage renal failure but the normal reciprocal relationship between NaE and plasma renin activity is frequently disrupted. In consequence, plasma renin activity (PRA) is often abnormally high for any given level of NaE loading. Cases of hypertension resistant to dialysis have the highest PRA levels and show the greatest improvement after bilateral nephrectomy. These observations strongly implicate the renin-angiotensin system and provide one of the main arguments in favour of bilateral nephrectomy.

1.1.3. *Other factors*

There is frequent abnormality of the sympathetic nervous system in end-stage renal failure, with elevation of plasma catecholamines in many cases. The complex interaction of the system with NaE, fluid load and PRA make it hard to assess the significance of this abnormality. The sympathetic system may also be influenced by changes of vascular tone and responsiveness in end-stage renal failure, as well as by other uraemic changes, such as raised parathormone and prostaglandin levels. Hypercalcaemia contributes to hypertension through increased TPR, while hypocalcaemia has the reverse effect. These changes are probably related to alterations in intracellular free cytosolic calcium, which promotes smooth muscle tone and reactivity and may be part of the "final common pathway" in the generation of hypertension. Changes in endothelin levels may be important in the same way. The role of these, and other, factors, such as natriuretic hormone (increased in uraemia), on vascular tone and TPR is not fully understood and is still the subject of much research. Many observed changes may be secondary to sodium retention and volume expansion, but this does not lessen their potential importance as guides to the development of new therapeutic agents.

2. Therapeutic approach to hypertension

2.1. *General measures*

Almost all end-stage renal failure patients with hypertension require both sodium and fluid restriction by the time they approach dialysis. A regime of "no added salt" may be appropriate since few people comply well with more severe restriction. Fluid restriction to 1000–1500 mls per day is often a useful target, but again is dependent on compliance. Thirst, related to raised PRA levels, hyperparathyroidism, diabetes or high dialysate sodium levels, can be a major challenge to resolve. Exercise training reduces blood pressure and allows medications to be decreased, both in uraemic patients and patients on dialysis. Unfortunately, many patients (over 70 per cent) display reduced exercise tolerance which lessens its practical value. Following EPO therapy, exercise tolerance may be expected to improve, although rising haemoglobin exerts its own effect on blood pressure.

2.2. *Dialysis*

Dialysis and its analogues, in all their forms, reduce blood pressure by removing sodium and water. Various studies claim control of hypertension in 65–80 per cent of patients if a satisfactory dry weight is achieved (i.e. the weight below which further dialysis causes unwanted hypotension). We have not achieved this level of success. Haemofiltration, which removes large volumes of fluid and NaE in exchange for a smaller replacement volume, can increase control where dialysis proves insufficient. Aggressive dialysis with concurrent ultrafiltration tends to produce regular hypotensive episodes. Sequential dialysis and ultrafiltration often produce the same effect as the two combined (but without hypotension) and are thus particularly suitable for haemodynamically unstable persons. Sequential ultrafiltration seems to work by preventing significant osmolar changes between extracellular and

Table 10. Factors influencing antihypertensive drug selection
in dialysis patients

Absorption
Pharmacokinetics
Mode of action
Interactions
Dialyzability
Accumulation of metabolites
Enhancement of risk factors e.g. atherogenic
                                   cardiac
                                   lipidaemia
                                   arrhythmia
Effectiveness
Unwanted effects
Compliance
Cost

---

intracellular fluid. The effect of dialysis and related processes on inter-dialytic blood pressure is not clear at present. It is obviously affected by compliance. Clinical studies suggest that CAPD and continuous cycling peritoneal dialysis (CCPD), because of their continuous or semi-continuous nature and greater capacity to remove sodium and water, achieve better pressure control than haemodialysis. In addition, hypertensive patients on CAPD show a decrease in left ventricular hypertrophy and an improved ventricular ejection fraction.

2.3. *Drug therapy*

In various studies, up to 35 per cent of the hypertensive dialysis population required antihypertensive drugs. In our experience at Belfast, the require-ment has been higher (over 50 per cent). The factors influencing drug selec-tion are shown in Table 10. A full knowledge of pharmacokinetics and drug interactions is desirable before prescribing, but is often lacking.

Diuretics have limited application, with risks of oto- and nephro-toxicity, but may be used to improve sodium and water loss in selected patients. Beta blocking agents have been criticised for their tendency to promote left ventricular failure. They also vary considerably in cardioselectivity as well as in their effects on sympathetic activity, blood sugar and lipid levels. However, they are valuable antihypertensives and have been widely used, particularly for younger patients and in long-acting forms. In the many dialysis patients who have associated cardiovascular disease, they are effec-tive as prophylaxis of recurrent myocardial infarction, as well as in the management of angina and many arrhythmias. Centrally acting agents (e.g. methyldopa, clonidine) are now less frequently used. This is partly due to a relatively high incidence of side-effects, notably postural hypotension. How-ever some effects which are normally unwanted may be beneficial in renal failure. For example, in patients nearing the need for dialysis, clonidine's tendency to lead to potassium loss may be usefully exploited. Calcium channel blockers (e.g. nifedipine, verapamil and diltiazem) rapidly lower TPR and mean arterial pressure. They can be used sublingually to control hypertensive crises without risk of postural hypotension, as well as being effective relievers of angina by this route. Vasodilators (e.g. prazosin, hydralazine, doxazosin) are effective for many patients. More potent forms, such as minoxidil, labetalol (which also has a beta blocking effect) diazoxide and nitroprusside can all be useful for hypertensive crises or in cases of serious resistance. They have considerable potential for unwanted effects.

2.4. *Therapeutic problems*

Hypertensive crises are mainly caused by fluid and sodium excess. Emergency dialysis and/or ultrafiltration may be essential. Blood transfusions or rising haematocrit due to EPO therapy may be the precipitating factors, in which case venesection should be considered. Resistant hypertension is common. Full investigation is important but is often omitted. The accuracy of readings, patient compliance, drug effectiveness and the emergence of factors such as renovascular disease or hyperparathyroidism should be considered. Fluctuating hypertension may be associated with autonomic dysfunction, especially if postural hypotension is also present. Full haemodynamic studies, using mainly non-invasive techniques, such as radionucleides and echocardiography, can give valuable information. In view of the prognostic importance of blood pressure control, there is a strong case for more active study of all the forms of dialysis hypertension and for the development of new methods of investigation and treatment.

3. Bilateral nephrectomy (BN)

There are two main arguments in favour of BN for hypertension in pre-transplant dialysis patients. First, it can be shown that, in most such patients, PRA (plasma renin activity) is abnormally high for any given degree of sodium load. Second, among hypertensive dialysis patients who have been successfully transplanted, the incidence of post-graft hypertension is lower in those patients who have first undergone BN. These observations suggest a contribution to continued hypertension from the patient's own kidneys. In Belfast, there was for many years a policy of BN in all cases of hypertension. Mortality was very low (under two per cent) and improved blood pressure control was observed in many cases, both before and after transplant. Nevertheless BN for hypertension is now less frequently performed, for several reasons:-

82

Table 11. Main grounds for considering bilateral nephrectomy/nephro-ureterectomy

Lesion	Specific Examples
1. Hypertension	Selected severe cases
2. Infection	Active e.g. TB
	pyonephrosis
3. Urological abnormalities	Gross ureteric reflux
	Megaureter
	Urinary diversion
4. Tumours	Malignant
	or recurring
5. Polycystic kidneys	Massive or persistently
	symptomatic
6. Calculi	Large and bilateral
7. Miscellaneous	Massive proteinuria

1. The complications, morbidity and long-term effects of the procedure itself;
2. The development of new, more effective drugs for blood pressure control;
3. The persistence of renoprival hypertension in over thirty per cent of patients following BN;
4. The absence of significant differences in atherogenic complications in the long term (five to ten years) between patients who had undergone BN for hypertension and those who had not.

There are a number of possible indications for the removal of the patient's own kidneys, with or without the ureters and other parts of the urinary tract (Table 11). Where appropriate, of course, *unilateral* nephrectomy may be the procedure of choice.

3.1. *Hypertension*

This has already been discussed. The criteria are listed in Table 12.

Table 12. Criteria for bilateral nephrectomy in hypertension

1. Severe hypertension on starting dialysis
2. Short preceding history of hypertension
3. Age under 40
4. No evidence of generalized atheroma
5. No major atherogenic factors (e.g. smoking, diabetes)
6. Recurrence of disease in graft unlikely
7. Early transplant probable (e.g. living related donor)
8. Good fluid compliance likely

3.2. *Infection*

Persistent bilateral infection related to factors such as calculi or obstruction is an indication for BN, particularly if severe associated structural change is present. In renal tuberculosis, BN removes major potential sources of recurrent mycobacterial infection. In hydronephrosis, hydro- or megaureter and reflux nephropathy, bilateral nephro-ureterectomy was for a long time regarded as necessary, whether or not there was evidence of recurring urinary infection. The danger of fatal or disabling post-transplant ascending infection was considered to demand the procedure. However, despite a clear increase of post-transplant urinary infections in non-nephrectomised patients, and occasional reports of infection-mediated graft damage, there is no compelling evidence to suggest increased mortality or graft loss in this group, at any rate when low dose immunosuppression policies have been followed. In many cases of lower urinary tract dysplasia, there are other causes of increased incidence of urinary infection after transplant (e.g. bladder abnormalities). Many such patients, who are often very young, are not hypertensive and have a well maintained urinary output. Bilateral nephro-ureterectomy transforms them into anuric hypertensive individuals, with a high risk of fluid overload and hypertensive encephalopathy (Figures 11, 12). A policy of selection thus seems appropriate, restricting surgery to patients with gross abnormalities, a history of serious infection, associated hypertension and absence of high urinary output or bladder abnormalities. In some cases of moderate ureteric reflux, submucosal teflon injections may prove effective in abolishing the lesion, without the need to consider bilateral nephro-ureterectomy.

3.3. *Obstructive and other urological abnormalities*

Provided all reversible factors have been completely excluded, these lesions, quite apart from their infective risk, may justify surgery if they are associated with severe pain or inconvenience (e.g. nephrostomy tubes, urinary diversions etc.). In some cases, diversionary surgery has been carried out many years before the development of renal failure, in the hope of preventing it. If this has happened, a complete bladder assessment regularly reveals that this organ is useable for transplantation. Occasionally (e.g. in cases of tumour, incontinence etc.) bladder use is impossible.

3.4. *Tumours*

Bilateral malignant tumours obviously require BN, although, in a few cases, partial salvage of one kidney, with successful autotransplantation, has been achieved. Renal carcinoma is the commonest indication. Benign or congenital

84

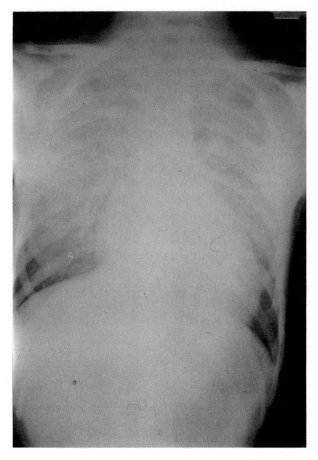

Figure 11. Pulmonary oedema due to fluid overload in an anephric patient. Hypertensive encephalopathy was also present. He was normotensive before bilateral nephro-ureterectomy for gross ureteric reflux.

tumours or malformations may justify BN for complications such as bleeding or pain. Malignant tumours of urinary tract epithelium have a strong tendency to recur. This can necessitate the eventual removal of the entire tract. BN and other surgery would of course be quite inappropriate in the event of metastatic spread, since in this situation transplantation should not be considered.

Many failed kidneys undergo cystic degeneration with time. Occasional instances of carcinomatous change have occurred (Figure 13). This is another argument in favour of BN, but the overall incidence of such tumours does not, of itself, outweigh other factors. However, there is a case for routine ultrasound screening of all non-nephrectomised patients five and more years after transplantation. All clinical symptoms and signs relating to the patient's native kidneys should be fully assessed.

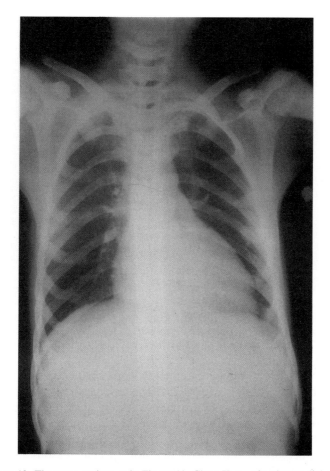

Figure 12. The same patient as in Figure 11. Chest X ray after haemodialysis.

3.5. *Miscellaneous*

Polycystic kidneys justify removal if they are excessively large or painful, or are associated with calculi or severe recurrent infection or haematuria. In practice many involute partially after successful transplantation. Routine removal is advocated by some, but is probably not essential, particularly since the kidneys often provide some benefit to the dialysis in the form of residual function and maintained EPO production.

Large calculi are usually best removed, with nephrectomy, if necessary. In addition to pain, they may lead to bacteraemic infection or carcinomatous change. A few cases of massive proteinuria (mainly in small children with congenital nephrotic syndrome) have been successfully treated by BN, followed by transplantation.

It has been suggested by some that BN is always justified because it is

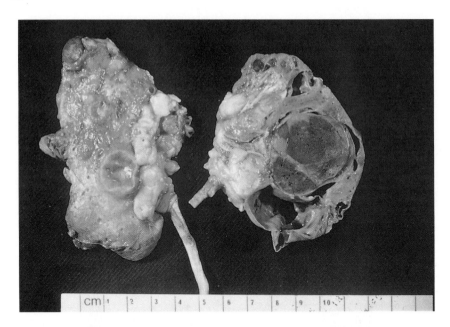

Figure 13. Renal carcinoma 10 years after transplant in a kidney which had developed cystic degeneration. The patient presented with hypercalcaemia related to secondary spread of tumour.

associated with lower rates of rejection and with better long-term graft function. The effect, however, is slight. The reason is unexplained, but could relate to higher post-graft blood pressure levels, or differing pre-transplant management, including the use of more blood transfusions for nephrec-tomised patients.

Uni-nephrectomy is often indicated for specific reasons (e.g. tumour, calculi or painful foci). The only general indication that we have noted is that uni-nephrectomy may be an effective way of "making space" for a graft in gross polycystic disease, without sacrificing the benefits to the patient of retaining some renal tissue.

3.6. *Operative technique*

Adequate pre-operative dialysis, particularly to control potassium levels and fluid overload, is necessary, since both can cause life-threatening post-operative problems. Full anaesthetic assessment is also important. However, if the patient's fitness for BN is in doubt, other than acutely, the suitability of transplantation should also be reconsidered.

Bilateral posterior incisions should be used where possible. Transverse or longitudinal abdominal incisions have a high morbidity and disrupt dialysis in CAPD cases. Occasionally however, (e.g. for removal of cystic

Table 13. Main benefits of bilateral nephrectomy

1. Improved blood pressure control
2. Better graft function (slight, over large series)
3. Less urinary infection
4. Avoidance of neoplastic change in native kidneys

hydronephrotic kidneys or when ureterectomy is also necessary) the posterior route is not practicable, and an anterior or lateral approach is required.

Effective destruction of native renal tissue without its removal ("medical nephrectomy") may be possible. In some cases of severe hypertension, bilateral renal artery embolization has proved successful. However, it has a number of complications and has not been entirely reliable in its effect. Indomethacin and similar drugs have also been used to produce the same result: one candidate is the renal failure patient who also has massive proteinuria, with consequent hypoproteinaemia, oedema and hypotension.

3.7. *Adverse effects of BN*

Early mortality of BN has ranged from zero to over 10 per cent and is higher in cases of anterior approach. Haemorrhage, profound hypotension, hyperkalaemia and intra-abdominal complications are the chief causes of death. Short-term morbidity, which is considerable, relates to these factors as well as to infection. Long-term mortality should not be overlooked: fatal late hyperkalaemia and fluid overload in renoprival patients have been recorded. Anaemia is exacerbated, although this is now reversible with EPO, and bone disease may deteriorate. The problems of the anephric patient are made worse if, due to difficulties of tissue matching for transplantation, or to a high level of cytotoxic antibodies, there is likely to be a prolonged wait for a donor kidney. It is true that some people adapt surprisingly well to the anephric state. For others, the quality of life is seriously reduced.

3.8. *"Cost-effectiveness" of BN*

BN must be judged in terms of its overall ability to prolong survival and improve quality of life. In a few cases (e.g. bilateral tumours) this is not in doubt. In most cases the essential question is whether its benefits after transplantation outweigh its immediate harmful effects. The main benefits are shown in Table 13. These are all desirable, once transplantation has been successfully performed. However, the first three benefits do not significantly improve length or quality of life. Cardiovascular disease, the greatest threat to the patient, relates best to duration and severity of hypertension at the time of starting dialysis. Neoplastic change, though preventible, is rare.

Taking into account the known mortality and morbidity of BN, it is best to perform it in selected cases only.

To maximize cost-effectiveness in appropriate cases, there is a case for increased use of BN after successful transplant as prophylaxis against neoplastic change: probably this approach has been inadequately used.

4. Lower urinary tract preparation

The various bladder abnormalities that may be encountered need not be a bar to successful transplantation, provided that the patient is otherwise suitable. Transplantation into an ileal conduit is quite feasible, with good results, although it is important that the conduit should have been constructed well in advance in order to lessen problems of infection and healing. Previous cystectomy for neoplastic disease is an obvious indication. However, in spite of defects of size or function, the bladder is usually satisfactory for the purposes of transplant, or can be made so by corrective surgery. It is probable that in the past more conduits have been constructed then was really necessary.

Case History

A 12–year-old boy with megacystis and megaureter had a urinary diversion into an ileal conduit "to protect his very tenuous renal function". Nevertheless, five years later he developed end-stage renal failure and, after a period of haemodialysis, a cadaver transplant was inserted into the conduit. The graft failed after six years for a number of reasons, including urinary infection. The patient returned to haemodialysis. Two years later, after resection of the donor kidney and the ileal conduit, a successful living related donor transplant was performed, using the patient's own enlarged bladder. Seven years after the operation he is well with normal renal function. There is no clinical evidence of bladder problems or of significant urinary infection.

Every candidate for transplantation should have a sufficient urological assessment. Many would contend that micturating cysto-urethrography is a minimum requirement, although in cases of known glomerular disease, without symptomatic lower urinary disorder, it is almost always normal. Ureteric reflux is the chief unsuspected lesion detected by this investigation. Further bladder studies include cystoscopy and urodynamic investigations. These help to determine bladder capacity, degree of trabeculation, presence or activity of infection, existence of diverticuli or stones and the extent of any bladder outlet obstruction. Severe obstruction should be corrected before transplantation. Prostatic hypertrophy amounting to acute urinary retention falls into this category, while minor problems can be corrected, if necessary, after successful transplantation. Bladder capacity can be increased by preliminary ileo- or caeco-cystoplasty if necessary.

However, even quite small bladders (capacity 120 mls or less) have proved functionally adequate after transplant. Some bladders, unused for a long time, have a low capacity, leading to irritating frequency following operation. This situation, in our experience, almost always reverses with time. Mega-cystis also produces surprisingly few problems, although it is associated with an increased risk of post-graft urinary infection. Neurogenic bladder, with inability to void urine, might seem to require diversionary surgery but has in fact been well managed by intermittent self-catherisation following trans-plant, without serious infection. Thus, although full assessment remains im-portant, there appear to be few cases in which the patient's own bladder is not more acceptable for transplantation than any form of urinary diversion.

5. Other surgical procedures

Pre-transplant splenectomy reduces rejection rates, but increases post-trans-plant mortality due to infection. Essentially it is a way of irreversibly increas-ing immunosuppression and should therefore be avoided in almost all cases.

Surgery for duodenal ulcer – e.g. vagotomy and pyloroplasty – was for-merly performed routinely at many centres to avoid steroid-induced exacer-bations. Since the advent of H_2 blocking agents, this should hardly ever be necessary.

A number of other preparatory surgical procedures are often advisable. They are related to the possibility of infection or other complications as a result of immunosuppression. Dental surgery is indicated in many cases. Other procedures depend on the clinical state of the individual patient. In Belfast some of the operations considered necessary have been: bowel resec-tion for complications of colonic diverticular disease; cholecystectomy; ap-pendicectomy; coronary angioplasty or by-pass surgery; cardiac valve surg-ery; tonsillectomy; and the removal of varied benign or potentially malignant skin, subcutaneous or breast lesions.

Further reading

Briggs, J. D. The recipient of a renal transplant. In *Kidney Transplantation*. Morris, P. J. ed, 3rd ed. Philadelphia, Saunders 1988: 71–92.

Heyka, R. J., Paganini, E. P. Blood pressure control in chronic dialysis patients. In *Replacement of Renal Function by Dialysis*. Maher, J. F., 3rd ed. Dordrecht, Kluwer Acad. Publishers, 1988: 772–787.

CHAPTER 7

Preparation for transplantation 3

J. F. DOUGLAS

1. Immunological preparation

Immunological preparation has a two fold purpose. First, it is necessary in order to define the patient's immunological status. Second, manipulation of that status can aid the eventual acceptance of a transplanted organ by the recipient's immune system.

1.1. *Blood grouping, tissue typing and immunological screening*

These procedures are all essential. ABO blood group compatibility is normally necessary for successful transplantation, although in a few cases of low donor antigenicity (such as in A2 kidneys) and/or recipient pretreatment, ABO incompatible grafting has proved successful. The source of incompatibility is thought to be graft vascular endothelium, which carries A and/or B antigens. Tissue typing must, as a minimum, cover the Class 1 antigens (at least A and B loci) and Class 2 (DR) antigens of the Human Major Histocompatibility System (MHS). Class 1 (C locus) and minor histocompatibility systems seem to be of lesser, though not negligible importance and can usually be ignored when considering the practical problems of acceptable "matching" between donor and recipient. It has been claimed that modern cyclosporin-based immunosuppression regimes render HLA and/or DR matching irrelevant, but this is not borne out by large-scale studies, which consistently show improved graft survival rates with close HLA matching on all forms of therapy. In addition, in the event of graft failure, close tissue matching reduces the difficulty of finding a second donor, since the number of potentially unacceptable donor antigens is kept to a minimum. In Belfast, it is our policy also to regard as generally unacceptable the incompatible HLA antigens of the marital partners of parous women, since the possibility of sensitization to these antigens by way of exposure to the foetus cannot be excluded.

Regular immunological monitoring for the development of cytotoxic

Mary G. McGeown (ed.), Clinical Management of Renal Transplantation, 91–106.
© 1992 *Kluwer Academic Publishers, Dordrecht. Printed in the Netherlands.*

antibodies is an important part of pre-transplant preparation. It allows a distinction to be made between patients who display little or no sensitization and those who are, or become, highly sensitized (over 90 per cent antibodies), due to previous failed grafts, pregnancies or transfusions. Such patients are difficult to transplant, since offers are fewer, positive cross-matches are more common and the risk of early, acute rejection may be greater. However, highly sensitized patients have often done well after transplant despite these problems. Close or "beneficial" matching (i.e. matching associated with a higher rate of graft survival) allows graft survival rates comparable to those of non-sensitized patients, while the UK Transplant Service policy of wide organ distribution increases the chance of finding a suitable kidney. Nevertheless, occasional patients may have to endure waiting times of up to ten years before a suitable opportunity occurs.

Antibody levels in highly sensitized patients may fall with time or following multiple blood transfusions and this can permit some successful transplants in patients who show a positive "historic" response (i.e. a positive reaction gained from a sample of serum taken in the past, sometimes several years earlier) but a negative response on current samples. Efforts to eliminate cytotoxic antibodies prior to transplantation have been made, with some success, using plasmapheresis and occasionally immunosuppressive drugs. Certain non-HLA and auto-antibodies may produce apparent sensitization responses, which can however be ignored in predicting graft outcome (Chapter 9). Their detection should be left to immunological laboratories but they should be suspected whenever "cytotoxic antibodies" emerge without any obvious predisposing reason.

Sensitization is a major problem for patients awaiting transplantation. In many centres, the numbers of patients with significant antibody levels is greater than 50 per cent. Sensitized patients tend to accumulate with time on waiting lists as non-sensitized ones are removed by successful transplantation. In caring for those whose antibody levels are as yet low or non-existent, every effort should be made to prevent their development. Unnecessary transfusions should not be given to patients with known antibody levels or (possibly) multiple pregnancies. Blood transfusions (apart from those given to promote graft acceptance by "enhancement" – see below) should only be given after thorough washing or filtration to remove leucocyte fragments. A policy of close or "beneficial" tissue matching should be followed as far as practicable, in order to minimize the problem of sensitization in patients returning to transplant waiting lists after the eventual failure of earlier grafts.

1.1.1. *Previous transplants*. Patients whose former grafts have failed figure increasingly in "on-call" lists. Early losses (within three months of operation) are usually due to acute rejection. Late losses (over one year post-transplant) have a wider range of causes but are most commonly due to chronic immuno-logically-mediated deterioration ("chronic rejection"). Previous transplants raise a number of issues.

1.1.2. *Risk of rejection*. Previous early rejection of a graft (under one year) by no means rules out successful later transplantation. However, repeated early rejections progressively decrease the prospects for later grafts, partic-ularly if the loss occurred despite the use of cyclosporin. In such situations, re-assessment of transplantability may be desirable. Late failure of grafts does not appear to influence the result of subsequent transplantation.

1.1.3. *Sensitization*. Graft loss is associated with a high incidence of sensi-tization, which may be exacerbated by transfusion and eventually reach high levels (over 90 per cent). Each failed graft, unless a "full-house" (i.e. identi-cal) match, also increases the numbers of unacceptable antigens, since, even if antibodies are currently undetectable, it must be assumed that exposure to the antigen of itself produces immunological "awareness" in the recipient. The policy of close and "beneficial" matching which underlies organ-sharing schemes such as that organized by UK Transplant Service is based on the idea that good matching both reduces graft loss and facilitates later trans-plantation. Belfast has adhered closely to this policy for many years.

1.1.4. *Graft nephrectomy*. Following early graft failure, nephrectomy should usually be performed promptly in order to prevent necrosis or infection and to lessen the risk of sensitization. It also allows immunosuppression to be withdrawn. Following late failure, the decision to operate is less straightfor-ward. Sensitization is already well established and the risks of necrosis or infection are usually less. The transplanted kidney, which has had a period of good function, is usually still producing a valuable urinary output. The operation itself is often much more difficult, due to the embedding of the graft and its blood vessels in fibrous tissue. Thus, while nephrectomy is desirable in many cases, it may be acceptable to proceed to a second trans-plant in some cases without removing the first kidney.

1.2. *Blood transfusion*

Blood transfusion improves the anaemia of chronic renal failure and has long been used for this purpose. There are disadvantages. First, transfusions may introduce infections, such as hepatitis B, human immune deficiency virus (HIV) and cytomegalic virus (CMV). Second, HLA and other antigens in transfused leucocytes may stimulate production of cytotoxic antibodies. Repeated transfusion can lead to a high degree of sensitization, particularly in parous women and previous graft recipients. Adequate filtration or saline washing of blood before transfusion greatly reduces the effect. However, in 1973, Opelz and Terasaki, from an analysis of large numbers of graft recipients, showed a surprising benefit of transfusion. This was a significant (15–20 per cent) improvement in graft survival at one year for transfused over non-transfused patients. The effect was shown to be dependent on the presence of leucocytes in transfused blood and was not related to transfusion at the time of transplantation. The mechanism of protection is unclear. It has been suggested that "selection out" of potentially sensitized individuals (who develop antibodies after transfusion and therefore are not exposed to them at transplantation) from non-sensitized individuals is important. However, experimental evidence suggests a process of active "enhancement", dependent on the activation of antigen-specific suppressor T cells.

The transfusion effect was most obvious in centres where graft survival rates were otherwise relatively poor. In recent years, overall improvement in graft survival, particularly in non-transfused patients, both with and without the use of cyclosporin, has reduced the transfusion effect to a factor of less than five per cent at one year and cast some doubt on its value. There is also evidence that only DR-mismatched grafts obtain a benefit. In consequence it has been argued that the balance of advantage no longer favours transfusion, in view of its sensitizing potential. However, a number of strategies may lessen unwanted effects. These include:- non-transfusion of patients at high risk of sensitization: restriction of transfusion to three units or less: partial DR-matching of transfused blood, which appears to reduce sensitization. At present, the Belfast policy is to continue with pre-transplant transfusions, while taking account of the above points.

In many centres, when there is a living related donor available, donor-specific transfusions have been used for haplo-identical pairs, with the effect of improving graft results to equal those of grafts between HLA-identical siblings. The risk of sensitization is up to 30 per cent. As with random transfusions before cadaver grafts, the effect has become less marked in recent years. In Belfast recipients of kidneys from living related donors are not usually treated in this way.

1.3. *Splenectomy*

Splenectomy has been performed in many centres, before, as well as at the time of, transplantation, with the object of improving graft survival. Significant improvement was observed in early studies in US but later reports did not confirm this. An alarming increase in mortality, mainly due to sepsis, has been reported (Chapter 15). It is clear, therefore, that splenectomy is essentially an extra and irreversible form of immunosuppression, which should generally be avoided. Two possible exceptions are:- hypersplenism, especially associated with severe leucopenia: and cases in which an ABO incompatible graft has been given inadvertently.

1.4. *Plasmapheresis*

Plasmapheresis, which has been used to treat acute, steroid-resistant rejection with a vascular component, has also been applied to the pre-transplant situation. First, it has been used in the preparation of recipients for successful ABO-incompatible living related donor transplants. Second, it has been used in highly sensitized dialysis patients to reduce titres and reactivity and pave the way for successful cross-match negative transplantation in these individuals. Some acceptable results have been achieved, but not without morbidity, especially where immunosuppressive drugs have also been used.

1.5. *Immunosuppressive agents*

Immunosuppressive drugs, including steroids, azathioprine and cyclosporin, have been used in the immediate pre-transplant period, particularly in the preparation of living related donor recipients. There is no evidence that pre-transplant immunosuppression significantly improves graft survival. The above agents, with the addition of cyclophosphamide, have also been used, as already noted, to reduce the level and range of cytotoxic antibodies in highly sensitized potential recipients.

2. Renal osteodystrophy

Renal osteodystrophy is a term used to describe the overall effects of renal failure upon the skeletal system. It includes the lesions produced by abnormalities of calcium and phosphorus homeostasis, as well as by other biochemical changes occurring in renal disease. Among these changes must be numbered the effects of dialysis itself and the toxic osteopathy (mainly caused by aluminium) which may be associated with it. Transplantation and immunosuppression further influence the evolution of renal osteodystrophy. This should be remembered when considering pre-transplant management (see also Chapter 8).

   The main pathological features of renal osteodystrophy are shown in Table 14.

2.1. *Osteomalacia*

The normal kidney metabolises precursor substances to biologically active calcitriol (1,25 dihydroxycholecalciferol: vitamin D3). Defective production of calcitriol in renal failure leads to impaired absorption of calcium (and to a lesser degree, of phosphate), reduced mineralization of osteoid tissue,

Table 14. Pathological lesions and clinical features of renal osteodystrophy

Lesion	Clinical features
Osteomalacia	Skeletal deformity Bone pain and tenderness Proximal myopathy Renal rickets (in children) Growth retardation (in children)
Secondary hyperparathyroidism	Skeletal deformity Bone pain Gastro-intestinal symptoms Extra-skeletal calcification Pruritis
Osteitis fibrosa	Pathological fractures Bone resorption on X-ray Slipping epiphyses (in children)
Osteosclerosis	Areas of increased density on X-ray
Avascular necrosis	Joint pain (NB hip) Typical areas of increased density on X-ray
Osteoporosis (osteopenia)	Pathological fractures Pain Skeletal deformities
Aluminium-induced osteopathy	Bone pain Deformities Pathological fractures Encephalopathy Microcytic anaemia
Extra-skeletal calcification	Pruritus Joint pain Peri-articular swellings Calciphylaxis Peripheral ischaemia Decreased peripheral pulses Cardiac and respiratory disorders

decreased responsiveness of bone to parathyroid hormone (PTH), retardation of bone growth, proximal myopathy, hypocalcaemia and increased secondary secretion of PTH.

2.2. *Secondary hyperparathyroidism*

Parathyroid hyperplasia and increased PTH production begin early in the course of renal failure and become more marked as it advances. The chief stimulus appears to be a reduced blood ionized calcium (Ca^{++}) level. This is in turn caused by the factors set out in Table 15.

While decreased calcitriol production and secondary hyperparathyroidism

Table 15. Factors contributing to reduced blood ionized calcium levels and increased PTH activity in chronic renal failure

Phosphate retention
Reduced calcitriol production
Decreased responsiveness to PTH
Impaired renal degradation of PTH
Reduced inhibitory effect of Ca^{++}
Absence of normal inhibitory effect of calcitriol on PTH production

are clearly central to the development of renal osteodystrophy, they and other factors are involved in such complex interactions from the earliest stages of renal failure that is is difficult to identify the initial defect(s) responsible for the pathogenic sequence. This knowledge is nevertheless important for the prevention and treatment of the disease. Current findings support the idea that phosphate retention in early renal failure increases the filtered load of phosphate in surviving nephrons and that the resulting increased phosphate concentration in proximal tubular cells inhibits 1-hydroxylation, thus reducing calcitriol production. If this sequence is correct, it is clearly important both to restrict phosphate intake and to use therapeutic calcitriol from the onset of renal failure.

2.3. *Osteitis fibrosa and osteosclerosis*

These conditions are found on histopathological examination often with typical radiological features (Figures 14, 16). In renal failure, they reflect continued secondary parathyroid hyperactivity. Osteitis fibrosa is characterised by increased osteoid formation and resorption rates, with evidence of peritrabecular fibrosis. Osteosclerosis arises from an increase in thickness and numbers of trabeculae in spongy bone. It is best seen in areas of primarily cancellous bone, such as the vertebral bodies, where it can produce the typical "rugger jersey" appearance of the vertebral column on X-ray.

2.4. *The role of aluminium*

Aluminium accumulates in chronic renal failure, causing encephalopathy, microcytic anaemia, hypercalcaemia and osteopathy. The sources of excess aluminium are chiefly diet, aluminium-containing oral phosphate binders and dialysis fluid contamination (from aluminium in the water supply). Raised blood aluminium levels are associated with histological localization of aluminium along the mineralization front of bone (Figure 17). A refractory "dialysis osteomalacia" develops, often with serious complications, such as pathological fractures. In addition to the presence of severe osteomalacic changes with osteitis fibrosa related to secondary hyperparathyroidism, there

98

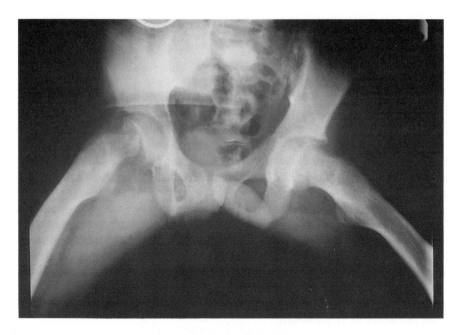

Figure 14. Severe bone resorption caused by secondary hyperparathyroidism in a boy of 16 with long-standing "megacystis-megaureter" and renal dysplasia. Note (1) Urinary diversion; (2) Femoral neck bone resorption; (3) Slipped right femoral epiphysis.

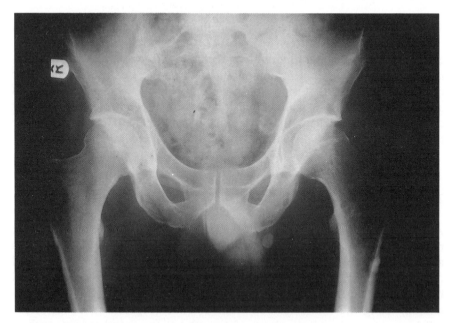

Figure 15. Same patient as Figure 14. Reversal of bone changes on X-ray two years after successful transplantation. The slipped epiphysis had been initially treated by (temporary) internal pinning.

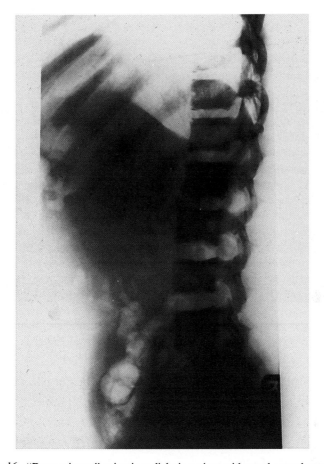

Figure 16. "Rugger-jersey" spine in a dialysis patient with renal osteodystrophy.

is also often evidence of osteopenia, whose relationship to the osteomalacia is uncertain. If aluminium accumulation is prevented, or reversed by chelating drugs (e.g. desferrioxamine), these lesions either fail to appear or improve.

2.5. *Osteoporosis or osteopenia*

Osteoporosis is a decrease in bone mass without specific pathological features. It is characterised by decreased bone density. The term "dialysis osteopenia" has been used to describe an apparent reduction in bone mass which is out of proportion to other evidence of renal osteodystrophy. Loss, or rarefaction, of cortical and trabecular bone, the development of pathological

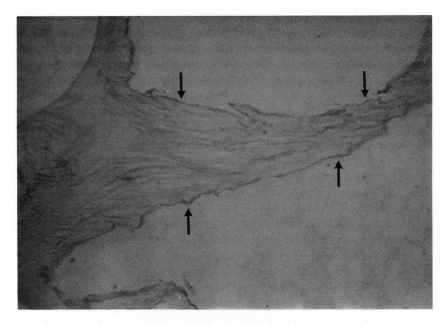

Figure 17. Bone biopsy from 56 year old man on dialysis, with high blood aluminium levels and history of pathological fractures. Dark line shows accumulation of aluminium at mineralization front.

fractures and a failure to respond to vitamin D therapy or parathyroidectomy are typical. A causative role for aluminium has been suggested, but is unproven.

2.6. *Miscellaneous factors*

Impaired collagen synthesis, producing osteopenia, and metabolic acidosis, contributes in some degree to the overall picture. Acute hypermagnesaemia suppresses PTH activity. In end-stage renal failure dialysis patients, chronic hypermagnesaemia is common. Magnesium accumulates in bone and promotes abnormal turnover. In this situation, magnesium in dialysis fluid should probably be reduced. Iron, silicon and sulphur also accumulate at the mineralization front, with uncertain results. Roles for fluoride (from dialysis fluid) and for heparin (used as an anticoagulant) in dialysis osteodystrophy have been suggested but not confirmed.

Oxalate deposition may occur, not only in primary oxalosis, but also, occasionally, in dialysis patients who exhibit raised plasma oxalate levels (aggravated by vitamin C therapy). Low PTH or phosphate levels, which may emerge following aggressive therapy for renal osteodystrophy, may lead to an exacerbation of osteomalacia, indicating the complexity of renal bone disease.

Long-term haemodialysis patients, especially if membranes of low biocompatibility are used, may develop dialysis-related amyloidosis. This is caused by the accumulation of a new amyloid protein, beta-2-microglobulin. Erosive arthritis occurs, with peri-articular bone cysts (probably amyloid deposits), pathological fractures and carpal tunnel syndrome. Haemofiltration and haemodiafiltration lower beta-2-microglobulin and may prove beneficial. It is not yet clear whether or not successful transplantation reverses the condition.

2.7. *Extra-skeletal calcification*

Soft tissue calcification is often first diagnosed radiologically. The chief predisposing factor is a high plasma calcium-phosphate product. Secondary hyperparathyroidism, hypermagnesaemia, severe metabolic acidosis and the presence of local tissue injury also seem important. Ocular, arterial, peri-articular, tumour-like, and visceral deposits (cardiac, pulmonary, renal etc.) are the lesions most commonly reported (Figures 18–20). Some calcification (e.g. peri-articular or tumour-like) can be reversed by medical management and dialysis, as well as by transplantation. Vascular calcification (particularly in the elderly) is difficult to reverse by any means, often hinders vascular access for dialysis and may persist after transplantation. It certainly contributes to an increased incidence of serious cardiac and pulmonary disease, which is usually refractory to all treatment, including transplantation.

Extra-skeletal calcification may be detected by simple X-ray but, for full assessment, computerised tomography and skeletal scintigraphy are more informative. In view of the increased mortality associated with visceral calcification, these techniques should be used freely in the assessment and preparation for transplantation of patients with extra-skeletal calcification.

2.8. *Paediatric renal osteodystrophy*

The pathogenic factors of renal osteodystrophy in children appear to be the same as in adults. However, the results in growing bone are more damaging, producing growth retardation, renal rickets, severe deformities of bone and joints and epiphyseal slipping. Because of this, the management of children is difficult and involves both more aggressive medical therapy and more frequent surgical intervention. The need for correction of abnormalities by transplantation is also usually more urgent.

2.9. *Clinical states of renal osteodystrophy*

Although almost all dialysis patients have some degree of renal osteodystrophy (secondary hyperparathyroidism is almost invariable), striking clinical

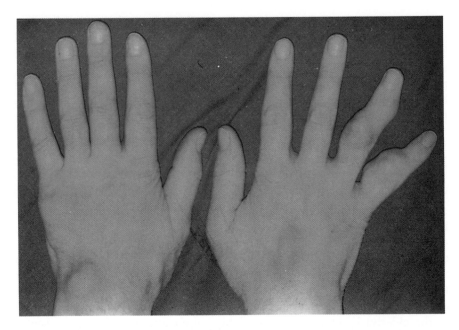

Figure 18. Peri-articular soft-tissue calcification in a patient on regular haemodialysis therapy.

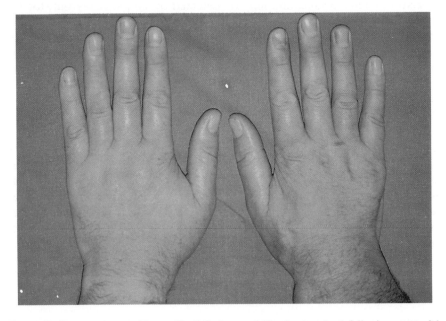

Fiugre 19. Same patient as Figure 18. Soft-tissue calcification resolved following successful transplantation.

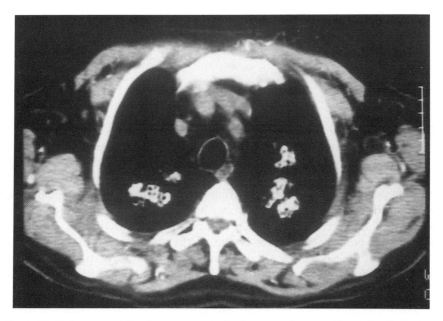

Figure 20. Pulmonary calcification on computerized tomography scan. The patient had a long history of phosphate therapy for hypercalcaemia prior to developing renal failure.

manifestations are relatively uncommon. Suggestive symptoms are:- persistent or recurrent bone pain, tiredness associated with muscle weakness, altered mood and intractable pruritis. It is easy to dismiss these as "just uraemic", although it is true that inadequate dialysis can make osteodystrophy worse. Evidence of soft tissue calcification may appear without clinical warning and invariably requires prompt corrective action. Fractures, loss of height or weight, increasing anaemia and cognitive or expressive disorders suggest aluminium toxicity. In older women on dialysis there is often significant underlying "non-renal" osteoporosis, while in all patients (particularly those at increased risk) severe atherosclerosis may be present. Both these states tend to aggravate osteodystrophy and extra-skeletal calcification. In children and adolescents, growth retardation is a serious problem, while renal rickets (whose commonest presentation is genu valgum) is often seen. Children with a long history of non-hypertensive high output renal failure are most at risk, since their decline into dialysis-dependence is very slow, allowing time for the progression of bone disease. Severe secondary hyperparathyroidism, with periosteal resorption, marked rickety changes and frequent slipping epiphyses, is common in this group, often requiring extensive corrective surgery.

Typical clinical syndromes (Table 14), biochemical changes and radiological findings can be observed in many cases of renal osteodystrophy. Where available, bone biopsy from the iliac crest, which is straightforward and safe, is valuable in detecting early changes, distinguishing the contribution of different factors, defining appropriate treatment and observing response to it.

2.10. *Relationship to transplantation*

Successful transplantation, by returning renal function to normal, eliminating hyperphosphataemia and restoring vitamin D metabolism, gradually reverses secondary parathyroid hyperplasia and the effects of renal osteodystrophy. The results are often dramatic (Figures 15–19). However, any complacency regarding the existence of osteodystrophy in patients awaiting transplantation is to be condemned. Poor control can have serious adverse effects in the post-transplant period. Active secondary hyperparathyroidism promotes post-graft hypercalcaemia. This is due to the return of normal vitamin D metabolism in the presence of continuing parathyroid hyperplasia. In many cases, calcium levels slowly return to normal as parathyroid tissue involutes, although a high percentage of patients, even if normocalcaemic, still have detectable increases in PTH levels up to three years after successful transplantation. In some cases, persistent "autonomous" overactivity leads to the need for parathyroidectomy. Poorly controlled osteodystrophy is associated with an increased rate of soft tissue calcification. Arterial calcification makes vascular anastomosis at transplantation much more difficult and, sometimes, impossible. Poorly controlled osteodystrophy is likely to exacerbate post-transplant bone disease. For example, avascular necrosis of bone is related to steroid therapy, but has also been recorded in cases of renal failure where no grafting or steroid therapy had been used. The incidence of the condition after transplantation is greater in the presence of severe prior renal osteodystrophy. In children, although growth may spurt dramatically after successful transplantation, especially on cyclosporin monotherapy or following human growth hormone treatment, failure to meet normal growth targets is at least partly attributable to the severity of pre-existing bone disease. Gradual improvement of aluminium-induced osteopathy has been observed after transplantation, with increased urinary excretion of aluminium. However, overall improvement is not invariable: some cases of progressive bone disease and encephalopathy related to aluminium have been recorded. Hypophosphataemia and steroid-induced osteoporosis (or osteopenia) after transplantation may produce serious and complex manifestations of bone disease, particularly in older persons.

Case history

A 65 year old woman with renal failure due to hypertensive nephrosclerosis also had some evidence of renal osteodystrophy, as well as marked postmenopausal osteoporosis. Dialysis could not be readily offered because of non-medical constraints but following successful transplantation her uncontrolled uraemic state improved rapidly. Unfortunately, a series of fractures, involving the femoral necks, the pelvis and the vertebral bodies greatly detracted from her quality of life until her death, four years later.

Secondary hyperparathyroidism, soft tissue calcification and hypercalcaemia are associated with an increased risk of hypertension as well as of cardiac and pulmonary disease. This can be observed in post-transplant, as well as in dialysis, patients. It is therefore important, following the "global" strategy of patient survival and well-being, to minimize risks from an early stage of the disease.

2.11. *Prevention and treatment of renal osteodystrophy*

The goal of management is fourfold:-
1. To maintain normal blood calcium and phosphorus levels.
2. To prevent or suppress parathyroid hyperplasia.
3. To prevent or reverse soft tissue calcification.
4. To prevent the accumulation of skeletal toxins, such as aluminium, or to eliminate them, if present.

Management is complex and difficult. Control of phosphate is essential. It is best achieved by dietary restriction, adequate dialysis and the judicious use of phosphate-binding agents. Dietary calcium supplements help to bind phosphate and to improve calcium absorption. Once phosphate levels are controlled, calcium can be normalized by the use of vitamin D sterols, notably 1-alpha-hydroxy- and 1,25 dihydroxycholecalciferol (calcitriol). Great care is needed to avoid hypercalcaemia from therapy with the risk of soft tissue calcification. Parathyroidectomy is of value for established and symptomatic secondary hyperparathyroidism with evidence of severe bone involvement, persistent hypercalcaemia, soft tissue calcification, calciphylaxis or unresponsiveness. Aluminium osteopathy is best prevented by use of an appropriate water purification system, which combines reverse osmosis with a deionization process. Dialysate water and patient blood levels of aluminium should be monitored regularly and aluminium-based phosphate binders used sparingly, if at all. Established aluminium toxicity has been shown to respond to chelation by desferrioxamine: this agent mobilizes tissue stores of aluminium into the blood and increases the ultrafiltrable fraction of aluminum in plasma, thereby improving its removal from the patient by dialysis. Control of the dietary and dialysate content of other potentially harmful substances, such as magnesium, fluoride and oxalate is also advisable. Drugs which interfere with vitamin D metabolism (e.g. anticonvulsants) should be avoided where possible. In long-standing dialysis patients, the use of highly permeable biocompatible membranes should be considered, in order to prevent or treat the accumulation in bone of β_2 microglobulin amyloid.

106

Further reading

Coburn, J. W. and Slatopolsky, E. Vitamin D, parathyroid hormone and the renal osteo-
dystrophies. In *The Kidney*, Brenner, B. M. and Rector, F. C. eds., 4th ed. Philadelphia,
Saunders, 1991; 2036–2120.
Llach, F. and Coburn, J. W. Renal osteodystrophy and maintenance dialysis. In *Replacement
of Renal Function by Dialysis*, Maher, J. F. ed., 3rd ed. Dordrecht, Kluwer Acad. Publishers,
1988; 912–952.
Strom, T. B. and Carpenter, C. Immunobiology of kidney transplantation. In *The Kidney*,
Brenner, B. M. and Rector, F. C. ed., 4th ed. Philadelphia, Saunders, 1991; 2336–2360.

CHAPTER 8

Renal osteodystrophy

A. P. MAXWELL

Renal osteodystrophy is a term used to describe disorders of bone occurring in patients with chronic renal failure. The different forms of bone disease encountered in uraemic patients are mainly the results of interactions between three clinically recognisable problems: hyperparathyroidism, reduced vitamin D metabolite production, and aluminium toxicity affecting bone mineralisation. Bone disease may be broadly divided into states of high bone turnover like hyperparathyroidism and low turnover states of impaired bone formation and mineralisation such as osteomalacia.

Bone turnover is a dynamic process influenced by the type of renal disease and the severity of renal failure, the type and duration of renal replacement therapy, and drug treatment (such as aluminium containing phosphate binders, steroids and vitamin D analogues). Although renal osteodystrophy is often subclinical it can result in substantial morbidity in some patients.

Bone disease may be suspected from clinical features and laboratory findings such as hypocalcaemia, hyperphosphataemia, high circulating parathormone (PTH) levels or high random aluminium levels. However, laboratory blood tests and radiological examination may be misleading in the evaluation of renal osteodystrophy. Bone biopsy remains the most accurate diagnostic procedure in elucidating the underlying bone disorder.

1. Pathophysiology

Bone is a vital component of the mechanical structure of the body but it also provides dynamic metabolic functions particularly for calcium homeostasis. Bone may be regarded both as a reservoir for calcium and an important buffer system involved in regulating acid-base balance. Bone is a complex milieu of specialised cells, intercellular matrix and mineral salts. Growth of bone is determined by active processes of modelling and remodelling normally involving approximately 20% of bone structure, the remainder being quiescent.

Osteoblasts and osteoclasts are the two main cell types involved in bone turnover and are believed to be derived from haemopoietic stem cells.

Mary G. McGeown (ed.), Clinical Management of Renal Transplantation, 107–113.

Osteoclasts are large multi-nucleated cells which actively participate in bone resorption and degradation. Osteoblasts are found on advancing bone growth surfaces and in contrast to osteoclasts secrete bone matrix and facilitate bone mineralisation. Osteocytes are osteoblasts which are buried in bone matrix and these cells can communicate via thin canaliculi in bone. Osteocytes are also involved in rapid calcium ion flux.

Receptors for PTH and 1,25 dihydroxyvitamin D3, the major bioactive metabolite of vitamin D, are present on both osteoblasts and osteoclasts. Local cytokines in addition to the systemic signals of PTH and $1,25(OH)_2D3$ regulate the activity of bone cells. Therapy aimed at altering the levels of PTH and $1,25(OH)_2D3$ will modulate the bioactivity of these bone cells.

Bone matrix consists of proteins and mineral crystals. Type 1 collagen is the predominant protein (>90%). The remainder are structural proteins like fibronectin, osteonectin and bone Gla protein (the most abundant non-collagenous bone protein). Crystals of calcium phosphate and calcium apatite form the major components of the inorganic mineral content of bone. Tetracyclines are used to assess the rate of mineralisation and bone growth. These antibiotics are incorporated into the bone mineralisation front and the tetracycline label is visible under fluorescent light microscopy. The mineralisation rate is determined by administering these drugs on at least two occasions prior to a bone biopsy. The resulting distance between the two areas of labelled bone is equivalent to the rate of mineralisation.

Renal failure may lead to a sustained loss of calcium from bone. Buffering of the metabolic acidosis accompanying renal failure may accelerate the loss of bone mineral content. Structural failure of bone resulting in deformity and fracture can subsequently occur. Renal bone disease develops in the early stages of renal failure and abnormal bone histology is seen in over half of the patients in whom the glomerular filtration rate has fallen to 50% of normal. Most patients with end stage renal disease have abnormal bone histology. Aluminium deposition in bone is a variable finding but is reported in up to half of long-term dialysis patients studied.

Virtually all types of metabolic bone disorder have been described in patients with renal disease. However renal osteodystrophy may be divided into three main histological groups:
1. hyperparathyroidism
2. low turnover uraemic osteodystrophy (osteomalacia and adynamic renal bone disease)
3. mixed uraemic osteodystrophy with features of both (1) and (2).

A variable amount of bone aluminium deposition may be seen in the three types of uraemic bone disease.

2. Hyperparathyroid bone disease

In this form of renal osteodystrophy there is a marked increase in bone turnover reflecting the effects of chronically elevated PTH levels on bone.

The increased PTH secretion is believed to be secondary to phosphate retention and decreased calcitriol ($1,25(OH)_2D3$) production. Elevations in serum phosphate and a reduction in nephron number accompanying renal failure combine to reduce the bioactivity of renal 1 alpha-hydroxylase. This enzyme catalyses the hydroxylation of 25 hydroxy-vitamin D in the proximal tubule resulting in the formation of the active vitamin D metabolite $1,25(OH)_2D3$ (calcitriol). The fall in calcitriol production can lead to secondary hyperparathyroidism by two pathways.
1. a decrease in plasma calcium resulting in a compensatory rise in PTH to restore calcium levels
2. loss of inhibition of parathyroid gland tissue by calcitriol.

Receptors for $1,25(OH)_2D3$ are present on parathyroid cells and calcitriol has a direct suppressive effect on PTH secretion by reducing parathormone gene expression.

Histologically hyperparathyroid bone disease is associated with an increase in both osteoclasts and osteoblasts in the numerous abnormal bone remodelling sites. There is an increase in osteoid primarily of a woven, irregular type. Overall bone formation rate is increased. This can be documented with tetracycline labelling. Mineralisation of the osteoid is increased but the deposition of calcium is irregular and disordered. Marrow fibrosis may be a prominent feature and in advanced cases pseudocysts are present.

3. Low turnover uraemic osteodystrophy

3.1. Osteomalacia

Osteomalacia represents a form of low turnover renal osteodystrophy and is characterised by a marked decrease in remodelling sites, an increase in unmineralised osteoid, and a decrease in both osteoclasts and osteoblasts. Tetracycline labelling demonstrates greatly reduced bone formation rates. The total bone volume is variable in osteomalacia but the mineralised bone volume is always reduced. The bone is subject to deformity and fractures.

3.2. Adynamic renal bone disease

In contrast to osteomalacia this form of low turnover renal osteodystrophy is characterised by both a reduction in osteoid and mineralisation resulting in a loss of bone volume. Risk factors for this condition appear to include diabetes mellitus, older age, CAPD treatment and prolonged duration of renal replacement treatment. It remains controversial whether this condition is idiopathic or represents a later stage in the treatment of renal osteodystrophy.

4. Mixed uraemic osteodystrophy

This is arguably the commonest histological finding in patients with end stage renal disease. There is no dominant underlying cause and features of both hyperparathyroidism and defective mineralisation are present. Bone formation rates and volume are variable and mixed uraemic osteodystrophy may reflect a transition between high and low turnover renal osteodystrophy.

5. Aluminium deposition in bone

Aluminium deposition has been reported in 90% of patients with low turnover uraemic osteodystrophy, 50% of patients with mixed uraemic osteodystrophy and in 10 to 15% of persons with hyperparathyroidism. Patients treated with haemodialysis were previously at considerable risk of developing aluminium toxicity from aluminium absorption during haemodialysis because of the high aluminium content of many local water supplies. With the advent of reverse osmosis treatment for water purification this problem has been largely solved. However aluminium intoxication still occurs from the ingestion of aluminium containing antacids used as phosphate binders.

Aluminium is deposited at the bone mineralisation front at the bone/osteoid interface leading to low bone turnover and a histological lesion typical of osteomalacia. Raised aluminium levels are associated with decreased PTH and calcitriol levels.

6. Clinical and biochemical features

Symptoms of abnormal bone and mineral metabolism are rarely present until advanced renal failure develops. Hyperparathyroidism may present with bone pain, proximal myopathy, pruritus, vascular and soft tissue calcification. In adults osteomalacia is associated with muscle weakness and spontaneous fractures. Osteomalacia in children may cause growth delay and in advanced cases bone deformity. Aluminium intoxication has been associated with encephalopathy, seizures, bone fractures and muscle weakness.

Soft tissue calcification may result in tumour like skin deposits described as tumoural calcinosis. Conjunctival calcification causes irritation and a "red eye syndrome". Soft tissue calcification is related to the magnitude of the calcium-phosphate (Ca × P) product and can improve with normalisation of calcium and phosphate levels. In contrast vascular calcification can progress despite correction of underlying abnormal biochemical values.

Unfortunately biochemical parameters are relatively insensitive diagnostic tools for the accurate diagnosis of the type and severity of renal osteodystrophy. Serum calcium and phosphate concentrations are poor predictors of the aetiology of underlying bone disorder. Hypercalcaemia may be a feature of aluminium overload, vitamin D analogue treatment or hyperparathyroidism. Hyperphosphataemia may develop in hyperparathyroidism partly due to increased intestinal absorption but also secondary to release from bone.

Aluminium intoxication may be suspected if random aluminium levels are high. A desferrioxamine (DFO) infusion test may improve the diagnostic accuracy of aluminium overload. Deferoxamine chelates aluminium and can mobilise tissue aluminium stores. A significant rise in plasma aluminium level after the administration of DFO is suggestive of aluminium overload. However a large number of false negative results are reported and bone biopsy with staining for aluminium remains the most reliable test (Chapter 7, p. 100).

Parathyroid hormone levels are higher in hyperparathyroid bone disease than in low turnover uraemic osteodystrophy and PTH concentrations appear to correlate well with bone turnover rates. In renal failure decreased clearance results in the accumulation of biologically inactive C-terminal fragments of PTH. N-terminal and mid-molecule PTH assays appear to be most clinically relevant in patients with renal failure. However there is still considerable overlap in PTH levels in patients with the various types of renal osteodystrophy.

Vitamin D metabolites may be assayed and in general levels of 25 (OH)D2 are normal whilst levels of $1,25(OH)_2D3$ are low. However measurements of vitamin D metabolites are of limited value in patients with renal failure unless it is suspected that liver disease, anticonvulsant therapy or nephrotic syndrome are influencing vitamin D metabolism.

Radiological examinations are frequently performed in patients with renal failure but the interpretation of abnormalities is difficult. Radiological abnormalities may be absent in early renal osteodystrophy or conversely obvious radiological lesions may reflect the predominent bone disorder that was present months or years earlier. Bone biopsy remains the most accurate method of determining the histological derangement present and guide appropriate treatment.

7. Treatment

Renal osteodystrophy develops insidiously as renal failure progresses and treatment is most effective if therapy is commenced early. Phosphate retention plays a key role in the development of renal osteodystrophy by reducing both calcium and calcitriol concentrations resulting in stimulation of PTH secretion. Management of patients with renal failure must include efforts to maintain normal calcium and phosphate levels and supplement deficient calcitriol production.

Hyperphosphataemia may be controlled by dietary phosphate restriction and a variety of phosphate binding drugs. Phosphate binders are taken with meals and combine with dietary phosphate to limit its absorption. The therapeutic dilemma is that none of the presently available drugs are ideal phosphate binders. Aluminium hydroxide-containing antacids are effective binders but aluminium toxicity and bone deposition make these compounds unsuitable as the sole long term therapy. Calcium salts have advantages as phosphate binders by reducing exposure to aluminium and supplementing calcium intake which may suppress PTH release. However calcium salts are relatively unpalatable as large doses (2–12 g/day) are required and there is the risk of hypercalcaemia particularly with concurrent calcitriol treatment. Dialysis also influences control of calcium and phosphate concentrations and lower dialysate calcium levels may be used to optimise the dosage of calcium salts used as phosphate binders whilst calcitriol therapy is maintained.

Vitamin D therapy appears to be particularly important in preventing or ameliorating secondary hyperparathyroidism. Indications for calcitriol administration include hypocalcaemia after plasma phosphate concentration has been normalised and hyperparathyroidism normalised. Low turnover uraemic osteomalacia may be refractory to calcitriol treatment if significant aluminium deposition is present in bone. Normally calcitriol is administered orally but there is evidence that intraperitoneal (with CAPD) or intravenous use may be more effective in suppressing PTH secretion.

In the majority of patients bone disease can be controlled by a combination of dietary phosphate restriction, phosphate binders and vitamin D supplements. Some individuals have accumulated a significant aluminium burden. When aluminium overload has been confirmed by bone biopsy or response to DFO it is important to discontinue aluminium hydroxide phosphate binders. Chronic administration of DFO has been used to mobilise tissue stores of aluminium, the resulting aluminium-DFO complex being removed by dialysis. If this therapy is successful bone turnover increases with enhanced activity of both osteoblasts and osteoclasts and improved bone growth. Deferoxamine administration is expensive. It is associated with a variety of side effects which include hypotension during infusion, acute mental changes, loss of hearing and visual acuity and increased incidence of Yersinia and mucomycosis infections.

Parathyroidectomy should be reserved for patients with predominantly hyperparathyroid bone disease refractory to conservative medical treatment. Careful assessment for aluminium overload is required since aluminium deposition increases substantially following parathyroidectomy if osteomalacia is also present. Parathyroidectomy is recommended for calciphylaxis, a rare and poorly understood syndrome associated with severe secondary hyperparathyroidism, characterised by vascular calcification and peripheral ischaemic necrosis.

Conclusion

Renal osteodystrophy represents a spectrum of bone disorders resulting from the complex interactions of bone metabolism with the pathophysiology of renal failure. The key to its management is accurate diagnosis of the underlying disorder coupled with a clear understanding of the pathogenesis of renal bone disease. The continuing challenge for physicians is provision of optimal, safe clinical care of renal failure patients including the prevention of disabling renal osteodystrophy.

Further reading

Andress, D. L., Endres, D. B., Malony, N. A. *et al.* Comparison of parathyroid hormone assays with bone histomorphometry in renal osteodystrophy. *J. Clin. Endocrinol. Metab.* 1986; 63: 1163–1169.

Fournier, A., Moriniere, P., Cohen Salal, M. E. *et al.* Adynamic bone disease in uremia: may it be idiopathic? Is it an actual disease? *Nephron* 1990; 58: 1–12.

McCarthy, J. T., Kumar, R. Renal osteodystrophy. *Endocrinology and Metabolism Clinics of North America* 1990; 19: 65–93.

Malluche, H., Faugere, M-C. Renal bone disease 1990: an unmet challenge for the nephrologist. *Kidney Int.* 1990; 38: 193–211.

Malluche, H., Smith, A. J., Abreo, K., Faugere, M-C. The use of deferoxamine in the management of aluminum accumulation in bone in patients with renal failure. *N. Engl. J. Med.* 1984; 311: 140–144.

Salusky, I. B., Foley, J., Nelson, P., Goodman, W. G. Aluminum accumulation in children and young adults with chronic renal disease. *New. Engl. J. Med.* 1991; 324: 527–531.

CHAPTER 9

Tissue typing

D. MIDDLETON

The tissue typing laboratory provides three main services for the renal transplant unit:
1. HLA typing and matching of recipients and donors. Matching in this sense means the sorting of the recipient list to identify those recipients who might have a transplant from a particular donor.
2. Screening of the recipients for antibodies.
3. Carrying out cross match tests between selected possible donor recipient pairs.

The tissue typing laboratory may be part of the blood transfusion service of the region, or may be an independent laboratory working within or without a university department. The Tissue Typing Laboratory in Belfast was originally set up within the general laboratory of the hospital to service the Renal Transplant Unit. It has developed into an independent Tissue Typing Laboratory serving not only the Renal Unit but the needs of the Province for other tissue typing services such as bone marrow transplantation, disease studies, etc.

An outline of the methods used and the reason for preferring certain techniques will be given in the Appendix to this chapter.

1. HLA typing

1.1. *Source of Donor*

Before December 1990 618 renal transplants were performed in the Renal Unit, Belfast City Hospital. 568 kidneys came from cadaveric donors and 50 from living related donors. Of the recipients transplanted from cadaveric donors 491 received their first transplant, 67 their second transplant and 10 their third transplant. In the recipients transplanted from related donors 44 received their first transplant, five their second transplant and one his fourth transplant.

Mary G. McGeown (ed.), Clinical Management of Renal Transplantation, 115–133.
© 1992 *Kluwer Academic Publishers, Dordrecht. Printed in the Netherlands.*

1.2. *Introduction to HLA*

HLA antigens are coded for by loci on the sixth chromosome and are classified into Class I (HLA-A,-B,-C) and Class II (HLA-DR,-DQ,-DP). Whereas Class I antigens are found on the majority of cells, Class 11 antigens are limited in their distribution and are found mainly on macrophages, monocytes, B lymphocytes and activated T lymphocytes.

1.3. *Matching policy*

Apart from trying to obtain a suitable match grade other factors have been considered when determining the matching policy. When a patient has had a failed graft, the mismatched antigens of the failed graft have been avoided in a subsequent graft. When a patient has been pregnant the paternal HLA-A,-B antigens present in the child and absent in the patient have been avoided. The crossmatch has been performed using historic sera as well as current sera. Either a current positive crossmatch or a historic positive crossmatch has been regarded as a contraindication to a transplant.

There have been occasions when the above policies have been reduced but only after the passage of time had shown that the continuation of the policy was preventing an individual patient from receiving a transplant.

We have also sought to avoid mismatching for antigens present at a high frequency in the population. This policy has been followed with a view to increasing the chance of a patient obtaining a subsequent transplant if the previous graft failed.

Before the introduction of prospective HLA-DR typing, kidneys were transplanted according to the best match, usually more than two HLA-A and -B mismatches being avoided. A retrospective analysis of HLA typing in 1985 showed a significant effect of matching on graft survival for HLA-DR antigens alone and for HLA-A and -B antigens combined. Since that analysis the policy at this Unit has been to ensure that a minimum of three antigens are matched between donor and recipient, including at least one HLA-DR antigen.

We have used blood group compatibility, rather than blood group identity, when the matching grade was better (Table 16). Although this has enlarged the pool of donors for blood group A recipients, these recipients have a lower percentage of transplants in which antigens are mismatched for zero or one HLA-A and -B antigens (33.7%) compared to blood group O recipients (45.3%). This reflects the fact that, at all times, more blood group O than blood group A recipients are waiting for a transplant. There was no difference in graft survival of blood group O kidneys whether they were transplanted into a blood group O or blood group A recipient.

Table 16. Blood group of recipient and donor in cadaver transplantation

	Blood Group	
Recipient	Donor	Number of Transplants
O	O	281
A	A	171
B	B	49
AB	AB	3
A	O	44
B	O	14
AB	O	2
AB	A	3
AB	B	1

1.4. *Tissue matching*

The matching used was as follows: Transplants 1–7 performed prior to 1970 were matched for blood group compatibility only. From 1970 onwards the HLA-A and -B locus antigens of all transplants were known prospectively and used for matching. The transplants which took place between 1981 and 1983 were typed by serological methods for HLA-DR retrospectively. Prospective HLA-DR typing was introduced in 1984 and subsequently used for matching in all transplants. Since May 1986 the HLA-DR antigens have also been typed by DNA techniques. These techniques have been applied retrospectively to cadaveric donors. However, since 1987 the HLA-DR type of the recipient has been performed prospectively by DNA methods in addition to serological methods. HLA-DP typing by oligonucleotide typing has recently been applied to stored material from recipients and donors of all cadaveric transplants that have taken place since May 1986.

1.5. *Exchange of kidneys*

Kidneys are exchanged in the United Kingdom and Eire under the auspices of the United Kingdom Transplant Support Service (UKTSS), Bristol. Of the 568 cadaveric donors used 334 were local and 234 were from other centres. As expected a better grade of matching is obtained using imported kidneys (Table 17). For first grafts there was no difference in graft survival between imported and local donors (Figure 21). We have previously shown that the graft survival of a kidney used for a Belfast recipient was superior to the survival of the other paired kidney regardless of whether the donor was from Northern Ireland or not. This shows that excellent graft survival rate has not been due to the selection of donors from the same, relatively homogeneous, population as the recipients.

There have been three distinct eras in our experience with exchange of

Table 17. Matching obtained in imported kidneys compared to local kidneys

Mismatch	% Imported Kidneys	% Local Kidneys
HLA-A,B		
0	14.5	8.2
1	33.8	28.7
2	36.8	47.0
3	13.7	14.3
4	1.3	1.8
HLA-DR		
0	46.8	29.8
1	46.8	63.4
2	6.3	6.8

kidneys. In each year from 1971–1977 60% of the kidneys used were from outside centres and 40% were kidneys from local donors. From 1978–1988 this trend was reversed. During this period 69% of kidneys used were from local donors with 31% of the kidneys coming from other centres. This change was due to an increase in the number of local kidney donors, the number of kidneys imported remaining similar throughout both periods.

Since January 1989 over 90% of the transplant units in the U.K. have agreed to contribute at least one kidney if there is a beneficially matched recipient in another centre. A beneficial match is defined as a maximum of one HLA-A or HLA-B mismatch and no HLA-DR mismatch. In this period 60% of kidneys used were from outside centres and 40% were from local donors.

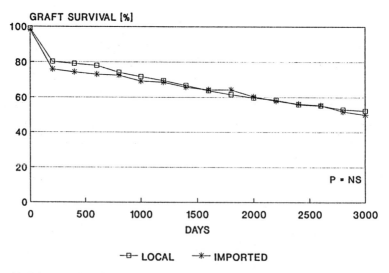

Figure 21. Primary cadaveric renal transplantation: actuarial graft survival and source of kidney.

1.6. *Organisation of cadaver typing*

Since 1971 an on-call service for tissue typing has been available 24 hours a day. Until 1988 plates containing all prospective recipients' sera were prepared and frozen. When a donor became available the donor was typed and crossmatched at the same time against all blood group compatible prospective recipients.

Since 1988 we have performed the above in two stages. The donor typing is performed and then suitable patients according to matching are selected. We have developed our own computer programmes for matching of cadaver donors with our recipients. The most suitable patients are then selected for crossmatching, which is usually carried out the next morning. This enables us to obtain from the prospective recipients fresh blood samples, only a few hours old at the time of transplant. It has also facilitated the organisation of the staff on-call rota and enabled more detailed crossmatching tests to be performed. The donor type is already known when the donor kidney is imported but we perform a check re-type. The patient for whom the kidney has been sent is crossmatched along with other suitable alternatives, during the time the tissue typing is performed.

1.7. *Management of patients on recipient list*

The laboratory is informed of new patients who are being prepared to go on the list of recipients awaiting transplantation. The laboratory arranges to obtain all blood samples required throughout the periods before and after tansplantation. The laboratory is responsible for registration of the patient on the UKTS waiting-list and arranges the updating of immunological details and matching criteria adjustments.

Results of typing patients and patients' sera screening are held in the laboratory, many on computer.

When a donor becomes available the donor is tissue typed and suitable recipients crossmatched. A list of suitable recipients in order of matching criteria is given to the consultant nephrologist who makes the final decision as to whom should receive the kidney.

1.8. *Results*

Patient and graft survival rates are shown respectively in Figures 22 and 23. Although not significant the results show that live transplants have the best graft and patient survival, that there is little difference between first and second transplants and that third transplants have the poorest graft and patient survival.

Figures 24, 25 and 26 show the graft survival in primary cadaveric trans-

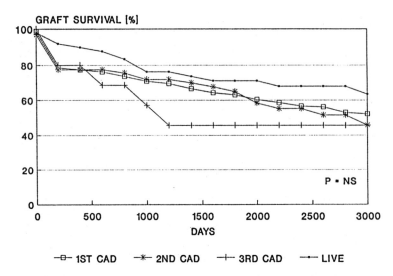

Figure 22. Actuarial graft survival in live, 1st, 2nd and 3rd cadaveric renal transplants.

plants for HLA-A, HLA-B and HLA-DR loci respectively. All primary cadaveric transplants, with the exception of the first seven transplants previously mentioned, were analysed for the effect of HLA-A and -B loci. All transplants since 1981 were analysed for the effect of HLA-DR matching on graft survival.

There was a significant benefit on graft survival of matching for the HLA-A locus but not for the HLA-B locus. Although not significant, analysis of matching at the HLA-DR locus showed a decrease in graft survival with

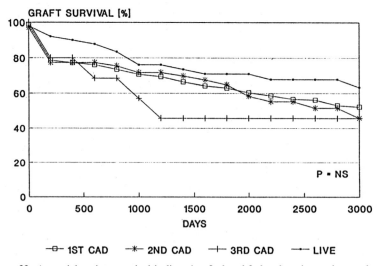

Figure 23. Actuarial patient survival in live, 1st, 2nd and 3rd cadaveric renal transplants.

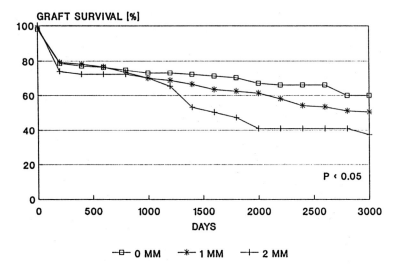

Figure 24. Primary cadaveric renal transplantation: the effect of HLA-A locus matching on actuarial graft survival.

increasing number of mismatches. In this series only 45 transplants have taken place with two mismatches at the HLA-DR locus. As previously discussed the policy has been to avoid two mismatched HLA-DR antigens since the findings of our retrospective analysis of HLA-DR matching. Since we commenced prospective HLA-DR typing only six transplants have been performed with the knowledge that two HLA-DR antigens were mismatched.

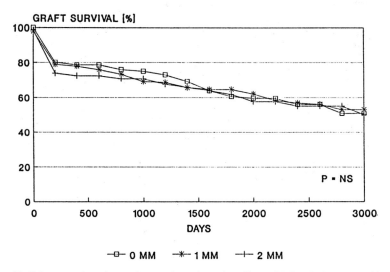

Figure 25. Primary cadaveric renal transplantation: the effect of HLA-B locus matching on actuarial graft survival.

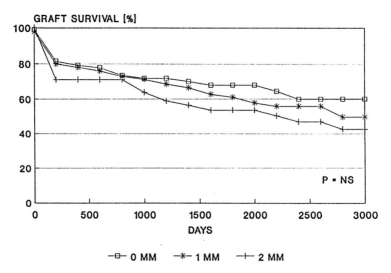

Figure 26. Primary cadaveric renal transplantation: the effect of HLA-DR locus matching on actuarial graft survival.

However, 10 transplants considered at the time of transplantation, by serology, to have only one HLA-DR antigen mismatched have been shown by DNA techniques to have two HLA-DR mismatches.

The numbers of second transplants are too small to analyse for the effect of HLA loci. However, it is of interest to note that 55% of second cadaveric transplants have zero or one HLA-A and -B antigens mismatched whereas 39% of primary cadaveric transplants have zero or one HLA-A and -B antigens mismatched. This reflects the better matching required in second transplants in order to obtain a negative crossmatch in this more sensitised group of patients.

When the accumulative effect of HLA-A, -B and -DR loci matching is analysed, transplants mismatched for one, two, three or four antigens have very similar graft survivals. However, although the numbers are small, transplants with zero mismatches have a significantly higher graft survival than transplants with five or six antigens mismatched (Figure 27).

2. Screening of recipients' sera for antibodies

2.1. *Testing of sera*

Clotted blood (10 ml) was collected from recipients on the following occasions: monthly and 14 days after transfusion prior to transplantation and at two, four, six and eight weeks after transplantation. All patients received at least two blood transfusions before transplantation. The sera were

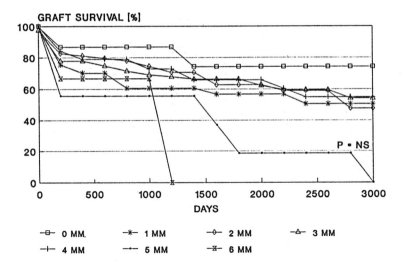

Figure 27. Primary cadaveric renal transplantation: the effect of matching for HLA-A, -B, -DR loci on actuarial graft survival.

separated and stored in aliquots at $-70\,°C$. For screening three panels of cells each consisting of 15 individuals were used. Recipient serum samples were screened monthly against one panel. Those samples which gave one positive reaction, regarded as questionable positive, were screened against the next two monthly panels and if there was still doubt, screened again against the original panel on the fourth month. The reactivity of a serum is represented by the panel reactivity antibody (PRA) i.e. the percentage of individuals with which a serum reacts. All sera were stored for a minimum of one year. After that time for each patient culling took place and many negative samples were discarded.

2.2. Autoantibodies

In some individuals the serum reacts with autologous cells indicating that autoantibodies are present. In patients whose serum reacts positively with panel cells further tests are necessary to determine whether or not the antibodies detected are autoantibodies. Positive samples are tested against autologous cells. All samples are also tested against lymphocytes from B cell chronic lymphocytic leukaemia patients (CLL) to give an indication of whether autoantibodies are present (samples positive against normal lymphocytes and negative against CLL cells have a higher probability of being autopositive). Samples are also treated with dithiothreitol (DTT) to see if there is a reduction in antibody activity. This is another indicator of autoantibodies. However, samples reduced by DTT treatment, which

Table 18. Level of panel reactive current antibodies in males and females prior to first and subsequent transplantaion

| | Level of antibodies | | |
	Negative	10–50%	60–100%
Males, 1st graft	288 (91.1%)	26 (8.2%)	2 (0.6%)
Females, non-pregnant, 1st graft	70 (86.4%)	7 (8.6%)	4 (4.9%)
Females, pregnant, 1st graft	89 (74.8%)	22 (18.5%)	8 (6.7%)
Males,> 1st graft	25 (48.1%)	24 (46.2%)	3 (5.8%)
Females, non-pregnant,> 1st graft	8 (50.0%)	7 (43.8%)	1 (6.3%)
Females, pregnant,> 1st graft	5 (33.3%)	6 (40.0%)	4 (26.7%)

removes IgM antibodies, are not used in the crossmatch. We have found only seven patients with autoantibodies.

In patients shown to have autoantibodies the serum sample is absorbed using lymphocytes of the patient as follows: 50 µl of serum is added to 5×10 patient's lymphocytes, mixed for 30 minutes at room temperature, and incubated at 4 °C for 30 minutes. After centrifugation this procedure is repeated twice with fresh lymphocytes, the last incubation being extended to 16 hours. These samples are then used for crossmatching.

2.3. *Antibodies due to pregnancy*

Sera samples were also tested from patients who had previously been pregnant, against the lymphocytes of the father of the child.

2.4. *Sensitisation levels*

The main causes of sensitisation are pregnancy and a previous transplant. Blood transfusion also contributes to some extent but has a greater effect in patients who have been stimulated previously by pregnancy or a failed transplant.

Table 19. Level of panel reactive historic antibodies in males and females prior to first and subsequent transplantation

| | Level of antibodies | | |
	Negative	10–50%	60–100%
Males, 1st graft	217 (68.7%)	88 (27.8%)	11 (3.5%)
Females, non-pregnant, 1st graft	53 (65.4%)	21 (25.9%)	7 (8.6%)
Females, pregnant, 1st graft	52 (43.7%)	48 (40.3%)	19 (16.0%)
Males,> 1st graft	12 (23.1%)	28 (53.8%)	12 (23.1%)
Females, non-pregnant,> 1st graft	5 (31.3%)	6 (37.5%)	5 (31.3%)
Females, pregnant,> 1st graft	3 (20.0%)	5 (33.3%)	7 (46.7%)

Tables 18 and 19 show the levels of current and historic antibodies respectively in patients before they were transplanted. The level of antibodies is similar in males and in females who have never been pregnant but is much greater in females who have had previous pregnancies. In all groups of patients the level of both current and historic antibodies is increased prior to a second or subsequent transplant, compared to the corresponding levels in patients prior to first transplantation.

The proportion of patients with high levels of antibodies has increased over the years. In December 1982 24% of patients on the Belfast waiting-list had a PRA greater than 50% whereas in December 1990 the corresponding figure was 38%. The percentage of patients waiting for a second or subsequent graft increases with time. The highly sensitised patients accumulate on the recipient pool. At December 1990 of patients waiting for a graft for more than two years 11 of 24 had antibodies with a PRA greater than 80% and only two had no antibodies. Of patients waiting between one and two years 6 of 13 had antibodies with a PRA greater than 80% and only two had no antibodies. In contrast, in patients waiting less than one year only 2 of 28 had antibodies with a PRA greater than 80% and 17 were negative. These antibodies were present at various times pre-transplantation.

2.5. *Graft survival compared to antibody levels*

There is no difference in primary cadaveric graft survival between patients without antibodies, either current or historic, and patients with antibodies prior to transplantation. However, a significantly higher graft survival is found in patients with a PRA of 0–50%, either current or historic, compared to patients with a PRA of 60–100% (Figures 8 and 9).

In an effort to reduce the problem of patients becoming sensitised by blood transfusions, recently blood transfusions matched for at least one of the patient's HLA-DR antigens have been used. The availability of a tissue typed bone marrow donor panel, compiled at this laboratory from blood donors has made this possible.

3. Crossmatching of recipients and donors

3.1. *Selection of sera used in crossmatching*

Sera of recipients are crossmatched against prospective donors. Sera are selected to include the current sample which should not be older than one month. As mentioned previously efforts are made to obtain a sample at the time of transplant. Historic positive sera chosen to represent peaks in antibody activity are always included. However, if a patient's antibody profile has remained unchanged throughout, samples are chosen at intervals during the time a patient was on dialysis.

126

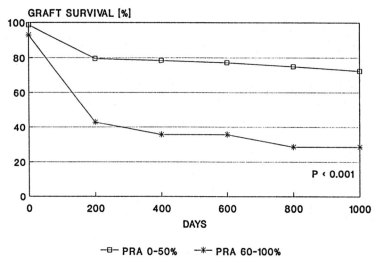

Figure 28. Primary cadaveric renal transplantation: the effect of current antibodies on actuarial graft survival.

3.2. *Historic sera*

It has been reported that a positive cross match with a historic serum does not prohibit transplantation. In Belfast the general policy of not transplanting when an historic crossmatch is positive continues. However, on seven occasions this policy was ignored for individual recipients as it continually

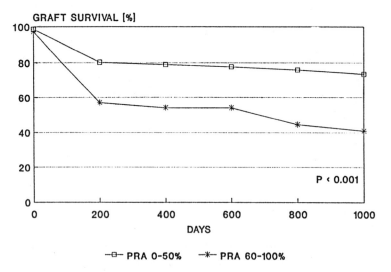

Figure 29. Primary cadaveric renal transplantation: the effect of historic antibodies on actuarial graft survival.

prevented the patient from receiving a kidney. Two of these patients received primary grafts which failed at 28 days and 31 days respectively. A third patient received a second graft, it failed at 83 days. The remaining four grafts continue to function, one primary graft after 2 months, three secondary grafts at 39 months, 60 months and 89 months respectively.

3.3. *SOS scheme*

It is difficult to obtain kidneys for highly sensitised patients. Many different schemes have been tried in the hope of solving this problem. For the last seven years Belfast has taken part in a SOS scheme organised by UKTS. Sera are submitted from patients with a PRA greater than 85%. These sera may be current or historic. The sera are then tested at UKTS to validate the antibody reactivity and then aliquots are distributed to each centre taking part in the scheme. Each centre undertakes to test the SOS sera against each of their blood group compatible cadaveric donors. The tests are performed in duplicate with one sample coded and only when both results are negative is the donor considered suitable. This ensures that highly sensitised patients are crossmatched against a large number of donors.

Apart from greatly increasing the chances of obtaining a crossmatch negative kidney for the highly sensitised patient, it also gives a clear indication of the feasibility of obtaining a suitable kidney for that patient. The historic sera preventing the transplant of patients who have been on the SOS scheme for more than two years, will be ignored.

The duration of each cycle of the SOS scheme is four months. The disadvantage of the scheme is the amount of sera required for distribution. Thus the volume of sera available is very quickly used up. 1.0 ml is required for the first cycle and 0.8 ml thereafter for each subsequent cycle (viral tests and antibody validation are performed on each serum when first received).

During the seven years of the existence of the SOS scheme, 12 Belfast patients have been transplanted with its help. The one year graft survival in these patients is 58.3%. During the same period suitable local kidneys have been found for seven other highly sensitised patients (who were on the SOS scheme at the time of transplantation).

4. Appendix. Techniques used in tissue typing

4.1. *Microlymphocytotoxicity test*

A two-stage microlymphocytotoxicity test is used for the serological identification of HLA-A,-B,-C and -DR antigens. Target cells for HLA-A,B,C typing are lymphocytes obtained from patient's blood, anti-coagulated with sodium citrate, by centrifugation on a density gradient. Since 1984 when prospective HLA-DR typing was commenced, when typing cadaveric donors, lymphocytes isolated from spleen or lymph node have been used. Before 1984 peripheral blood was used as the source of lymphocytes for local donors and spleen or lymph node for imported kidneys.

HLA-DR typing requires the isolation of B lymphocytes. The preparation of B lymphocytes was initially performed by the elimination of T lymphocytes, using sheep red cells rosetting. The quality of B lymphocytes isolated has been greatly improved during the last three years by the use of magnetic beads coupled with a monoclonal antibody to Class II antigens. Trypan blue is usually used for identification of the dead cells. However, since the introduction of magnetic beads for the isolation of B cells we have used fluorescent dyes to determine the viability of cells. Live cells are visualised with acridine orange and stain green while dead cells take up ethidium bromide and stain orange. Since 1990 we have typed cadaver donors using magnetic bead isolation from peripheral blood, both for B lymphocytes and for T lymphocytes, the latter used for Class I antigen typing. This technique has been trouble-free and will be very beneficial for typing multi-organ donors, enabling prospective matching to be performed for heart and liver transplantation.

4.2. *Complement*

Rabbit complement is used in the microlymphocytotoxicity test. It is very important to control the quality of this reagent. In earlier years we bred our own rabbits but recently, because of the small size of the pool of these rabbits, it was decided to purchase commercial complement. We obtain samples of various batches of complement, test these samples and choose a suitable batch (i.e. non-toxic, of good titre, comparable to complement in use). It is important to test complement for both Class I and Class II antigens. It may be necessary to obtain a separate batch of complement for Class I and Class II antigens. Some commercial complements are not of high quality. We have found that some complement batches give false negative results for Class II typing.

4.3. *Automation*

A semi-automated method of reading the microlymphocytotoxicity test has been used. This enables results to be recorded immediately. An automated technique for the addition of sera and target cells to the typing plates is also in use.

4.4. *Freezing and thawing of lymphocytes*

Lymphocytes for freezing are suspended at a concentration of 4.0 × 10/ml in Roswell Park Memorial Institute 1640 medium (RPMI) containing 25% foetal calf serum (FCS). A volume of 1.0 ml is cooled to +4 °C in a cryotube and an equal volume of RPMI/25% FCS with 20% dimethyl sulphoxide (DMSO), previously cooled to +4 °C, is added drop by drop with thorough mixing. The cryotubes are placed in a polystyrene box at +4 °C and the box transferred to −70 °C overnight. The cryotubes are transferred to liquid nitrogen the following working day.

To retrieve the lymphocytes the cryotube is thawed at 37 °C ensuring that the temperature of the contents does not rise above +4 °C. The contents are then added to 4 ml of RPMI/50% FCS, previously cooled to +4 °C, and centrifuged at 2,000 rpm for 5 min. The lymphocytes are resuspended in complement fixing buffer with 20% FCS and the viability checked before use.

4.5. *Procurement of HLA reagents*

Accuracy in typing has always been a prominent aim of this laboratory. There are many ways to promote accuracy which mostly depend on the enthusiasm of the laboratory staff. The Belfast laboratory takes part in quality control schemes run by UKTS. In addition it has always been the policy to check on the tissue type of donors typed at another centre. Any differences in typing results are investigated and the source of HLA sera giving these results examined.

A local tissue typing plate is used in Belfast – the samples of serum used for the plate come from many sources using the best sera obtainable for each antigen. There is a programme by which serum samples collected from pregnant women are screened for antibodies to HLA-A, -B, -C, -DR and -DQ loci. When a suitable antibody is found the lady is approached either by her doctor when a small volume of blood (60 ml) is required, or plasmapheresis is arranged when a larger volume (up to 500 ml) is needed. The smaller amounts are sufficient for the Belfast plate and for exchange with other laboratories, the larger amounts are needed for contributing serum to UKTS, Eurotransplant, Collaborative Transplant Study, Heidelberg (CTS) and to International Histocompatibility Workshops. In many women the antibody disappears from the circulation within months of delivery, but good typing sera have been found in women years after the last childbirth. Suitable HLA sera can also be obtained by screening female blood donors who have previously been pregnant.

The screening, obtaining and exchanging of sera are very time consuming. However, they are necessary in order to obtain good sera. It is a more economic and accurate way of typing than the use of commercial plates. The heterogeneity of our population is much lower than some populations e.g., in the USA. Therefore typing in Belfast does not require sera which recognise antigens unique to certain races. However it has never been found more difficult to type for imported kidneys than local donors.

An added difficulty is that a majority of patients with Class II antibodies also have antibodies to Class I. These sera need to be absorbed with pooled platelets to remove the Class I activity.

For screening of sera we use as target cells lymphocytes from the blood of staff, of families of renal patients and of patients typed for disease studies. The tissue types of relatives of prospective renal recipients are determined for several reasons: when live transplantation is contemplated; for proof of homozygosity at an HLA locus of a patient; and when aid in the detection of a patient's antigens becomes necessary, for example in those instances where the combination of antigens makes the identification of the individual antigen very difficult.

When blood is obtained from any of the above the lymphocytes are frozen in liquid nitrogen to give a convenient supply. As far as possible all the HLA antigens are covered in as few members of a panel as possible, therefore the panels chosen are highly selective, not random. In screening for Class II antibodies cells from patients with chronic B cell lymphocytic leukaemia (CLL) are used.

4.6. *Analysis of sera reaction*

A computer programme has been developed to aid analysis. Obviously new HLA sera obtained either from our own screening or from an outside source are extensively tested before routine application. Records are kept of the results of sera so that a comparison may be made of their performance on different typing plates. It is important to remember that the activity of a sera can change on long-term storage. Unexpected reactions by a serum can reveal extra or even new specificities. The two × two contingency table has been used to establish and document a serum's pedigree. The four components of the table contain the number of concordant antiserum/panel cell antigen positive (+/+) negative (−/−) reactions, the number of missed reactions (+/−) and the number of extra reactions (+/−). From these data the correlation coefficient R can be obtained. The quality of a serum increases as the R value approaches unity. For common specificities an R value of 0.95 is sought but for rare specificities the only sera available may have a lower R value.

When there is conflict between the results of four sera, supposedly recognising the same antigen, reference can be made to previous results in an attempt to explain these discrepancies (i.e. a serum known to have the tendency to either have false positive or false negative reactions). A further important point is that sera to be exchanged must be tested for viruses such as hepatitis A and HIV.

4.7. *Restriction fragment length polymorphism (RFLP)*

During the last three years the techniques of molecular biology have been introduced to this laboratory. These methods have many advantages for Class II typing. They enable homozygosity to be proven without resorting to family members, new splits of antigens may be identified, discrepancies between this method of typing and the serological type may be shown (further aiding in sorting out the quality of the HLA sera used) and the HLA-DQ type of the recipient and donor can be determined. The latter was previously impossible to perform because of lack of reliable sera. We have used the enzyme TaqI and sequential probing with DR/β, DQ/β and DQα probes to ascertain the HLA-DR and -DQ type using restriction fragment length polymorphisms (RFLP).

The discrepancies between the serological type and the RFLP arise in two ways. In some instances an incorrect antigen is defined by serology and in other instances the serology has failed to define an antigen. We have recently taken part in a a study under the auspices of the Collaborative Transplant Study Heidelberg, whereby samples of donor and recipients from 82 centres world-wide were RFLP typed. It has been shown that by serology 31% of recipients and donors are incorrectly typed for HLA-DR. For purposes of this study samples typed as the broad antigen by serology and the corresponding split antigen by RFLP were not counted as discrepant typings. The rate of discrepancies found in this study is much greater than in our own centre showing the worthwhile benefit of having good HLA sera.

The disadvantage of RFLP typing is the time required to perform the test, thus the test is not applicable to prospective cadaver donor typing. However since 1986, we have typed the donors retrospectively. During this period ten primary cadaveric transplants which had been performed on the assumption that, by serology, there was only one HLA-DR mismatch, have been shown in fact to have two mismatches. On eight occasions the extra mismatched antigen was due to the donor having a different split than the recipient, of a broad HLA-DR antigen. These differences could not be detected by serological methods. On the other two occasions the donor was shown to have an extra HLA-DR antigen by RFLP.

The homozygosity rate of HLA-DR antigens for our cadaver donors is 12.4%, for recipients 10.8% and for normals 12.7%. As the population of Northern Ireland is relatively homogenous the homozygosity rate in other centres should not be any greater than these figures. If it is, this suggests that some HLA-DR antigens are not being detected.

4.8. *Oligonucleotide typing*

More recently the technique of oligonucleotide typing has been introduced after amplification of DNA by the polymerase chain reaction, for HLA-DP typing. This method enables detection of a one base difference in the sequence of an allele. Much work is needed before this method can be used to type cadaver donors prospectively for Class II antigen. Improvements in typing to this level of specificity will probably not be necessary for renal transplantation as improved immunosuppressive drugs and new methods of inducing tolerance are found. However these methods will improve the accuracy of testing and end the reliance on HLA sera.

An influence of HLA-DP matching on graft survival has not been demonstrated in this unit. The actual graft survival at 6 months was 82.6% (19/23), 77.5% (69/89) and 80.0% (28/35) for patients with zero, one and two HLA-DP mismatches respectively. At present we are typing for HLA-DP, recipients and donors of transplantations which have occurred with no mismatching at the HLA-A, -B, -DR and -DQ loci. These samples have been obtained from the CTS, showing again the value of co-operation in tissue typing.

4.9. *Crossmatching technique*

Crossmatching is performed using a two-stage microlymphocytotoxicity method. All tests are performed in triplicate. Cells and sera are incubated for one hour at 22 °C, followed by the addition of rabbit complement and a further incubation at 22 °C for two hours. Crossmatching is also performed using a washed technique i.e., at the end of the first incubation the serum is removed, the cells washed twice before the addition of rabbit complement. This has the benefit of removing anti-complementary effects of the sera which interfere with the test.

Three sets of spleen and lymph node are taken from each local donor, one set to accompany each kidney and the other set used for typing in this laboratory. For crossmatching we use spleen. We have reasoned that by using lymphocytes isolated from spleen there would be a higher percentage of B lymphocytes and since there is a higher preponderance of HLA antigens on the surface of the B lymphocyte the test would be more sensitive. The spleen or lymph node is collected in phosphate buffered saline, cut up and the cells teased out. Lymphocytes are then isolated as usual on a density gradient. On all occasions lymphocytes from spleen or lymph node are stored in liquid nitrogen for retrospective studies. DNA is also isolated from spleen and stored at −70 °C.

Acknowledgements

The contribution of staff past and present is gratefully acknowledged, in particular Mrs. J. Martin for help in developing the serological techniques and Mr. D. Savage and Mrs. C. Cullen for developing the DNA techniques. The latter also helped to develop the computer programme for analysis of results. I would like to thank all donors of antibodies and cells without whose help the laboratory could not have been developed.

CHAPTER 10

The cadaveric donor

G. LAVERY

The transplantation of organs has been one of the most notable advances in medicine in the last 30 years. Indeed, kidney transplantation has become so frequent and so successful that it is viewed as almost routine. Today the public expects that any suitable patient requiring a renal transplant will receive one after an acceptable waiting period. There are, however, still 8,000 patients in the UK on dialysis and the waiting list for transplants has increased from around 2,500 to over 4,000 in the last 5 years. It is therefore imperative that the number of kidneys available for transplantation is maximised and the quality optimised. This chapter will deal with the subject of kidney retrieval from the cadaveric donor. Since kidney retrieval is increasingly accomplished as part of multiple organ retrieval, it will be considered in that setting.

1. Identification of the potential donor

With the exception of corneas and the situation of live related donation, organs for transplantation may be retrieved only from individuals who are receiving mechanical ventilation in an intensive care unit (ICU). Table 20 lists the situations in which cadaveric organ donation may be considered. Kidneys and other organs may be retrieved for transplantation only when
1. brain stem death has been diagnosed.
2. the kidneys/organs are suitable for transplantation.
3. consent has been obtained from the next-of-kin.
4. the coroner (if appropriate) has agreed to organ retrieval.
   Brain stem death will be discussed at length later in this chapter. When deciding whether the kidneys would be suitable for transplantation the past medical history of the patient and the illness or events which led up to brain stem death must be considered. The contraindications to kidney donation are summarised in Table 21. Acute episodes of hypoxia or hypotension in the hours or days preceding brain stem death may also be a contraindication to organ donation. In general, a normal plasma urea and creatinine and a

Mary G. McGeown (ed.), Clinical Management of Renal Transplantation, 135–151.
© 1992 *Kluwer Academic Publishers, Dordrecht – Printed in the Netherlands.*

Table 20. Situations in which cadaveric organ donation may be considered

---

1. Severe head injury
2. Subarachnoid haemorrhage
3. Other cerebrovascular accident
4. Cardiac arrest with associated brain stem death
5. Primary (non-malignant) brain tumour

---

good urinary output are a reasonable guide to renal function. If there is doubt it is legitimate to follow the protocol for kidney retrieval and establish organ suitability by renal biopsy and histological examination. The age limits for donation in the past have been 2–60 years of age. Today individuals of up to 70 years of age may become kidney donors.

2. Brain stem death

Brain stem death (BSD) is a product of modern techniques of resuscitation and intensive care medicine. Before such techniques were available, BSD due to local injury or ischaemia was followed almost immediately by cardiac and/or respiratory arrest. Conversely, if cardio-respiratory arrest occurred then BSD occurred soon afterwards. Such modes of death were understood by everyone – medical and lay person alike. Today the respiratory and circulatory functions can be maintained for prolonged periods after death of the brain stem. The clinical dilemma is this: how can the individual who is brain stem dead and maintained by mechanical ventilation be distinguished from the individual who is in a state of deep coma and who may, given time, show some neurological recovery.

The concept of BSD is not new. It was first described in 1959 and termed "apnoeic coma". At the time the implications of apnoeic coma were unknown and the usual practice was to ventilate these individuals until another event caused "cardio-respiratory" death. Studies in the 1970's showed that apnoeic coma or brain death was inevitably followed by cardiac arrest even when cardio-respiratory support was maintained.

In 1979 the Conference of Medical Colleges and their Faculties in the UK published "Diagnosis of Brain Death". This laid down criteria for the diag-

Table 21. Contraindications to kidney donation

---

1. Major systemic sepsis
2. Present or past history of malignant disease (excluding primary brain neoplasm)
3. Primary renal disease
4. Hypertension
5. Positive serology for –
   Hepatitis B surface antigen
   HIV antibody

---

nosis of BSD and stated "brain death represents the stage at which the patient becomes truly dead". In January 1980 a further communication entitled "The removal of cadaveric organs for transplantation" was circulated to all hospital doctors. This and its update of 1983 is the code of practice governing the diagnosis of BSD and the subsequent retrieval of organs today.

2.1. The diagnosis of brain stem death

The diagnosis of BSD should be considered in any patient who is:
1. deeply comatose;
2. receiving positive pressure ventilation;
3. has suffered a condition known to be capable of causing BSD, e.g. trauma, intracranial disease, severe cerebral ischaemia or hypoxia.

Brain stem death should be diagnosed by two medical practitioners who have expertise in this field. One should be a consultant and the other a consultant or senior registrar. These two doctors must be "clinically independent" – that is they must not belong to the same team. In the absence of a consultant, a doctor who has been fully registered for at least 5 years and who is experienced in this branch of medicine may make a diagnosis of BSD. Each doctor involved must convince himself that the preconditions (Table 3) have been satisfied. The Code of Practice suggests that an adequate interval be allowed for drug effects to be excluded. It does not quantify the time period nor suggest the use of plasma drug levels. When considering metabolic or endocrine disturbances which might contribute to prolonged coma, no limits are set. Judgement should be used to decide whether an abnormality might mimic BSD (Table 22). Failure to satisfy the preconditions can have unfortunate sequelae (see later).

Having satisfied the preconditions, the two doctors perform a number of simple bedside tests. These must be carried out on two occasions by each doctor. They may perform the tests together or separately. The period between each test is at the discretion of those involved but should be long enough to be acceptable as two separate testings by all those involved and

---

Table 22. Preconditions for diagnosis of brain stem death

1. The patient must;
   be deeply unconscious
   be receiving mechanical ventilation
   have an injury/disorder capable of causing brain stem death
2. The following must be excluded as causative/contributary factors;
   depressant drugs
   hypothermia
   neuromuscular blocking agents
   metabolic or endocrine disturbances

Table 23. Tests of brain stem function

Stimulus	Response	Pathway
light shone into each eye	pupillary constriction	II-midbrain-III
stroke across each cornea	contraction orbicularis oculi	V-pons-VII
press supra-orbital nerves	facial grimace limb movement	V-pons-VII V-bs-cord
side rotation of head	compensatory eye movements	VIII-bs-III + VI
20 ml iced water in ears	nystagmus retching	VIII-bs-III + VI
Tracheal suction movement ET tube	gag/cough	IX-med-X
Apnoea until pCo > 6.65 kPa	respiratory effort	direct-med-cord -periph nerves

II, III etc. – cranial nerves; bs – brain stem; cord – spinal cord; med – medulla.

short enough to avoid unnecessary prolongation of the process. In practice the period varies from 20 minutes to 24 hours.

The tests are designed to ensure that all brain stem reflexes are absent (Table 23). Some practical points must be borne in mind when performing these tests. When testing the oculo-vestibular reflex it is important to visualise the tympanic membrane. An external auditory canal blocked with wax or clotted blood will prevent ice cold fluid stimulating the VIII nerve. The apnoea test must always be performed last, lest the hypercarbia that it causes might produce detrimental effects in a patient who is not, in fact, brain stem dead. During this test adequate oxygenation must be maintained. Rather than using an anaesthetic circuit (Figure 30(a)) it is recommended that oxygen be insufflated at 6 l/min through a narrow bore tube (such as a nasogastric tube) which has been passed through the endotracheal tube to a level just above the carina (Figures 30(b)). This produces much better oxygenation than the use of a conventional anaesthetic circuit (Figure 31).

The apnoea test supports the diagnosis of BSD when no respiratory movements occur following disconnection from mechanical ventilation and an increase in arterial carbon dioxide tension above the threshold for stimulation of respiration (usually this requires an apnoeic period of 5–10 min). The code of practice stipulates that the PaCO should rise to about 6.65 kPa (50 mm Hg). Many individuals will not have spontaneous respiration with PaCO levels of 50 mm Hg. It is therefore the practice in many units to ensure that, during the apnoea test, the PaCO reaches at least 9 kPa (65–70 mm Hg).

There may be circumstances in which it is impossible to carry out all of the tests mentioned above (e.g. severe trauma to the eyes may rule out

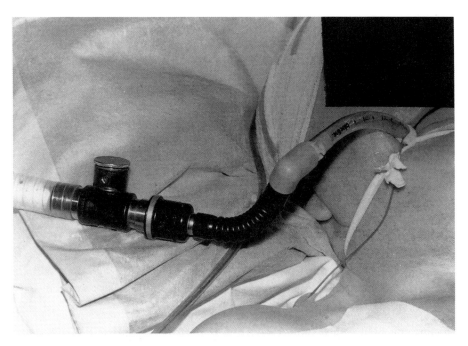

Figure 30(a). Oxygenation during apnoea test via anaesthetic circuit.

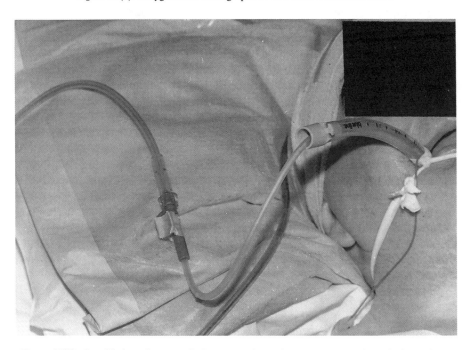

Figure 30(b). Insufflation of oxygen during apnoea test via a tube passed through the endotracheal tube to a level just above the carina.

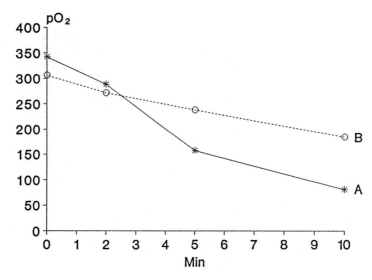

Figure 31. Oxygenation during apnoeic period. A oxygenation via anaesthetic circuit; B insufflation via tube passed through the endotracheal tube.

testing the light reflex and corneal reflex; perforated tympanic membranes may make testing of the oculo-vestibular reflex inadvisable). The code of practice is a set of guidelines drawn up after much discussion, not a set of inflexible rules. The doctors involved must decide whether the diagnosis of BSD can be supported in the absence of one or more of the signs. It is important to realise that the presence or absence of spinal cord reflexes have no bearing on the diagnosis of BSD. Indeed they are often present in such individuals.

The tests above are all simple procedures which can be carried out at the bedside. They do not require the support of complex investigation. The use of an EEG is not necessary for the diagnosis of BSD. EEG testing was suggested in a 1968 paper from Harvard but rejected by a further publication from the same institution 12 months later. Similarly, neither cerebral blood flow studies nor angiography play any part in the diagnosis of BSD.

The diagnosis of BSD should not be considered until the patient has been in coma for at least 6 hours. If the coma has followed a cardiac arrest, then 24 hours should be allowed to elapse after restoration of the circulation. Since a patient must be assumed to be alive until BSD is confirmed, the time of death is recorded as the point when the second set of brain stem tests are completed.

2.2. *Brain stem death – prognostic significance*

It might appear unnecessary to discuss prognosis when the brain stem no longer functions. It is useful, nevertheless, to acquaint those who have no difficulty in accepting the concept of BSD with the experience gained before that concept had widespread support. This is particularly true today when the diagnosis of BSD leads directly, at some point, to the discontinuation of mechanical ventilation. Familiarity with the lessons of the past also help when confronted with those who refuse to accept BSD as "real" death.

In the late 1960's, despite the existence of the Harvard criteria, many ICU physicians still ventilated patients in "apnoeic coma" until cardiac arrest occurred. In 1970, a neurosurgical study from France linked absence of brain stem reflexes and asystole in 70 comatose patients receiving full ventilatory support (Gaches et al., 1970). Further studies confirmed this connection and, in 1979, the code which still guides our practice today was published. Even then the practice of discontinuing ventilation after BSD had been confirmed did not gain acceptance immediately. Today we can compile evidence from more than 1000 cases of BSD which shows that, despite full medical support, BSD always leads to cardiac arrest (Pallis, 1983). This occurs a variable time after the onset of apnoeic coma but always within a few days (Jorgensen, 1973).

There have been claims that individuals have survived and even recovered after death of the brain stem. Pallis (1980) discredited the most notorious claims made in the British media and later a retraction was published (Paul, 1981). Pallis has also developed a series of questions which are invaluable when assessing such worrying claims.

Is this a real clinical case or a scenario developed for the purposes of debate?

Are all the details of the case available from a reputable source?

Was the patient in coma and receiving mechanical ventilation?

Was the effect of drugs specifically excluded?

Was the timing of brain stem testing appropriate (could the patient's physiological state have contributed to the absence of brain stem reflexes)?

Did the tests for apnoea constitute an adequate stimulus for spontaneous respiration?

3. The medical management of the potential donor

The diagnosis of BSD is, of course, a completely separate issue from that of organ retrieval and transplantation. Once BSD has been established it is legitimate to consider the BSD individual as a potential organ donor. Furthermore it is reasonable to maintain mechanical ventilation and other forms of organ support to optimize the condition of those organs. It may become necessary to increase the level of organ support or to change the management priorities completely in an effort to obtain organs suitable for transplantation. Thus, after BSD has been diagnosed, the ICU staff are no longer treating a patient but rather attempting to maintain a normal environment for organs which may be suitable for transplantation.

The clinician responsible for the potential kidney donor faces a number

Table 24. Potential problems occurring after brain stem death

1. Hypotension
2. Hypothermia
3. Diabetes insipidus
4. Oliguria
5. Pulmonary dysfunction
6. Cardiac dysrhythmias

of hurdles which must be overcome to allow successful organ retrieval and subsequent transplantation. When BSD is confirmed the question is "Are the kidneys suitable for transplantation?" The contraindications are as listed in Table 21. Three hurdles then remain:
1. maintaining the organs in an optimum condition
2. obtaining consent for kidney retrieval and
3. successfully carrying out the retrieval procedure.
Since many vital centres are situated in the brain stem it is not surprising that BSD is associated with a number of physiological disturbances. In a potential kidney donor, ICU management should attempt to minimize these disturbances and thereby reduce deterioration of renal function. The potential problems which may occur are listed in Table 24 and will be discussed below.

3.1. *Hypotension*

This is said to occur in 75% of patients with BSD. A major underlying factor is usually hypovolaemia following deliberate dehydration or the use of an osmotic diuretic in an attempt to control intracranial pressure before BSD occurred. The onset of diabetes insipidus may also predispose to hypovolaemia. Another factor is the lack of vasomotor tone following death of the brain stem. This will produce generalized vasodilation and venodilation. The result is a fall in peripheral resistance, relative hypovolaemia, venous pooling and a decrease in venous return resulting in decreased cardiac output.

Treatment is based on the infusion of fluid to restore an adequate circulating blood volume. This may require central venous (CVP) or pulmonary capillary wedge pressure (PCWP) monitoring. If infusion of fluids is not sufficient, an inotrope may be added to increase cardiac contractility and, therefore, cardiac output. Dopamine is probably the inotrope of choice in this situation. Vasoconstrictors without inotropic effect are contraindicated as they will improve blood pressure only by increasing peripheral resistance thereby decreasing organ perfusion still further.

3.2. *Hypothermia*

Hypothermia occurs in 60% of patients with BSD. It is common for core temperature to fall below 34 °C. There are four underlying factors (Table 25). Vasomotor centre dysfunction produces generalised vasodilatation and excessive heat loss through the skin. The presence of hypotension and/or diabetes insipidus may require the infusion of large volumes of fluid which are usually relatively cold. Muscle inactivity leads to reduction of heat generation. Hypothermia is best treated by anticipating it. Warming blankets should be used as soon as body temperature starts to fall, intravenous fluids should be warmed and the temperature of inspired gases may be increased using a heated humidifier.

Table 25. Causes of hypothermia after brain stem death

1. Dysfunction of temperature regulating centre
2. Dysfunction of vasomotor centre – increase in peripheral heat loss
3. Infusion of large volume of relatively cold fluid
4. Lack of muscle activity

3.3. *Diabetes insipidus*

Diabetes insipidus may occur in 90% of cases of BSD and is caused by a lack of anti-diuretic hormone (ADH). It is important to differentiate diabetes insipidus from other causes of polyuria. Hyperglycaemia is not uncommon in patients with BSD and can cause an osmotic diuresis. The osmotic diuresis caused by mannitol can also mimic diabetes insipidus especially when, prior to BSD, it has been used in large amounts in an effort to control raised intracranial pressure. The result of poorly managed diabetes insipidus is hypovolaemia and hypotension leading to ischaemia damage of transplantable organs. Hypernatraemia and hypokalaemia are the usual associated electrolytic abnormalities.

Diabetes insipidus should be suspected in any individual who has an "at risk" history and who is polyuric in the absence of the factors mentioned above. The finding of a very low urinary specific gravity (<1.005) and low urinary osmolality (usually <200 mOsmol) associated with a normal or high plasma osmolality (often >330 mOsmol) and a rising serum sodium level will confirm the diagnosis.

The treatment of DI is based on the assumption that:
1. hypovolaemia already exists
2. the urinary loss of sodium is low
3. hypokalaemia will occur secondary to the diuresis.

Inappropriate use of fluids will produce hypernatraemia. Colloids, which are relatively rich in sodium, may have been used to correct acute falls in blood pressure. Established hypovolaemia needs to be corrected by a bolus of crystalloid and/or colloid. On-going losses should be replaced mainly with fluids low in sodium, such as 5% dextrose. Potassium should be infused at approximately 20 mmol per litre of crystalloid given.

When urinary output reaches a level (>500 ml/hr) with which it becomes difficult to keep pace, exogenous ADH should be given. This is particularly useful when there is co-existing hypovolaemia and a need to restore circulating blood volume. Desmopressin can be given subcutaneously (2–8 I.U.) or intravenously. Since it is a potent vasoconstrictor especially of the splanchnic vascular bed, it should ideally be administered by a controlled infusion with an initial rate of 0.1 IU/min. The object is to reduce urinary output to a level compatible with intravenous fluid replacement.

3.4. *Oliguria*

This is much less common than diabetes insipidus and when it occurs it is almost always due to hypovolaemia and/or hypotension. Treatment is, of course, infusion of fluids. As discussed earlier, this may require CVP or PCWP monitoring. If oliguria persists renal perfusion may be improved by giving an intravenous infusion of dopamine (2–3 μg/kg/min) or dopexamine. Higher doses of dopamine may be used to improve cardiac contractility and therefore arterial pressure and perfusion. One should be wary, however, of using dopamine in doses exceeding 10 μg/kg/min since this may cause vasoconstriction due to alpha agonist activity and thus reduce organ perfusion.

3.5. *Pulmonary dysfunction*

Severe hypoxaemia is common after BSD and often necessitates an increase in respiratory support. Many of the problems are those occurring in all intubated and mechanically ventilated patients.

Pulmonary atelectasis can be reduced by the use of positive end expiratory pressure (PEEP), regular tracheo-bronchial suction and chest physiotherapy. Many ICUs discontinue these measures after BSD has been diagnosed. This is ALWAYS a mistake especially when the organ retrieval is delayed, as sometimes occurs particularly in multiple organ retrievals.

Rapidly advancing pulmonary infection has been described after BSD. A "normal" chest X-ray may progress to severe bilateral patchy opacification due to bronchopneumonic consolidation within a few hours. This may represent a dysfunction of the immunological system in association with the other abnormalities described above. If a patient has been on antibiotic therapy prior to BSD occurring then this should be continued. Failure to do so may result in florid infection which may compromise organs for transplantation.

Pulmonary oedema, due to fluid overload, may result from attempts to ensure adequate urinary flow. It may be due to administration of excessive doses of mannitol prior to BSD. The use of large volumes of crystalloid in patients with diabetes insipidus may also predispose to pulmonary oedema. Pulmonary oedema may occur in this group of patients without obvious cause. This has been called "neurogenic pulmonary oedema". It should be viewed as a diagnosis of exclusion. It may be due to abnormalities in vasomotor control resulting in failure of the pre-capillary sphincters to protect the pulmonary capillaries from the high hydrostatic pressure in the arterioles. This upsets the normal balance in the pulmonary capillary bed and results in a net outward flow of plasma water. Treatment is symptomatic. Inspired oxygen concentration and PEEP may have to be increased.

During mechanical ventilation, the pressure applied to the airways falls to zero at the end of expiration. If a positive pressure is applied to the airways at this stage of the respiratory cycle it is referred to as positive end expiratory pressure (PEEP). PEEP causes an increase in functional residual capacity of the lungs (FRC). FRC is known to decrease in the supine patient and with advancing age as well as in many pathological conditions e.g. adult respiratory distress syndrome, abdominal distention. When FRC falls below a critical volume, known as the closing volume (CV) then small airways close on expiration and may not re-open. This produces distal atelectasis which results in non-aerated but perfused alveoli and a functional right to left shunt causing arterial hypoxaemia. By maintaining FRC above CV, PEEP reverses or prevents this process and so "recruits" alveoli which would otherwise be non-functional.

When the alveolar sac contains pulmonary oedema fluid, the alveolar-capillary diffusion distance is increased. PEEP causes a redistribution of this fluid by distending the alveolus (thereby increasing the surface area) and compressing the fluid around the alveolar wall. This reduces the alveolar-capillary diffusion distance towards normal again. PEEP does not reduce the amount of alveolar fluid (it may in fact cause a slight overall increase) but it reduces its adverse effects.

3.6. Dysrhythmias

Following BSD, even in the presence of continuing maximal physiological support, cardiac arrest will occur after a variable period of time. It is therefore not surprising that, in the period between BSD and organ retrieval, cardiac dysrhythmias are common. They will occur more frequently in the presence of the physiological disturbances discussed above. Electrolyte disturbances are common, hypokalaemia, in particular, causing dysrhythmias. Arterial hypotension reduces coronary perfusion pressure and myocardial blood flow and therefore results in myocardial hypoxia and acidosis. Raised intracranial pressure can cause dysrhythmias by direct pressure on the brain stem centres which control heart rate. The use of large doses of inotropes in an (often inappropriate) attempt to maintain perfusion and arterial pressure often results in tachyarrhythmias.

4. Consent – approaching the family

One of the reasons for failing to retrieve organs from potential donors is the refusal of consent by next-of-kin. This may be due to inadequate public education about transplantation, but may also be due to an inappropriate approach to the families. Requesting consent for organ retrieval, at a time of family grief and turmoil, is a difficult task. Each ICU should have several members of staff specifically identified for this task. These individuals should be chosen, not by status, but for their abilities to communicate with relatives and their commitment to organ retrieval. If a transplant co-ordinator is available then he or she may shoulder much of this workload or support the ICU staff.

Many individuals hesitate to ask for organs due to a fear of making bereavement worse. An interesting quote from the young wife of a trauma victim was "My husband has just died. How can anything make it worse"? Families will often be "emotionally numb" at the time when consent for retrieval is sought but will derive some benefit from the act of donation weeks or months later.

The next-of-kin should be approached after the first set of brain stem tests, informed of the findings and that the second testing may confirm the diagnosis of brain stem death. The concept of organ donation may be raised although no attempt to obtain consent should be made at this time. This allows a period for discussion between members of the family and others whose views they value. The possession of an organ donor card, although useful in establishing the intent of the potential donor in life, has little relevance. It would be a courageous clinician who proceeded to organ retrieval from a donor card holder against the wishes of the family. In practice, it is the next-of-kin who decide which organs, if any, should be retrieved.

Consent should be obtained from the nearest relative but does not have to be agreed by all the relatives. When no relatives can be traced, the clinician in charge should ascertain if there is any evidence regarding the deceased wishes i.e. donor card or religious beliefs which might preclude donation. If no obstacle to donation is uncovered then it may be possible to proceed to organ retrieval. If a family does refuse to give consent for organ retrieval, it is inappropriate to ask the reason as this may make them feel under pressure and convey disapproval.

After consent has been obtained and recorded in the patient's chart, the wishes of the family should be carried out as far as possible. They should be allowed to say their "goodbyes", preferably in the ICU. They should be encouraged to ask questions rather than "wonder in silence". It is important that the process of organ retrieval does not materially hold up the arrangements for burial which must be made at this time. In many units the policy is that retrieval must occur so that, on the morning after the diagnosis of brain stem death, the body is available for autopsy or removal from the hospital mortuary.

Within a few weeks the next-of-kin should be informed, by letter, of the fate (in general terms) of the organs retrieved. A transplant co-ordinator can also help the family in the longer term, if needed, by the use of counselling and support groups. The wisdom of this is questioned in some quarters as it may hinder the normal grieving process. If counselling is given, it is important to remember the need to preserve the confidentiality of the recipient.

5. The process of retrieval

Having diagnosed BSD in a potential organ donor and been able to maintain the organs in a stable physiological environment, the practical problems associated with an organ retrieval must now be addressed.

Some of the steps should be initiated a little earlier. After the first testing for brain stem death (assuming this supports the diagnosis of BSD), it is reasonable to send blood for hepatitis B, HIV and CMV tests. The United Kingdom Transplant Support Service (UKTSS) in Bristol should be informed about the potential organ donor and of the organs which are potentially suitable for transplantation. This is best done through the local transplant co-ordinator. The next-of-kin should be kept abreast of the situation. Good communication will prepare the family for the distressing period ahead and will improve their rapport with the ICU staff.

The results of the second set of brain stem tests will confirm (or refute) the diagnosis of BSD. If BSD is confirmed, the family should be informed and consent for organ retrieval sought. The doctor obtaining consent should record this carefully in the notes. The code of practice does not require that a consent form be signed and witnessed. However, many regional health authorities having taken legal advice, recommend this. After consent has been obtained, UKTSS should be informed.

The code of practice "Removal of Cadaveric Organs for Transplantation" states that death is only conclusively established when BSD criteria have been satisfied on two successive occasions. Thus, when BSD is diagnosed, the time of death must be recorded as the time when the second set of tests were completed by both doctors involved. Up to that point, death has not been conclusively established and the patient must be presumed to be alive.

The smoothness with which organ retrieval proceeds depends on communication and anticipation of the problems. The operating theatre co-ordinator/senior sister should be notified of the potential donor, which organs are being offered for retrieval and at what time retrieval is likely to begin. As further information is obtained, via UKTSS or direct from units interested in the potential donor, this should be relayed to the ICU and theatre staff in the donating hospital and to any other retrieval teams already involved. A common question from the theatre staff at this time is "Do we need to supply a scrub nurse?" Meanwhile the ICU staff need information for their own needs and for liaison with the next-of-kin.

The potential organ donor, as we have discussed, may be on a high inspired oxygen concentration, significant PEEP, receiving inotrope infusions and suffering from diabetes insipidus, electrolyte disturbances and cardiac dysrhythmias. In the operating theatre during organ retrieval the haemodynamic and respiratory monitoring instituted in the ICU should be continued.

A possible source of anxiety is the haemodynamic responses (an increase in arterial pressure and tachycardia) which may be exhibited by brain stem dead organ donors. They are not uncommon and may necessitate the use of a volatile anaesthetic agent. They do not mean that the diagnosis of BSD is incorrect. They may be due to an effect similar to the "mass effect" noted in quadriplegics, to spinal reflexes or to release of catecholamines mediated by spinal reflexes via pre-sympathetic fibres.

Potential organ donors may be unsuitable for donation of any organs due to the presence of a medical contraindication, the refusal of family to give consent, lack of co-operation by the coroner or failure to maintain the organs in an acceptable state. If this occurs then, after informing the family, supportive treatment should be stopped and cardio-respiratory arrest allowed to occur. The family must understand that they are merely being informed, not being asked to make a decision regarding "life support". A family which feels that it has chosen to "switch off" their relative may carry an unnecessary burden of guilt for many years.

6. Future developments

In the years ahead efforts must be made to improve the number of kidneys and other organs available for transplantation. The stimulus to do this will be two-fold. Firstly, the present trend to widen the indications for renal transplantation will continue and, secondly, public expectation will be such that any other treatment for chronic renal failure will be viewed as unacceptable. A number of approaches are being planned or implemented at present.

6.1. Audit

Audit will play an increasing role in identifying the deficiencies in our present practice regarding cadaveric organ donors. In 1989 an audit of all deaths occurring in ICU units in England was initiated and the first year's findings have recently been made available. Already it has settled one area of disagreement by showing that failure of ICU staff to request consent for organ retrieval from a suitable donor is uncommon. It did reveal that refusal to give consent was a significant factor in reducing the number of organs available for transplantation. In future audit should help to identify strategies which may be effective in improving organ donation.

6.2. *Alternatives to the donor card system*

Major problems with the present card system are that it is not always carried by victims of trauma and that it expresses an intent only – the family may refuse organ donation irrespective of the deceased's wishes. In this grey area, it is always wiser to accept the view of the living.

Another strategy which has been suggested to increase the number of organ donors is "required request" in which it would be compulsory for medical staff to request consent for organ retrieval from the next-of-kin in all suitable cases. This scheme is already in operation in some areas of the USA but it would appear to have little to offer if applied to major ICU units in the UK. It is possible that such a scheme might help if applied to units which infrequently identify potential donors.

"Lifeline Wales" is an attempt to avoid this situation. This is an "opting in" system on a computerized system which can be accessed round the clock. Such schemes have also been tried in Manchester and Glasgow but attracted too few participants to become useful. Another suggested scheme is "opting out" in which everyone is viewed as a potential donor unless they have registered to the contrary. This type of arrangement would seem to be less acceptable than "opting in".

6.3. *Transplant co-ordinators*

In future, it will be imperative to improve public knowledge about transplantation and to make medical and nursing staff more aware of, and more enthusiastic about, organ retrieval. These activities fall within the brief of transplant co-ordinators who have been introduced gradually to almost every region of the UK. Most co-ordinators hold nursing qualifications and are expected to fulfil the following roles:
1. to assist the transplant unit team in successfully running the transplant programme.
2. to help bring about an increase in the number of organs available for transplantation.
3. to give support, advice and information in all aspects of organ donation and transplantation to medical, nursing and other staff, patients, relatives and the general public.

The transplant co-ordinator role has evolved alongside the practice of multiple organ retrieval in which the amount of organisation, communication and trouble shooting have become unmanagable for clinical staff with other priorities within the ICU. The ideal transplant co-ordinator should be physically present in the unit during the preparation for organ retrieval, should liaise with the next-of-kin, obtain (or help to obtain) consent for donation, inform UKTS, ensure that the necessary paperwork and blood tests are completed, communicate with all groups involved and deal with unexpected problems as they occur. It is likely that, in future, their role as educators of the public and medical/nursing staff will be expanded and more finance will be provided for this. Another advance, achieved largely through the work of the United Kingdom Transplant Co-ordinators Association (UKTCA), is the evolution of support groups for the next-of-kin of organ donors.

6.4. The "Exeter Protocol"

A more controversial method for increasing the supply of organs for transplantation has been adopted by Feest and colleagues (1990). They set out to identify patients with cerebrovascular disease in general wards who would potentially fulfil the criteria for brain stem death within a relatively short period of time. These individuals, with the consent of the next-of-kin, were transferred to ICU for elective ventilation. If BSD was later confirmed then consent for organ donation was requested. The study ran for 19 months and identified 11 patients who fulfilled the criteria for transfer to ICU of whom 9 were actually transferred. As a result, the hospital's donor rate increased to 2.5 times the UK average. The study did, however, raise ethical as well as logistic problems. Due to the small numbers involved in the study one major question was unanswered. How many patients will be managed according to the "Exeter protocol" and fail to become an organ donor?" The paper is excellent if viewed as a pilot study and has shown the way for further research.

6.5. Reimbursement

It is widely appreciated that resources at donor hospitals are strained, particularly operating theatre staff, ICU beds and ICU staff. Since critically ill patients must continue to take priority over brain stem dead organ donors, this must reduce the rate of organ donation or favour single (kidneys) organ retrieval when a more complex (and time consuming) multiple organ donation was possible. The whole system of organ retrieval still relies heavily on the resources of the donating hospital and the enthusiasm of its staff.

The proposals of a working party of the Royal College of Surgeons and the College of Anaesthetists to improve this state of affairs includes the reimbursement of donor hospitals for costs involved in ICU management and the operative costs of organ retrieval. This must be seen clearly as a reimbursement of real costs and NOT payment for organs retrieved.

6.6. *Regional retrieval teams*

The present retrieval system may involve drawing together as many as four different surgical retrieval teams. This complex system often leads to delays if one team arrives late. The working party mentioned above has proposed the establishment of two organ retrieval teams for the UK, capable of retrieving all transplantable organs. Each team would have a cardiothoracic surgeon, an abdominal surgeon, an anaesthetist and a scrub nurse. The teams would be based near transplant centres and airports. Cambridge has been suggested as the base to serve the southern half of the UK, Manchester or Birmingham would serve the north. This would be less expensive than the present system when several retrieval teams may converge on the donating hospital from various parts of the country.

Further reading

Bodenham, A., Berridge, J. C., Park, G. R. Brain stem death and organ donation. *Br. Med. J.* 1989; 299: 1009–1010.

Cadaveric organs for transplantation. Working Party of the Department of Health. London, HMSO, 1983.

Feest, T. G. Riad, H. N., Collins, C. H. et al. Protocol for increasing organ donation after cerebrovascular deaths in a district general hospital. *Lancet* 1990; 335: 1133–1135.

Gaches, J., Caliscan, A., Fundji, F. et al. Contibution à l'étude du compasse et de la mort cerebral (étude de 71 cas). *Sem Hôp Paris* 1970; 46: 1487–1497.

Gentleman, D., Easton, J., Jennett, B. Brain death and organ donation in a neurosurgical unit: audit of recent practice. *Br. Med. J.* 1990; 301: 1203–1206.

Jennett, B., Gleave, J., Wilson, P. Brain death in three neurosurgical units. *Br. Med. J.* 1981; 282: 533–539.

Jorgensen, E. O. Spinal man after brain death. *Acta. Neurochirurg.* 1973; 28: 259–273.

Lavery, G. G., Coppel, D. L., Johnston, J. R., Lowry, K. G. An audit of organ retrieval – Could we do better? *Journal of the Irish College of Physicians and Surgeons* 1991; 20: 78.

Odom, N. J. Organ donation. *Br. Med. J.* 1990; 300: 1571–1575.

Pallis, C. Medicine and the media. *Br. Med. J.* 1980; 281: 1029.

Pallis, C. The ABC of brain stem death. British Medical Association, London, 1983.

Paul, R. Survival after brain death: withdrawal of allegation. *Lancet* 1981; i: 677.

Report of the Working Party on the Supply of Donor Organs for Transplantation. Conference of Medical Royal Colleges and their Faculties in the United Kingdom, 1987.

The removal of cadaveric organs for transplantation. A code of practice. Working Party of the Department of Health, London, HMSO, 1979.

CHAPTER 11

Retrieval and preservation of the kidney

J. A. KENNEDY

The ultimate success of renal transplantation depends on many controllable factors. The procurement of healthy viable renal tissue, with an adequate vascular pedicle and urinary drainage system was recognised as a key element in transplantation in a very early stage of our experience in the Belfast Unit.

The vast majority of transplant recipients rely on cadaveric grafts because of the unavailability of medically and immunologically suitable living related donors. Successful transplantation with the lowest possible recipient morbidity and mortality requires meticulous attention to technical procedures. At the outset and before the clinical program began, retrieval and insertion operations were performed on cadavers, so that the details of the surgical technique were perfected.

More than 20 years ago, it was common surgical practice to remove kidneys from cadavers after the cessation of cardiac action. Such practice was fraught with grave risks. The tissue to be transplanted was exposed to a dangerous partially anoxic warm environment before removal. The retrieval team assessed each individual donor situation. The records for the hours before death of urinary output, peripheral capillary circulation, as well as pulse and blood pressure readings were carefully studied. This pre-retrieval assessment reduced the risks of taking tissue likely to be non-viable after exposure to a warm anoxic environment.

With the wide acceptance of brain stem death (Chapter 10) many of the difficulties encountered in the early days have disappeared. "Multiple organ retrieval" poses its own difficulties but the integration of the technical procedures of the cardiac and renal surgeons has simplified the latters' tasks in such cases.

1. Surgical technique

Following removal of the kidney and simple perfusion with a cold lactate solution, the presence of a "full drip chamber stream" of fluid at a height of 1.5 metres above the kidney was a reliable sign that the vascular tree

Mary G. McGeown (ed.), Clinical Management of Renal Transplantation, 153–159.
© 1992 *Kluwer Academic Publishers, Dordrecht – Printed in the Netherlands.*

was free from agonal spasm. The presence of agonal spasm was frequently associated with micro-clotting problems. Now the cadaveric donor is given heparin intravenously to protect the renal circulation. In addition a potent alpha-blocker, phenoxibenzamine (100 mg) is given intravenously about 15 minutes before vascular disconnection is carried out.

2. Exposure and perfusion technique

The laparotomy is carried out through a long mid-line transperitoneal incision with lateral extension incisions into both flanks at the level of the umbilicus. After incision of the peritoneum on the left lateral margin of the gut, the left colon is retracted to the right giving access to the distal aorta for cannulation. The left ureter is easily identified as it crosses the first large branch of the common iliac artery. The ureter is carefully dissected free, sweeping the loose vascular tissue from its lateral side to just above the bladder where it is divided. This dissection is carried out proximally on the aorta, so as to avoid damage to the longitudinal ureteric vascular channels during the aortic cannulation.

Two tapes are placed around the lower aorta, the upper being placed well below the renal arteries. A small incision is made on the front of the aorta between the tapes to permit the insertion of a modified Foley catheter, which is then advanced upwards so that the balloon is placed above the renal arteries. The balloon is inflated. With the aorta occluded above and below by the double tapes, and the distal end of the catheter occluded, the opening just below the balloon permits *in situ* perfusion of the isolated aortic segment and renal arteries to achieve rapid cooling of the renal parenchyma. This allows extra time should the donor nephrectomy prove to be unusually difficult, as for example when multiple vessels are present.

The genital and adrenal veins which drain to the left renal vein can be ligated and divided at this stage and an adequate length of left renal vein divided between ligatures, as close as possible to the vena cava. The front of the aorta is now free and clearly visible permitting a detailed assessment of the arterial supply to both kidneys. Small single left polar vessels may be ligated safely but judgement is required as to whether a particular vessel should be retained for later bench surgery to avoid necrosis of a renal pole.

3. Vascular connections

When the artery to the left kidney is single it can be separated easily from the aorta using a suitably curved vascular clamp to produce a disc (Carrel patch) of aorta adequate for anastomotic purposes. Although the kidneys have been cooled, unnecessary handling of the organ should be avoided as far as possible. Traction should be avoided, prior to dividing the arteries, as the intima is easily torn and such an intimal arterial tear is a well known cause of failure to revascularise initially after the clamps have been released following insertion. In addition, such tears may cause late thrombosis after apparently successful revascularisation.

The procedure for removing the right kidney involves the same principles, displacing the right large bowel to the left, to expose the duodenum and inferior vena cava. Because of the restricted length of the right renal vein it has been our practice to excise a patch of inferior vena cava, using the curved vascular clamp.

A single renal artery on the right side can be separated from the aorta to provide adequate length. If multiple renal arteries are found to either kidney, it is best to remove that particular kidney en-block with aorta, after washout and perfusion have been performed. The kidney is subsequently transplanted using a Carrel patch carrying the multiple vessels. If bilateral multiple arteries are present, the aorta is cross-clamped. Both kidneys are removed en-block. The separation of both organs is then completed by surgical division of the aorta on the bench.

4. The ureter

The importance of the preservation of the blood supply of the ureter cannot be overstressed.

The intact ureter receives its blood supply by three main routes, that is by branches from the inferior renal artery, the lumbar arteries and unnamed but consistent vessels which are branches of either the common iliac or internal iliac arteries. The main venous drainage is through a network of vessels in the delicate surrounding parenchymal tissue, which must be meticulously and widely removed with the ureter, as a "surrounding" mantel. It is essential that dissection is not performed in the area of the renal pelvis or hilum of the kidney. There may thus be a large mass of peripelvic ureteric fatty tissue remaining with the kidney and ureter (Figure 32).

Any vascular insufficiency or venous congestion may cause failure of primary healing of the ureter in the transplant recipient. Urinary extravasation in the immunosuppressed patient has a very significant morbidity or even mortality. The incidence of ureteric or urinary leaks in the immediate post-transplant period is a good indication of the skill of the operating team and their appreciation of these points.

5. The living donor

It is essential to carry out bilateral renal arteriography before considering removing a kidney from a live donor. Statistically, most donors have a single renal artery to at least one of their kidneys. Should a related living donor

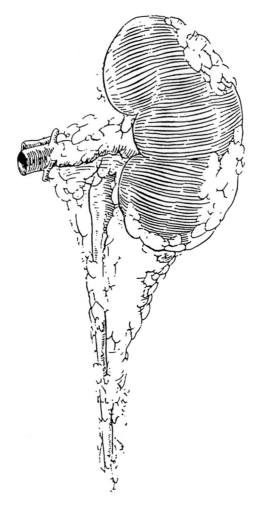

Figure 32. Fatty tissue surrounding the kidney and ureter, which should be left undisturbed. Taken from *Campbell's Urology*, Vol. 3, 5th edn., p. 2542, fig. 66, 4. Acknowledged from the *Journal of Urology*, 112: 445, 1974.

be demonstrated to have multiple renal arteries on both sides the patch technique is not appropriate because of the totally unacceptable risk to the donor. Particular care is required with the dissection so as to obtain the maximum length of vessel should it be necessary to use a donor kidney with multiple arteries. The anomaly may then be corrected on the bench prior to implantation.

Multiple renal veins are more often encountered on the right side but additional veins can always be safely ligated, provided a small cuff of donor vena cava is removed. The donor cava is then over-sewn with a running 5/0 vascular suture to ensure complete and safe haemostasis. The preservation of ureteric vascularisation is as essential in the living donor as in the cadaver. Even greater care is necessary to preserve the vascular envelope around the ureter down to the level of the pelvic vessels. It must be remembered that in the living, donor nephrectomy is being carried out not for a disease process but so that its anatomical integrity and function will be preserved in the recipient.

6. Preservation of the donor kidney

The donor kidney must be preserved long enough to provide time for the arrangements surrounding transplantation into a suitable recipient to be made. When a living donor is to be used many of the arrangements can be made in advance – the donor has been fully investigated and pronounced free from malignancy or any disease which might be transmitted to the recipient (including HIV, hepatitis B and CMV); the recipient has been fully investigated and both parties have had the blood group carried out, full tissue typing and the cross match test have been performed. When the donor is a cadaver the blood group and tests for HIV, hepatitis B and CMV can be carried out in advance but the tissue type is usually deferred until spleen or lymph nodes are available after removal of the organs. Exclusion of malignancy must await the autopsy. The recipient will be chosen from a pool of patients on computer, only a few of whom will be geographically near to the donor centre. Once selected for suitability, including the blood group and tissue type, the kidney, spleen and blood samples must be transported to the recipient's centre and the cross match carried out. Time may be required to prepare the patient selected, including time for dialysis if necessary before surgery. The cross match may turn out to be positive and another patient may have to be chosen.

When circulation ceases tissues soon undergo ischaemic damage, but there is considerable variation for different organs in the time within which this occurs. The brain becomes irreversibly damaged within a few minutes while skin will survive several hours without oxygen. The kidney will tolerate much longer periods of ischaemia than the brain but not nearly as long as skin. The ischaemia time tolerated may be prolonged by cooling. A wide variety of perfusion fluids have been used over the years, from simple electrolyte solutions to much more complex mixtures containing colloids. Table 26 shows the composition of some solutions now used widely. We use isotonic citrate (Marshall's) solution. University of Wisconsin (UW) preserving solution (Table 27) is used widely for preservation of liver, heart and heart lung; some use it for kidneys. We have found the simpler and cheaper Marshall's solution satisfactory for kidneys.

Complete ischaemia of the kidneys for 30 minutes in animals and in man causes temporary loss of function in a high proportion of cases. The shorter the ischaemia the more rapid the recovery, and after ischaemia for longer

Table 26. Solutions in common use for flushing of kidneys

	Collins'-C2	Euro-Collins'	Euro-Collins' mannitol	Sacks'	Hypertonic citrate	Marshall's isotonic citrate
Sodium (mmol l^{-1})	9	10	10	14	78	78
Potassium (mmol l^{-1})	108	108	108	125	84	84
Magnesium (mmol l^{-1})	30	–	–	8	40	40
Bicarbonate (mmol l^{-1})	9	10	10	20	–	–
Chloride (mmol l^{-1})	14	15	15	15	1	1
Phosphate (mmol l^{-1})	47	60	60	60	–	–
Sulphate (mmol l^{-1})	30	–	–	–	40	40
Glucose (mmol l^{-1})	126	180	–	–	–	–
Mannitol (mmol l^{-1})	–	–	180	200	200	100
Osmolarity (mmol kg^{-1})	320	340	340	430	400	300
pH	7.0	7.3	7.2	7.0	7.1	7.1

than 30 minutes recovery is often delayed for 10 days or longer. Functional recovery after ischaemia of longer than 60 minutes is likely to be incomplete. Nevertheless there are several patients in Belfast whose kidneys continue to function excellently after almost 20 years although they (the kidneys) were not perfused until 60–80 minutes after circulation ceased.

Table 27. Solution for flushing organs, containing additional buffer potassium lactobionate, energy sources, synthetic colloid, anti-microbial agent

University of Wisconsin (UW) Preserving solution	
Sodium (mmol l^{-1})	30
Potassium (mmol l^{-1})	120
Magnesium (mmol l^{-1})	5
Sulphate (mmol l^{-1})	5
Lactobionate (mmol l^{-1})	100
Phosphate (mmol l^{-1})	25
Raffinose (mmol l^{-1})	30
Adenosine (mmol l^{-1})	5
Glutathione (mmol l^{-1})	3
Allopurinol (mmol l^{-1})	1
Insulin (U l^{-1})	100
Dexamethasone (mg l^{-1})	8
Bactrim (ml l^{-1})	0.5
Hydroxyethyl starch (g l^{-1})	50
Osmolarity (mmol kg^{-1})	320
pH	7.4

Ischaemia time is described being made up of three periods: initial warm ischaemia time, cold ischaemia time and operative ischaemia time. The sum of the three periods is referred to as total ischaemia time, initial warm ischaemia and operative time are sometimes summed to give total warm time. Initial warm ischaemia times in excess of 30 minutes are not now generally regarded as acceptable because of the high incidence of delayed function. The operative ischaemia time is very variable, depending on the difficulties encountered with the vessels of the donor and recipient, and the skill and experience of the surgeon. It may vary from less than 30 minutes to 70 minutes or even more. The longer operative ischaemia times are often associated with delay in onset of function. Cold ischaemia time is less critical and it is commonly 30 to 40 hours, while satisfactory function has been reported even after 70 hours.

Kidneys are flushed initially with the chosen perfusion fluid chilled to 4°C until the effluent is no longer blood stained. This may be done after removal from the body via a carefully inserted cannula (great care must be taken to avoid damage to the intima of the renal artery), or better, as described above by direct perfusion through the aorta before removal. This initial flush washes out blood and particulate matter as well as cooling the kidney to reduce the metabolic rate. The preferred temperature appears to be the lowest obtainable without actually freezing the organs. Once the effluent is clear the kidneys should be immersed in an icy slush of the perfusion fluid in a sterile plastic bag, surrounded by a second sterile bag, then stored in a styrofoam container of crushed ice. They can then be transported as required.

A few centres in the United States use machine preservation but the vast majority of centres use simple manual perfusion. At an early stage we noted that good perfusion and rapid cooling of the organ demonstrated by a clear venous effluent was an excellent forecast of early renal function. We found that kidneys which were slow to perfuse did not function for longer than usual periods of time. Mechanical pulsatile flow techniques appeared initially to give extended preservation times, but are not now widely used. Grafts may be lost because of faults in perfusion and their use does not seem to improve long-term graft survival.

Conclusion

The primary result to be attained is the rapid revascularisation of the kidney and insertion of the ureter into the recipient's bladder. Even before reimplantation of the ureter the ultimate functional result may be anticipated by the observation of recovering peristalsis and even flow of urine from the ureter.

Further reading

Pegg, D. E. Principles of tissue preservation. In *Progress in Transplantation*. Morris, P. J., Tilney, N. L. eds. Edinburgh, Churchill Livingstone; 1985; 2: 69–105.

Salvatierra, O., Jr. Renal transplantation. In Campbell's *Urology*. Walsh, P. C., Gittes, R. E., Perlmutter, A. D., Stamey, T. A. eds. Philadelphia, Saunders; 1986; vol 3: 2534–2557.

CHAPTER 12

The living donor

B. G. WILSON, W. G. G. LOUGHRIDGE and S. R. JOHNSTON

On December 23 1954 the first successful renal transplant was performed, the donor and recipient being identical twins. In the Western world up to 20% of kidneys transplanted continue to come from live donors, the remainder from cadavers. However, in certain cultures the use of a cadaver kidney is not acceptable and live donation is essential.

1. Advantages of live donation

Long term graft survival (5–10 years) is better with a live donor kidney than with a cadaveric organ. Until very recently short term survival was also better. However, with the use of CYA particularly as triple or quadruple therapy, the differences are now minimal. There are however disadvantages of such heavily immunosuppressive protocols, particularly the risk of malignancy.

Transplantation can be performed as an elective procedure, limiting the length of time the recipient has to spend on haemodialysis with its inherent risks.

The supply of cadaveric kidneys, while increasing, is still less than the demand.

2. Disadvantages of live donation

These are to the donor. While the risk of mortality is small at 0.1%, there is the 1–2% risk of morbidity which occurs with any surgical procedure. In the long term, while there should be virtually no adverse effect on life expectancy, there is at least a theoretical risk of hyperfiltration damage to the remaining kidney. Should the transplant fail for whatever reason, there may be significant mental trauma to the donor and the recipient. If the donor is in employment significant financial loss may occur.

Mary G. McGeown (ed.), Clinical Management of Renal Transplantation, 161–165.
© 1992 *Kluwer Academic Publishers, Dordrecht – Printed in the Netherlands.*

3. The suitability of an individual to become a live donor

Many factors influence the decision as to whether a particular donor may be used. In general the donor should be genetically related to the recipient. Under current United Kingdom legislation relatives of full blood or half blood out to first cousins are generally acceptable. Proposals for donation from more distant relatives and unrelated persons must be submitted to the Unrelated Live Transplant Regulatory Authority (ULTRA) for approval (Chapter 2). Donors not genetically related, such as a spouse or partner, must be able to prove a long-term stable emotional relationship with the recipient. All donors must understand the nature of the medical procedure and the risks involved in donating the kidney. The donor's consent must not have been obtained by offer of reward of any sort or by coercion. The donor should also understand that consent can be withdrawn at any time.

Possible contra-indications for live donation are shown in Table 28. A living minor may not be used as a donor with the exception of providing regenerative tissues (under national law). While no upper limit exists, increasing age increases the risk of morbidity to the donor. Because of perfusion problems the donor kidney is less likely to be successful.

The presence of urinary tract disorders including proteinuria, haematuria, urinary stone disease, congenital anomalies such as polycystic disease, duplications and reflux or horse shoe kidney generally excludes donation. Some of these abnormalities do not absolutely prohibit donation and after appropriate investigation and treatment it may still be possible to consider the donor. More detailed investigations will then be required. Other potential donors if available may need to be similarly assessed before a final decision is made.

Table 28. Contraindications for live donation

1. Age
2. Pre-existing cardiovascular disease
3. Metabolic disorders especially diabetes
4. History of urinary tract disease
5. Pre-existing neoplasia

4. Pre-operative assessment of a potential living donor

The prospective donor must be interviewed in private. The recipient or other family members must not be present. If the donor is unrelated the regulations require a report from an independent third party who has interviewed both the donor and recipient and who is acceptable to ULTRA for this purpose. In general, to be acceptable to ULTRA the person making the report should be a physician, surgeon or psychiatrist of NHS consultant or equivalent professional status who is not otherwise party to the transplant proceedings, nor a close associate of one who is. He or she should not be practising in the fields of renal medicine or renal transplantation.

ULTRA has prepared a leaflet describing unrelated live donor kidney transplantation suitable for giving to the prospective donor.

In addition to a full routine physical examination and preoperative assessment including sedimentation rate, full blood picture, bio-chemical profile, routine urine test and culture, chest x-ray and electrocardiogram, additional special investigations should be carried out. These include coagulation screen, testing for hepatitis B, tests for venereal disease and of HIV and CMV status.

An intravenous urogram is required to ensure that there are two functioning kidneys with normal anatomy. On viewing this it is important to exclude any suggestion of delay in drainage at the pelvi-ureteric junction as such drainage problems may be accentuated following transplantation. However while the intravenous urogram is excellent at demonstrating anatomy it is less satisfactory for indicating precisely the relative function of the two kidneys. A much more accurate assessment of differential renal function is obtained by a dimercaptosuccinic acid radio-isotope scan.

Arteriography is essential to demonstrate the details of the arterial supply. Of particular importance is the number and size of arteries coming from the aorta since it is clearly not possible to take an aortic patch which is the usual procedure in the cadaver donor. The left kidney is normally preferred because of the longer vein, which makes insertion of the kidney technically easier. However if the arterial anatomy is more suitable on the right (a single artery) the right kidney will be selected despite the shorter vein.

5. The donor nephrectomy

The donor nephrectomy is carried out as a planned procedure. Preferably the retrieval and transplant operations are carried out in adjacent theatres. This allows the two operations to be co-ordinated, and ischaemic time to be kept to a minimum. Two surgical teams are preferable. If that is not possible it is quite acceptable that the two operations are performed sequentially. The small prolongation of cold ischaemia time will not affect ultimate function of the kidney. The recipient is not anaesthetised until the donor team is certain that there is a viable kidney to transplant.

The surgical approach to the donor kidney is a matter of the surgeon's preference taking into account the physical build of the patient. It may be through the loin or through an anterior transperitoneal approach. There are several points of difference between the approach for a donor nephrectomy and that of a standard nephrectomy. It is vital that the arteries, including polar vessels, are identified and carefully dissected to their origins. Obtaining the maximum length of vessel makes the transplant easier. It may be necessary on occasions to do a formal closure of the aorta or vena cava using a non-absorbable suture. Prevention of arterial spasm by gentle dissection and avoidance of traction on the vessels is important.

It is important to identify and ligate the gonadal and adrenal arteries and other small tributaries from adjacent tissues as they are encountered. This will minimise troublesome bleeding on release of the clamps following transplantation.

It is important to preserve the peri-ureteric sheath of tissues by careful dissection to ensure viability of the ureter. After transplantation the ureter depends on the renal artery for its sole blood supply. Stripping of the ureter impairs the blood supply to the distal ureter, hazarding viability and leading to failure of the uretero-vesical anastomosis. This may result in either stenosis or a urinary leak. It is also important to dissect an adequate length of ureter, usually by taking it down to the level of the pelvic brim. This will allow trimming of the ureter subsequently to the shortest appropriate length without tension.

It is important to dissect the kidney as cleanly as possible keeping close to the capsule. Care should be taken to avoid injuring the capsule. While this does not in itself harm the kidney, it may lead to increased blood loss by oozing during and after the transplant.

The perfusion technique is essentially the same as that described for a cadaver donor (Chapter 11) except that perfusion of the kidney *in situ* is clearly not possible.

6. Transplantation of a kidney from a live donor

The basic technique of transplantation is exactly the same as for a cadaver donor. However, the absence of an aortic patch in a kidney with multiple vessels, may require some further initial preparation of the donor organ prior to the actual transplant. If two arteries are present relatively close together and of good length, it is usually possible to carry out an anastomosis between these two vessels. However, particularly if there is a polar vessel at some distance from the main artery, it may be necessary to perform two arterial insertions. Similarly if duplex ureters are present it is usually preferable to anastomose these on the bench to allow one uretero-neocystostomy to be performed. As with the cadaver donor ureteric stents are not normally employed.

7. Post-operative care of the donor

This is the same as that for any patient who has had a nephrectomy. Similar complications may arise, such as deep vein thrombosis, pneumothorax or atelectasis. Heparin administration is recommended as prophylaxis against deep vein thrombosis.

The donor may need additional support as attention tends to be concentrated on the recipient. It is only at the post-operative period that the donor may appreciate fully the true significance and implications of the decision to donate a kidney. The donor does not experience the usual post-operative sense of relief at being cured of a disease and may need additional analgesia as well as emotional support during this early difficult period.

The donor should be kept well informed of progress of the recipient and of the transplanted kidney. If problems with the kidney arise it is important that the information is conveyed tactfully and consistently. To ensure this, such information should be conveyed only be the most experienced medical staff and preferably by those involved in pre-operative counselling. Good news of the recipient and transplanted kidney may speed recovery.

CHAPTER 13

Insertion of the kidney

P. F. KEANE and R. KERNOHAN

1. General principles

There are certain general principles which should be followed during the
insertion of the kidney (Table 29).

2. The standard kidney transplant operation

With the exception of patients receiving a kidney from a live donor, the
transplant patient is normally 'on call', and living at home. When a donor
kidney becomes available and the tissue type results are known, the patient
will be notified by phone to come immediately to hospital. Occasionally
when the donor tissue type matches more than one patient several patients
may be prepared, pending the cross-match results. Almost all of these patients are receiving either haemodialysis or continuous ambulatory peritoneal
dialysis (CAPD) and it is sometimes necessary to give a period of dialysis
immediately pre-operatively to correct electrolyte and fluid imbalances in
order to minimise the risks of surgery.

The operation of kidney transplantation is performed under general anaesthesia, although it would be technically possible to perform it under epidural
anaesthesia. As these patients will receive immunosuppressive drugs, it is
important that the highest standards of sterility are maintained to avoid
complications of infection. The bladder is catheterised under strict aseptic
conditions using a size 16 Ch. silastic catheter (silastic catheters have a lower
incidence of infection compared to ones of latex) and the bladder drained
of urine. The anastomosis of the ureter to the bladder is facilitated if the
bladder is partly distended and it is customary to fill the bladder with 100 ml
of saline. The catheter is spigotted for the duration of the surgery.

The abdomen is prepared with savlon, spirit and iodine and draped. It is
customary to place a right kidney into the left iliac fossa and a left kidney
into the right iliac fossa as this positions the kidney with the renal pelvis
anterior to the artery and vein. It is then easier to puncture or explore the

Mary G. McGeown (ed.), Clinical Management of Renal Transplantation, 167–179.

Table 29. General principles of insertion of the kidney

1. Surgical technique should be meticulous to avoid early post-operative morbidity and achieve the best long-term results.
2. The kidney should be placed in an accessible position for subsequent percutaneous procedures, e.g. biopsy or nephrostomy.
3. There should be easy access to an adequate arterial supply and adequate venous drainage.
4. The kidney should be placed as close to the bladder as possible to keep the ureter short and minimise the risk of vascular insufficiency and stricture formation.
5. The anastomosis of the ureter to the bladder should be performed in such a way as to minimise bleeding and the anastomosis should have anti-reflux properties.
6. Drains should be avoided – they provide a portal for the entry of infection and tend to hinder the post-operative mobility of the patient.

renal pelvis subsequently which is occasionally necessary in the treatment of complications such as the development of a stricture at the ureteric-bladder anastomosis. However, either kidney can be placed in either iliac fossa should the need arise, e.g. when a patient is having a second or third transplant. Occasionally, when it is important to keep the pelvis in the anterior position, the ipsilateral kidney can be placed in the iliac fossa in the upside down position without impairment of urine drainage. However, in this position the ureter is of necessity considerably longer than when the kidney is in the normal transplanted position.

The incision is made 2–3 cm above and parallel to the inguinal ligament extending from the midline to opposite the anterior superior iliac spine. The external oblique aponeurosis, internal oblique and transversus abdominus muscles are divided to reach the surface of the peritoneum. The peritoneum is swept medially, lifting it off the lateral pelvic wall muscles. This is usually accomplished by a minimal amount of sharp dissection, sweeping the peritoneum medially by hand. In a thin patient the external iliac artery and vein are immediately seen lying on the psoas and illiacus muscles. Care should be taken to avoid entering the peritoneal cavity. This has become increasingly important as many of the patients undergoing kidney transplantation are receiving peritoneal dialysis, which may have to continue in the post-operative period. A suitable self-retaining retractor is placed into the wound to allow adequate exposure of the iliac vessels from the bifurcation of the common iliac and internal iliac to the inguinal ligament. Some surgeons expose the entire common iliac artery up to the bifurcation with the aorta. The common iliac vessels are intimately associated with lymphatic vessels running over their anterior surfaces. During mobilization of the vessels some surgeons carefully identify and ligate these lymphatics to prevent the formation of a lymphocele. In Belfast we do not routinely mobilise the common iliac artery and vein, but mobilise the external iliac vessels along their entire length. We do not routinely ligate lymphatics and have not found a high incidence of formation of lymphocele.

When the vessels have been exposed the kidney is removed from the ice pack. The ends of the donor artery and vein are tidied and inspected for

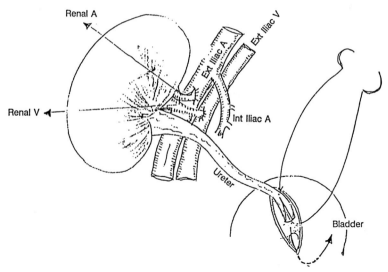

Figure 33. Renal transplantation: the renal artery has been anastomosed to the external iliac artery and the renal vein to the external iliac vein. The ureter is spatulated. Note that the needles are passed in the direction of the arrow.

inadvertent damage during organ retrieval; any open branches are tied and if metal clips have been used for haemostasis they are replaced by ligatures which we feel are more secure. Occasionally, if the artery is very long it may be shortened. This means sacrificing the aortic patch making the anastomosis slightly more difficult. However, redundant artery may lead to kinking and altered blood flow.

The kidney is placed in the wound in the position in which it is most likely to lie post-operatively and the best positions for the vascular anastomoses are noted. The kidney is removed from the wound to prevent excessive warming and suitable vascular clamps (Swinney clamps) are placed on the artery and vein. We do not routinely heparinise the distal femoral artery and vein and have not found this to be necessary. The kidney is clipped with artery forceps to the side of the wound in a position to allow best access for performing the vascular anastomoses. Either the arterial or venous anastomosis can be performed first depending on the preference of the surgeon and the anatomy of the vessels.

A suitable venotomy and arteriotomy are made with a fine scalpel and vascular scissors. The vein is sutured end to side using a continuous 5/0 polypropelene (Prolene) suture. The artery is anastomosed on its patch to the external iliac artery using a 6/0 polypropelene suture. On completion of both anastomoses (Figure 33) both clamps are released and any leaks identified and ligated. It is important that the anaesthetist is told when the clamps are about to be released as immunosuppressive drugs may need to be administered before the kidney is perfused and there is usually a reduction in blood pressure. On releasing the clamps the kidney usually perfuses immediately,

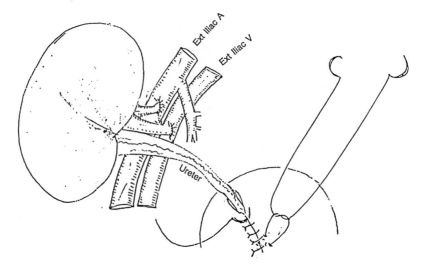

Figure 34. Renal transplantation: the muscle layer is approximated over the ureter.

changing from pale buff to pink in colour, becoming up to 30% larger in volume and pulsatile. If perfusion is sluggish this may mean a problem with the anastomosis, or spasm in the renal vasculature. The latter sometimes responds to an intravenous bolus of frusemide.

The next stage of the operation is to implant the ureter into the bladder. It is best to implant it in a position where the bladder is easily accessible and where the ureter can be kept reasonably short thereby maximising the blood supply to its end. The ureter is usually implanted onto the dome of the bladder in an anterolateral position. The bladder can be clearly identified by blunt dissection which has been facilitated by prior instillation of saline into the bladder. The dome of the bladder is held up between two stay sutures. With very careful use of diathermy, a 4 cm incision is made through the bladder muscle in the longitudinal or oblique plane. Careful dissection allows the bladder mucosa to bulge into the myotomy. The ureter is trimmed to a suitable length, and any bleeding points carefully ligated. The end of the ureter is spatulated over a distance of 1 cm and a double ended suture of polyglactin 2/0 is passed through the distal end of the ureter as shown in the diagram (Figure 34). A small hole is made in the bladder mucosa at the caudal end of the muscle incision and the needle coming through nearest to the spatulated part of the ureter is inserted through the hole in the bladder mucosa to enter as far as possible into the bladder. The needle coming through the distal end of the ureter is inserted through the hole in the bladder to exit from the bladder 1 cm proximal to the first needle. The ureter is passed through the hole in the bladder mucosa and pulled tight with this double ended suture. The suture is tied with the knot on the outside of the bladder. This causes the spatulated end of the ureter to assume the shape of an everted nipple. The muscle coat of the bladder is sutured over the reimplanted ureter to form a sub-muscular tunnel thus providing the anti-reflux mechanism. The urethral catheter is left to drain the bladder for five days.

This method of ureteric implantation is known as the modified Lich technique and its advantages over other methods are that the bladder is approached from the outside avoiding a cystotomy, bleeding is minimal and therefore there is little risk of catheter blockage in the post-operative period. The anastomosis is anti-reflux due to the submucosal tunnel and is very leak resistant. The technique is simple, quick and easy to perform.

Although in the past we routinely performed a capsulotomy and drained the retroperitoneal space with a tube drain we have not employed these measures for the past 18 months with no detriment to our results.

It is essential that surgical technique is meticulous with great attention paid to adequate haemostasis. The wound is closed in layers using absorbable sutures and a sub-cuticular skin suture.

3. Variations in technique

3.1. *Arterial anastomosis*

When the donor kidney is received without a patch of aorta or in the case of a live donor kidney, it is sometimes necessary to perform an end to end arterial anastomosis to the internal iliac artery (Figure 35). In some centres

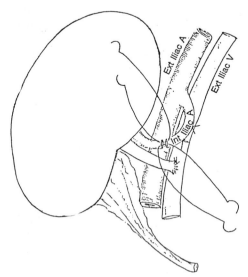

Figure 35. Renal transplantation: variations in technique: End-to-end anastomosis of the renal artery to the internal iliac artery.

172

this is the preferred technique for all transplants, but this necessitates a more extensive dissection to mobilise the internal iliac artery and swing it forwards into a suitable position.

3.2. *Multiple renal arteries*

It is not uncommon to transplant a kidney with more than one renal artery. If the origin of the arteries are close to each other on the aorta and are contained on a single patch, this can be anastomosed to the external iliac artery in the normal way (Figure 36). If there are several arteries without a patch then the options are to individually anastomose each artery to the external iliac artery or to anastomose the renal arteries to each other before transplanting the kidney (Figure 37). This latter technique has the advantage that it can be done on the bench thus reducing warming of the kidney. If there are two arteries of equal size then the ends can be spatulated and anastomosed to form a single ostium which can be anastomosed to the external iliac artery (Figure 38). Small upper polar arteries supplying less than 10% of the renal substance can be ignored and ligated. Lower polar arteries can contribute a significant proportion of the blood supply to the ureter and it is important to try and preserve these to safeguard the ureteric blood supply.

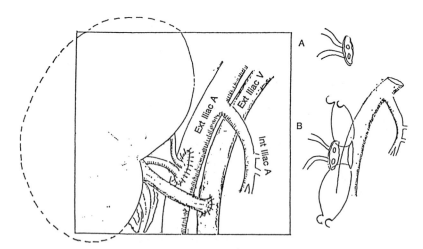

Figure 36. Renal transplantation: variations in technique: Carrel patch with two renal arteries anastomosed to the external iliac artery.

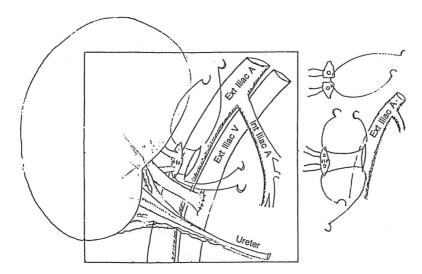

Figure 37. Renal transplantation: variations in technique: Two renal arteries on separate patches, patches are joined together, then anastomosed on one patch to the external iliac artery.

3.3. *Abnormalities of the veins*

Multiple venous drainage of the kidney is common. As there is adequate venous communication within the kidney the main draining vein is usually used for the anastomosis, the others being ligated.

3.4. *Transplantation in patients who have had multiple previous transplants*

Occasionally it may be necessary to anastomose donor kidney vessels onto the recipient aorta and vena cava. This may occur in spina bifida patients who have dysplastic lower limbs and in some patients who have had two previous transplants. In this instance a mid-line incision is made. The aorta and both common iliac vessels are identified and clamped. The vena cava and both common iliac veins are identified and clamped and if necessary lumbar veins posteriorly are also clamped. The operation is then carried out as described above and the ureter is reimplanted into the bladder in the same way. The kidney in this situation lies in the peritoneal cavity and may have bowel between it and the abdominal wall thus making biopsy more hazardous.

174

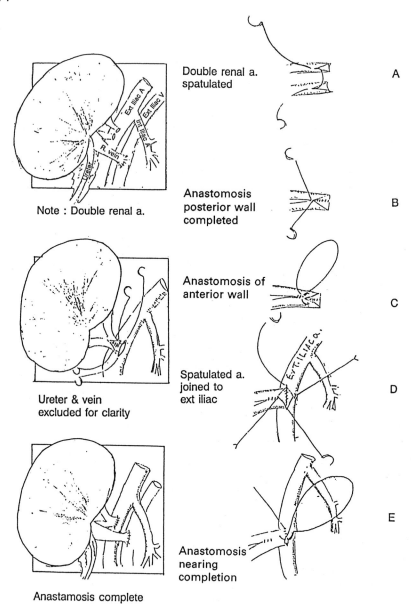

Note : Double renal a.

Ureter & vein
excluded for clarity

Anastamosis complete

Double renal a.
spatulated

A

Anastomosis
posterior wall
completed

B

Anastomosis of
anterior wall

C

Spatulated a.
joined to
ext iliac

D

E

Anastomosis
nearing
completion

Figure 38. Renal transplantation: variations in technique: Steps of anastomosis of double renal arteries to one another and to the external iliac artery. A double renal arteries spatulated; B anastomosis of the posterior wall of artery completed; C anastomosis of the anterior wall; D the spatulated artery joined to the external iliac artery; E the anastomosis nearing completion.

3.5. *Alternative techniques for reimplanting the ureter*

There are many methods of ureteric reimplantation which may be employed; while some have advantages over others most operating surgeons have their own preference. Techniques include a "drop in" technique where the ureter is simply inserted into the bladder with 1–2 cm lying free in the bladder and the ureter secured to the bladder mucosa with 3–4 chromic catgut sutures. The Politano-Leadbetter type of reimplantation implants the ureter as close to the trigone as possible while forming a submucosal tunnel to prevent reflux. Both these techniques require a large cystotomy with the attendant risk of bleeding and catheter blockage.

The "lay on" technique involves suturing the mucosa of the ureter to the mucosa of the bladder after making a small cystotomy in the dome of the bladder. The bladder muscle is then sutured loosely over the anastomosis and distal 2 cm of the ureter to form an anti-reflux valvular effect.

The modified Lich technique as already described above and the "lay on" technique avoid formally opening the bladder and there is a lower incidence of bleeding and catheter blockage.

Occasionally the donor ureter has been damaged. In this case the patient's own native ureter can be used. An anastomosis can be formed between the donor renal pelvis and the recipient's ureter. However, the rate of anastomotic failure with this technique is much higher than reimplantation of the donor ureter into the bladder.

4. Post-operative care

In Belfast the patients are nursed in a purpose designed transplant unit complete with positive pressure ventilation etc. The staff are required to change into theatre garb. The patient's visitors are not allowed direct access to the patient but can see and communicate with him through a clean/dirty corridor arrangement. While it is accepted with current knowledge that these restrictions are excessive, we feel that it helps to maintain high standards of patient care and restricts the number of personnel coming into contact with the patient thus reducing the risk of infection.

The surgery is carried out in an operating theatre dedicated to transplantation and related procedures. It is situated within the transplant unit. On transfer to the ward routine observations are made, which include quarter hourly pulse, blood pressure and hourly estimations of CVP and urine output measurements. There may be occasional bleeding from the end of the implanted ureter. It is important that the catheter does not become blocked and if this occurs it should be cautiously washed out with saline, so that the anastomosis is not compromised.

Usually the patient can take oral fluids and medication after 24 hours and can take a normal diet on the second post-operative day. The patient should be encouraged to become mobile as quickly as possible and should sit out of bed on day one. In this regard we have found that the abandonment of drains has been most beneficial.

5. Transplantation in children

Transplantation in children is more difficult than in adults and this bears a direct relationship to the age of the child. A fifteen year old is technically little different from an adult and presents little difference from an anaesthetic point of view, however, a two year old child presents more surgical and more anaesthetic problems.

Until recently transplantation in children younger than five years has shown poor results. Trumpeter et al. reported on 16 transplants performed in 15 children less than five years old in Guys Hospital, London. The mean follow up was 1–2 years with a 25% death rate.

The results of transplantation in children less than one year old remain poor and several centres have stopped transplanting children of this age, maintaining them on CAPD until they are old enough to reduce the risks. Miller et al. from Minnesota consider that live related donor transplants in the 1–5 age group give better results than cadaver transplants. Reports on these patients exhibiting catch-up growth remain at present contradictory.

5.1. *Problems in the under five age group*

The problems which may be encountered in children under five years are summarized in Table 30.

Table 30. Problems encountered in transplantation in children under five years

---
1. There will probably be disparity in size between the donor kidney and the recipient vessels and vice versa.
2. Vascular anastomosis is technically more challenging due to the small vessel size.
3. The kidney cannot usually be placed retroperitoneally in the pelvis due to inadequate space.
4. Fluid balance, particularly during initial perfusion of the kidney is more critical than in the adult due to the smaller intra-vascular volume and limited cardiac output in the small child.
5. Small children pose more difficult anaesthetic problems.
6. Post-operative care is more demanding than in adults.
7. Biopsy of the graft can be more hazardous due to the intra-peritoneal position of the graft.
8. Immunosuppression in children may lead to a greater incidence of malignancy.
9. Post-transplant hypertension is common.

5.1.1. Disparity in size between the donor kidney and the recipient. It is possible to transplant an adult kidney into a baby less than one year old. The kidney must be placed intraperitoneally and because the baby's iliac vessels are of small calibre it is necessary to anastomose the graft vessels onto the aorta and vena cava. The anastomosis of the ureter to the bladder is not usually a problem and the same technique is employed as in adults.

Conversely a donor paediatric kidney 18 months old can be transplanted into an adult subject to the surgeon's ability to anastomose the small graft vessels satisfactorily. It is generally thought that a kidney from a paediatric donor older than 1.5 years can provide adequate function for an adult recipient. Kidneys from donors less than one year old should probably not be used routinely in adults due to the technical problems of vascular anastomosis.

5.1.2. *Vascular anastomosis*. When an adult kidney is transplanted into a child vascular anastomoses do not pose any technical difficulties, provided the graft vessels are anastomosed onto suitable sized recipient vessels such as the common iliacs, aorta or vena cava. However, it is good practice to use interrupted sutures rather than continuous so that the anastomosis can grow with the child.

When a paediatric kidney is transplanted into an adult the vascular anastomoses are usually straightforward provided that patches of aorta and vena cava are present on the donor vessels. If there are no patches difficulties can be encountered due to the small size of the donor vessels and artheroma in the recipient vessels. When a paediatric donor kidney becomes available for use in an adult it is important to transplant it into a relatively young adult to minimise the technical problems.

5.1.3. *Placement of the kidney*. In children the pelvis is shallow and underdeveloped. This means that generally, even in older children there is insufficient space to place the graft in the usual retroperitoneal position in the iliac fossa. This can result in compression and kinking of the vessels especially the vein resulting in graft thrombosis. The loss of some kidneys in children in Belfast was thought to be due to this cause. It is therefore advisable to place the kidneys intraperitoneally to avoid this risk.

5.1.4. *Fluid balance*. In babies and very young children where it is necessary to anastomose the graft vessels to the aorta and vena cava, it is usually necessary to cross clamp the abdominal aorta during the anastomosis. When the kidney is perfused metabolites from the ischaemic lower limbs are released into the circulation causing vaso-dilatation and relative hypovolaemia. In addition an adult kidney when reperfused will take up 250 mls of blood which in a baby represents a significant proportion of the blood volume. These two factors can cause significant hypotension and fall in cardiac output on reperfusion of the kidney. This can be counteracted by ensuring that there is adequate fluid replacement as judged by the central venous pressure before the kidney is perfused. If this is neglected the kidney may initially perfuse but the perfusion may not be maintained therefore placing the graft at risk of thrombosis.

5.1.5. *Anaesthetic problems.* Babies and small children pose significant anaesthetic difficulties which are discussed elsewhere.

5.1.6. *Post-operative care.* Babies and small children should be nursed in a paediatric intensive care unit to facilitate the monitoring of central venous pressure, arterial pressure etc. In general, while it may seem appropriate to perform the surgery in an adult transplant unit, there can be difficulties in the post-operative management of babies and small children mainly because the staff in an adult transplant unit do not have the requisite experience in managing paediatric cases. In Belfast, transplants under five years of age are performed in the Royal Belfast Hospital for Sick Children where adequate post-operative care facilities are available.

5.1.7. *Biopsy of the graft kidney.* When grafts are placed intraperitoneally, loops of bowel may lie anteriorly and may pose a problem when needle biopsies are performed. In general we have not found a problem in practice and would not regard intraperitoneal placement as a contraindication to routine biopsy when indicated. It has been said that grafts placed intraperitoneally may have a high incidence of ureteric complications due to the inability of the ureter to pick up a collateral blood supply from the peritoneum and some surgeons tunnel the ureter behind the peritoneum before implanting it into the bladder. As the ureter usually has an adequate blood supply from the blood supply to the kidney, this seems no more than a theoretical point. In Belfast we do not tunnel the ureter behind the peritoneum in intraperitoneal grafts and have not encountered an undue incidence of ureteric problems.

5.1.8. *Immunosuppression in children.* In children with kidney transplants receiving immunosuppression there have been a few cases of malignant lymphomas. This is of course worrying, but further experience and long-term follow up will be required before this can be evaluated.

5.1.9. *Post-transplant hypertension.* Hypertension in the immediate post-transplant period is common in paediatric recipients. The mechanism causing this is at present unclear. It would be tempting to believe that an adult kidney transplanted into a small child may suffer from relative ischaemia due to under perfusion. However, graft renal vein renin sampling has not shown this to be the case and at present the cause is undefined. In most patients hypertension is transient and responds to the new anti-hypertensives such as nifedipine.

Further reading

Morris, P. J. ed. *Kidney transplantation: principles and practce*. 3rd ed. Philadelphia, Saunders; 1988.

Bishop, M. C. Renal transplantation. In *Textbook of genito-urinary surgery*. Whitfield, H. N., Hendry, W. F. eds. London, Churchill Livingstone; 1985; 2, 1236–1257.

CHAPTER 14

Management of the recipient during operation

J. P. ALEXANDER

Kidney transplantation has been performed successfully for over two decades and now lacks the newsworthiness of transplantation of other organs. Yet renal transplantation, when successful, is probably the most satisfying of all transplant procedures and can make remarkable improvements in the health of the patient and growth of the child which cannot at present be achieved by dialysis. In addition, transplantation for end-stage renal disease is much more cost effective than long-term dialysis. In an institution where multiple transplantation operations are performed simultaneously, responsibility for the conduct of the anaesthesia for renal transplantation may have to be delegated to relatively junior anaesthetic staff.

1. Historical

Early attempts to transplant kidneys were fraught with difficulties and frustration. Facilities for dialysis were limited and enthusiastic clinicians were forced to manufacture dialysis catheters in their spare time. Organs were removed after the donor heart had stopped and organ preservation was rudimentary, as was tissue typing. Little was known about immunosuppression and rejection was common. Operations were lengthy due to the time required to establish suitable vascular anastomoses, and the muscle relaxants used during anaesthesia were either gallamine or tubocurarine and either of these drugs may cause prolonged post-operative neuromuscular blockade. Although regional anaesthesia avoided some of the difficulties, patients found it unacceptable.

2. Pharmacokinetics in renal failure

A number of factors alter drug disposition in end-stage renal failure patients.

Mary G. McGeown (ed.), Clinical Management of Renal Transplantation, 181–199.
© 1992 *Kluwer Academic Publishers, Dordrecht. Printed in the Netherlands.*

2.1. *Protein binding*

Protein binding is probably the most important factor in determining drug distribution in that a protein-bound drug is inert. There is decreased protein binding in renal failure because a relative hypoalbuminaemia allows more unbound or free drug to exist. Highly bound drugs are most likely to demonstrate overdose effects since a relatively small change in binding will lead to a large increase in unbound drug. Cardiac glycosides, benzodiazepines, anticonvulsants, hypoglycaemic agents and neuromuscular blocking drugs all demonstrate this effect. When protein-binding is decreased, more free drug is available to distribute to sites of action. Because distribution is increased, plasma levels are lower, yet more drug has passed to receptor sites where a greater response may be observed than the low serum levels would suggest. Thus low serum levels may not indicate subtherapeutic amounts. Lower protein-binding will make more drug available for elimination; in renal failure this will have to be by the hepatic route unless the molecular size allows removal by dialysis.

2.2. *Metabolic acidosis*

Metabolic acidosis also affects protein binding. Endogenous organic acids accumulate in uraemia, and bind to plasma proteins, thus displacing protein-bound drugs.

2.3. *Ionization*

Ionization affects distribution, particularly where cellular membrane permeability is considered. Non-ionized molecules like narcotic drugs are lipid-soluble and more readily pass through the blood-brain barrier. Muscle relaxant drugs are highly ionized and water soluble, and have a limited volume of distribution.

2.4. *Dialysability*

The ability to dialyse a drug depends on three factors:-

2.4.1. *Molecular size.* Large molecules like morphine, dioxin, erythromycin and vancomycin are poorly dialysed.

2.4.2. *Water-solubility.* Many sedative and hypnotic drugs are small molecules but are not water-soluble. The majority of hypnotic drugs are lipid-soluble and readily pass through membranes. This means that their volumes of distribution are large (large reservoirs in major organs and peripheral tissues) and are difficult to remove by dialysis.

2.4.3. *Protein Binding.* Again, highly bound drugs are difficult to remove by dialysis.

3. Drugs used in anaesthesia in the renal failure patient

The importance of over- and under-hydration, electrolyte shifts and acid-base disturbances on the pharmacokinetics of drug action cannot be over-emphasized. Drugs which act mainly on the central nervous system must be fat-soluble and hence are normally reabsorbed during passage through the kidneys. The duration of action of such agents therefore depends on redistribution, metabolism or excretion via the lungs (for volatile agents), and not on renal function. This applies to the intravenous induction agents, narcotic analgesics and inhalational agents, but not to the water-soluble non-depolarizing muscle relaxants which are highly ionized at body pH.

3.1. *Pre-operative medication*

Virtually all the standard premedicant drugs have been used, although the dosage schedules may need to be modified in view of the increased sensitivity to the undesirable effects of medication that is seen in renal failure patients. When oral diazepam is used the amount of unbound drug is increased and the clearance of a single dose decreased. In spite of these theoretical disadvantages the drug has been widely used. The shorter acting temazepam or triazolam, may have some advantages. In view of their occasional unpredictable effects, narcotic drugs, in particular morphine, may be best avoided. Pethidine should also be avoided. Metoclopramide and cimetidine or ranitidine may be given. The latter does not interfere with the cytochrome P 450 hepatic metabolism of certain drugs.

3.2. *Induction agents*

At one time it was thought that the dose of thiopentone necessary to induce sleep was about half that required in the normal subject. However, with a relatively slow rate of drug administration in line with modern practice, the dose required for induction is only slightly less than that required in healthy patients, because the free drug volume of distribution and drug clearance are unchanged. The induction dose of other agents, and of hypnotic and sedative drugs may need to be reduced. The response to neuroleptic agents appears to be normal. Propofol has a profound effect on arterial blood

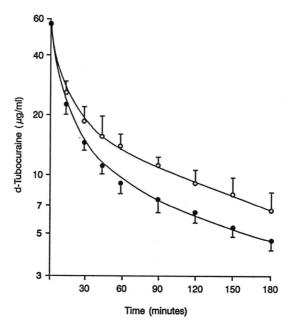

Figure 39. Renal disease slows the rate of decline in plasma concentrations of d-tubocurarine (From Miller *et al.* (1977) *J. Pharmacol. Exp. Ther.* 202, 1–7, reproduced with permission). Open circles refer to renal failure patients.

pressure in ill patients and cannot be recommended in conventional induction doses.

3.3. *Choice of muscle relaxant*

Although gallamine has been used successfully in renal failure patients there have been a number of reports of prolonged curarization and its use cannot be recommended. It relies entirely on renal excretion for its elimination. Tubocurarine has been widely used in renal failure patients. Although normally excreted by the kidneys, an alternative excretory pathway exists via the liver and biliary systems. However, postoperative respiratory failure due to recurarization can occur (Figures 39 and 40) and hypotension secondary to ganglion blockade in the recently dialysed patient has been described.

Both alcuronium and pancuronium have been satisfactory in clinical practice. Normally 50% of a given dose of the latter can be recovered from the urine, but in renal failure its mode of excretion is similar to that of tubocurarine (Figure 41). There have been isolated reports of prolonged curarization following the use of pancuronium in renal failure. It should be noted that acidosis slows down the metabolic degradation of non-depolarizing relaxants.

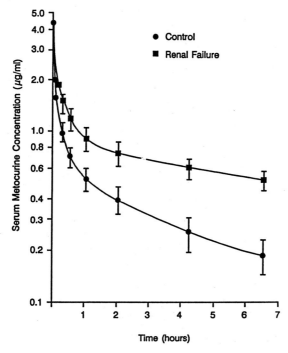

Figure 40. Effect of renal disease on plasma concentration of the muscle relaxant metocurine which has a similar pharmacokinetical profile to d-tubocurarine. (From Brotherton *et al.* (1981) *Anesthesiology*, 55, 273–6, reproduced with permission).

In the early 1980s, two new muscle relaxants were introduced into anaesthetic practice. Vecuronium has a similar chemical structure to pancuronium with an acetylcholine fragment on the D-ring of the steroid nucleus which is required for neuromuscular blockade, but without the acetylcholine fragment on the A-ring of the latter which is responsible for the vagolytic and sympathomimetic effects. Only 15–20% of a dose of vecuronium is excreted by the kidney. The primary means of elimination is the bile and rapid hepatic uptake and biliary excretion account for the more rapid clearance and shorter elimination half-life seen with vecuronium than pancuronium in normal and renal failure patients.

Atracurium is the other recently introduced drug. In 1851, Hofmann described the spontaneous degradation of a curare-like molecule, petaline, in mild alkali. Atracurium is the result of modern pharmacological engineering in pursuit of the ideal muscle relaxant. When injected into the blood stream, atracurium undergoes spontaneous degradation by the "Hofmann elimination reaction". Ester hydrolysis may also be involved. The effects of both vecuronium and atracurium may be mildly to moderately prolonged in renal failure (Figure 42). Both drugs may occasionally cause profound bradycardia, particularly when used in conjunction with synthetic opioid

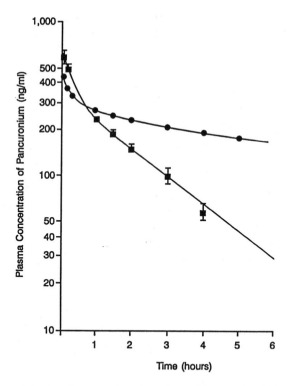

Figure 41. Pharmacokinetics of pancuronium in patients with normal and impaired renal function (From McLeod *et al*. (1976) *Br. J. Anaesth.*, 48, 341–5 reproduced with permission). Closed circles refer to renal failure patients.

drugs such as fentanyl and alfentanil. Hepatorenal failure does not prolong the plasma elimination half-life of atracurium so that it is the only available neuromuscular blocker that is unaffected by this condition. Laudanosine is a major metabolite of atracurium and is known to cross the blood-brain barrier and to have central nervous system stimulant properties in animals. Laudanosine is a monoquaternary amine and is normally excreted by the kidneys. Higher plasma concentrations are found in renal failure patients and the conventional view is that even prolonged infusions of atracurium in those patients will not produce levels of laudanosine which are likely to be epileptogenic. The author's experience in intensive care is at variance with this view. We have observed epileptiform seizures in two critically ill patients who were anuric and had cerebral irritation, which were only controlled by discontinuing the atracurium infusion.

Renal failure prolongs the duration of action of the anticholinesterase agents neostigmine, pyridostigmine and edrophonium by at least 100%, since they are excreted mainly by the kidney. This will enhance their pharmacological effect (Figure 43).

Patients with chronic renal failure have normal serum cholinesterase

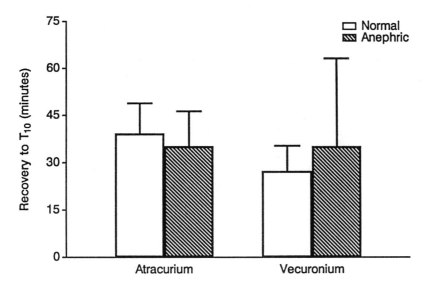

Figure 42. Time of recovery of twitch response to 10% of control after intravenous administration of atracurium (0.5 mg/kg) or vecuronium (0.1 mg/kg) to normal or anephric patients
during nitrous oxide-fentanyl-thiopentone anaesthesia. Absence of renal function does not
prolong the duration of action of either drug, although there was greater variation in response
to vecuronium. (From Hunter *et al.* (1984) *Br. J. Anaesth.*, 56, 941–50, reproduced with
permission).

unless there is atypical cholinesterase inheritance, so that there is no
contraindication to the use of suxamethonium provided serum potassium
levels are not greater than 5.5 mmol/l. However, the serum potassium level
is critical and will almost certainly rise during surgery. The use of suxamethonium for rapid-sequence induction can cause a 0.5–1.0 mmol/l increase
in the concentration of serum potassium and with preoperative concentrations above 5.5, the level may rise sufficiently to cause arrhythmia. Second
doses are reported as being particularly dangerous. Prolongation of action
of suxamethonium due to decreased levels of pseudocholinesterase in haemodialysis patients is clinically unimportant.

3.4. *Inhalation agents*

Anaesthesia with all inhalational agents temporarily depresses renal blood
flow, glomerular filtration rate and urine production, but there are usually
no lasting effects. Halothane, in low concentration, has been widely used in
renal failure and transplant patients. Patients given isoflurane demonstrate
no renal impairment following anaesthesia. Either drug can be recommended
although, where available, isoflurane will probably be preferred. Isoflurane
acts primarily on the peripheral vasculature and helps to control intraoperative hypertension. Halothane may cause potentially undesirable depression
of myocardial contractility. Nevertheless, halothane was used for years in

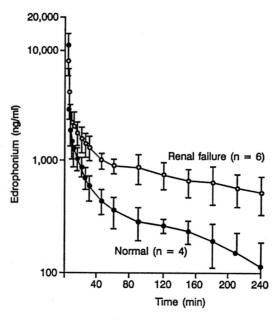

Figure 43. Plasma concentrations of edrophonium decline more slowly in renal failure patients than in normal patients. Delayed clearance of all anticholinesterase drugs parallels delayed clearance of non-depolarizing muscle relaxants. (From Morris *et al.* (1981) *Br. J. Anaesth.*, 53, 1311–3, reproduced with permission).

our institution in patients having multiple operations without adverse effects. These volatile agents have the additional advantage of potentiating the neuromuscular blocking action of many non-depolarizing muscle relaxants, especially vecuronium and atracurium, so that dosage of the latter can be reduced. This effect is particularly noticeable with isoflurane and with enflurane. However, metabolic break-down of the latter releases inorganic fluoride ions and, although peak levels of these ions in blood do not produce clinically significant postoperative impairment of renal function in normal patients, there may be a transient impairment following enflurane anaesthesia. This is evident where the duration of anaesthesia exceeds 2–4 hours of minimum alveolar concentration (2–4 MAC hours). There have been isolated reports of acute renal failure following enflurane anaesthesia in patients with pre-existing renal disease and its use in renal transplant surgery should probably be restricted or perhaps avoided.

3.5. *Analgesic drugs*

Nearly all the major analgesic drugs cause a fall in urine production and a rise in circulatory ADH levels. Fentanyl or derivatives may be the analgesics of choice in renal failure. Fentanyl can be given as an initial bolus dose of

100 μg with supplementary doses of 50 μg as required. Alfentanil can be given as an initial dose of 1 mg and a constant infusion of 50–100 μg/kg/h and the effect is alleged to be more predictable than that of fentanyl in that its elimination is less variable. Sufentanil is popular in North America, although respiratory depression due to unexpected high levels has been described. Norpethidine, the metabolite of pethidine, accumulates in renal failure and has an excitatory effect on the nervous system. Prolonged effects of narcotic analgesics in anuric patients have been described and accumulation of the narcotic or its metabolites or enterohepatic recirculation postulated. Evidence that the kidney has an important role in the elimination of opioid narcotics is accumulating. Peak concentrations of the metabolites of morphine, morphine-3-glucuronide and morphine-6-glucuronide are greater in renal failure patients and the latter is an active metabolite which relies on renal excretion. Previous and inaccurate reports of morphine accumulation during renal failure were probably artifactual due to the use of radioimmunoassays which did not distinguish between morphine and morphine-6-glucuronide. Uraemic patients appear to be exceptionally susceptible to the adverse effects of intrathecal narcotics.

3.6. *Immunosuppression*

Patients receiving a renal transplant require long-term immunosuppression and azathioprine which inhibits purine synthesis may be given (see Chapter 15). In current practice, cyclosporin A (CYA), an alkylating agent with less hepatotoxicity, is often used in preference to azathioprine. Cyclosporin A is an effective immunosuppressant but nephrotoxicity is a problem; hepatotoxicity, altered glucose tolerance, reduced prednisolone metabolism, increased serum cholesterol and triglyceride levels and many other side effects have been described with long-term use.

3.7. *Local anaesthetic drugs*

The local anaesthetic esters procaine, 2-chloroprocaine and tetracaine, undergo enzymatic hydrolysis with plasma cholinesterase. The toxicity of these agents is inversely proportional to their rate of degradation. The metabolism of the amide-type drugs (bupivacaine, etidocaine, lignocaine, mepivacaine and prilocaine) is more complex. Inactive metabolites formed in the liver are normally excreted by the kidney. Accumulation of metabolites is minimized by the use of the longer-acting bupivacaine and etidocaine, which are both highly bound to protein when in the blood stream. Bupivacaine cardiotoxicity has been reported in a patient with renal failure. Although renal failure will delay the excretion of the metabolites of lignocaine, problems are unlikely to arise unless significant hepatic dysfunction is also present.

3.8. *Colloidal plasma substitutes*

The clinical effects of infusing commercially available preparations of hydroxyethyl starch, dextran 40 and gelatine on plasma volume have been compared in healthy patients and in those with end-stage renal failure on chronic maintenance haemodialysis. As would be expected, increases in plasma volume were greater in the renal failure patients and lasted twice as long. Although low molecular weight dextrans do not appear to be nephrotoxic if given in recommended doses to patients with normal hydration and normal renal function, acute renal failure may be precipitated if shock or hypovolaemia is present. The renal tubular cells become grossly swollen with vacuoles containing dextran. With current knowledge of the fate of these substances in the body, their use in patients with poor renal function or those receiving a kidney transplant is not recommended. However some European transplant units use liberal quantities of dextran to maintain adequate plasma volume (lg/kg of dextran -40, -60 or -70).

4. Anaesthetic management of the living donor

It is important that the donor's pre-anaesthetic condition is optimal and the anaesthetic management flawless. These patients should be in good health, with good bilateral renal function. Donors should be encouraged to stop smoking and obese patients to be not more than 20% over ideal weight at the time of the surgery. The risk of serious peri-operative complications to the donor is small but real. The death rate has been reported to be of the order of 0.5%. Deaths from halothane hepatitis and from pulmonary embolism have been described. Major post-operative complications occur in about 4%, while about 25% suffer minor problems. One of our patients required prolonged mechanical ventilation and 42 days in intensive care for severe postoperative chest infection. The lateral jack-knife position favoured by some surgeons may lead to venous pooling and severe hypotension and has been known to damage the dependent kidney. Another of our donors developed acute renal failure in the remaining kidney and required haemodialysis support for 4 weeks and renal function remained subnormal.

Premedication is determined by the donor's level of anxiety. An intravenous infusion is started the night before surgery at a rate appropriate to provide optimum hydration of the donor on the morning of surgery. Non-invasive monitoring with electrocardiogram, automatic blood pressure recording, end-tidal carbon dioxide and pulse oximeter are routine.

The general anaesthetic technique used for this procedure is not critical and depends on the preference of the anaesthetist but is likely to include thiopentone and an intravenous narcotic for induction followed by either pancuronium, vecuronium or atracurium. It is advisable not to administer drugs eliminated predominantly by the kidney as there will be an acute 50%

loss of renal tissue. In animals the decrease in renal blood flow and in glomerular filtration rate is proportional to the mass of kidney excised and persists for 12–24 hours. After intubation, maintenance is with nitrous oxide in oxygen and a volatile agent, probably isoflurane. Some anaesthetists prefer to avoid the use of nitrous oxide since high dissection and rib removal may breach the pleura and give rise to pneumothorax. The patient is turned into the lateral position with the operation side uppermost. Intravascular volume is well maintained to ensure a urine output of 1.5 ml/min.

Maintenance of normocapnia is important, since both hypo- and hyper-capnia cause renal artery constriction. Vasopressors should be avoided if possible. The anaesthetist should be prepared to administer mannitol and frusemide prior to cutting of the ureter, and heparin prior to clamping of the renal artery.

During wound closure, diaphragmatic and pleural leaks should be excluded. Early postoperative clinical examination of the chest followed by x-ray should be routine to detect any pneumothorax. Demand for postoperative analgesia may be greater than expected.

5. Anaesthetic management of the cadaveric donor

With the diagnosis of brain-stem confirmed, and permission for organ donation received, the anaesthetist should check that consent allowing donation has been properly recorded in the case notes. Investigations which may be required by the nephrectomy or transplant teams should be complete. The donor's cardiac and pulmonary function is being supported in the intensive care unit and ventilation with oxygen will continue during transport to the operating theatre. The "rule of 100's" should be the aim, that is a systolic blood pressure greater than 100 mm Hg, urine output greater than 100 ml/h and the arterial oxygen tension (PaO_2) greater than 100 mm Hg (13 kPa). Management difficulties may include cardiovascular instability requiring volume infusion with or without inotropic drug support, pulmonary dysfunction secondary to thoracic trauma or neurogenic pulmonary oedema, diabetes insipidus, electrolyte abnormalities, anaemia secondary to blood loss and temperature instability. Intravascular volume is best monitored by a central venous pressure catheter. If a vasopressor is necessary, dopamine in the minimal dose necessary (not more than 10 μg/kg/min) is the drug of choice. Vasopressin to control diabetes insipidus is best discontinued prior to going to the operating theatre. Pre-nephrectomy hypotension and the use of dopamine or vasopressin increases the incidence of acute tubular necrosis and graft failure. The combined use of dopamine and vasopressin up to the moment when the aorta is clamped results in 20% of transplanted kidneys failing. Other vasopressors should be avoided. While many centres use mannitol or frusemide to promote diuresis, we have not found them necessary.

Controlled ventilation with 100% oxygen is provided during the surgical procedure. Non-invasive monitoring with electrocardiogram, blood pressure, pulse oximeter and end-tidal carbon dioxide measurement are routine. Arterial and central venous cannulae may be *in situ*. Muscle relaxants are used to aid surgery and to blunt spinal reflexes. A high proportion of cadaveric organ donors respond to surgical incision with abdominal muscle contraction (a spinal arc reflex) and autonomic nervous system responses, suggesting that even though irreversible brain-stem damage has occurred from which death is inevitable, some brain-stem function remains. The surgeon may call for a bolus dose of phentolamine shortly before the aorta is clamped. When this is done, the time is noted, monitors and infusions are turned off and the donor disconnected from the ventilator.

6. Anaesthetic management of the recipient

Successful renal transplantation is very dependent on haemodialysis which allows preoperative preparation to be accomplished rapidly, particularly in the patient who has been maintained on a chronic dialysis program. Unlike other major organ transplants, the patient can be maintained in reasonable health if the graft is slow to function or fails.

6.1. *Pre-anaesthetic evaluation*

Management of the recipient is similar regardless of the source of the donor. With improved techniques for preservation of the graft, the need to perform the operation as an emergency has passed. One noticeable recent trend has been to extend the transplant program to include the quite young and the relatively elderly, and to include patients with severe chronic disease of other organs. These require careful evaluation. Behavioural, mental or neurological changes and peripheral neuropathies are all common.

6.2. *Fluid and electrolyte status*

Most centres prepare recipients for live donor transplants with dialysis 12–24 hours prior to surgery. The recipient of a cadaver kidney is dialysed for several hours before the operation. If this is not done, there may be a certain amount of fluid retention, not necessarily disadvantageous, because patients dialysed to "dry weight" may respond to induction of anaesthesia with vasodilatation and associated hypotension.

Metabolic acidosis should not be a problem in the patient maintained on an adequate dialysis regimen. The serum potassium level is critical. Apart from dangers associated with the use of suxamethonium, potassium can be released from ischaemic muscle if the external iliac artery is used for vascular anastomosis and from the donor kidney if Collin's solution has been used as the preservative fluid. The danger period in both these instances is when the vascular clamps are released. Tall peaked T waves on the electrocardiogram may be noted. Severe hyperkalaemia produces a flat P wave, atrial asystole, intraventricular block with wide QRS complexes, and eventually ventricular asystole.

Hyperventilation and small bolus doses of sodium bicarbonate (50–100 mmol) will assist redistribution of potassium from serum to cells, but caution is required if hypernatraemia is present. Soluble insulin (10–20 units) administered with 25 ml of 50% dextrose intravenously will have a similar effect. Intravenous infusion of calcium salts (1 g of gluconate or chloride) will antagonize the cardiotoxic effects of potassium without altering serum levels. Removal of potassium from the body can be achieved by the use of cation-exchange resins given orally or rectally without resorting to dialysis in the immediate postoperative period.

6.3. *Anaemia*

Anaemia is a universal feature in end-stage renal disease. Haemoglobin levels of 6–8 g dl (haematocrit 20–25%) are common and patients compensate with a raised cardiac output and hyperdynamic circulation. Haemoglobin levels lower than 6 g dl are unacceptable and should be corrected with packed red-blood cells preoperatively or early in the operative period. With the increasing use of recombinant human erythropoietin very low haemoglobin levels will be seen less commonly in chronic renal failure. Preoperative heparin dialysis does not usually cause intra-operative bleeding problems. Untreated uraemia causes platelet dysfunction which is corrected by adequate dialysis.

6.4. *Drug therapy*

Patients requiring transplants have a high incidence of peripheral vascular disease and left ventricular dysfunction. The majority are hypertensive. Where this is not the case, one should suspect profound extracellular volume depletion, excessive antihypertensive medication, or occasionally previous bilateral nephrectomy or rare salt-losing nephritis. Patients commonly receive centrally acting antihypertensive agents, beta-adrenergic-receptor blockers, direct arterial dilators, calcium channel blockers or angiotensin-converting enzyme (ACE) inhibitors. Current advice is that patients should be maintained on their anti-hypertensive therapy up to the time of operation. This will reduce the harmful responses to laryngoscopy, intubation and the stresses of surgery. Significant coronary artery disease is becoming commoner as older patients are referred for transplantation. Some patients suffering from end-stage renal disease have accelerated atheroma formation; some workers routinely perform coronary arteriography and will consider coronary artery bypass grafts in selected patients prior to transplantation.

6.5. *Diabetes*

An increasing number of diabetics with end-stage disease are being offered transplantation. The diabetic state which may be destabilized by steroids requires careful control. Regular injections of insulin can be stopped on the day of surgery and replaced by an infusion of 5–10% dextrose containing 10–20 units of regular insulin per litre. This is infused at a rate of 100 ml/h in a modified Alberti regimen that does not include the use of potassium, combined with frequent measurement of blood sugar. Fine control over blood sugar can be achieved using a sliding scale of additional insulin administration (Table 31).

A high incidence of difficult laryngoscopy may be anticipated in diabetic patients who have limited joint mobility. This joint rigidity is probably due to glycosylation of tissue proteins from chronic hyperglycaemia and may involve laryngeal and cervical areas.

Table 31. The sliding scale of insulin dosage. Blood glucose is measured 2- or 4-hourly as appropriate.

Blood glucose mmol l^{-1}	Soluble insulin dosage
0–10	Nil
10–15	5 units subcutaneously
15–20	10 units subcutaneously
20 or more	Intravenous bolus of 5 or 10 units or constant infusion at 1–2 units hourly

6.6. *Monitoring*

Apart from the presence of a skilled and vigilant anaesthetist, certain basic monitoring procedures are considered necessary for all patients undergoing anaesthesia and surgery. Major surgery demands more sophisticated techniques. The single precordial lead electrocardiogram gives information on the heart rate, cardiac rhythm, and conduction disturbances. The CM5 configuration may give early warning of myocardial ischaemia. Modern automatic non-invasive blood pressure recorders measure systolic, mean and diastolic blood pressure at regular intervals. They can be set to cycle at one minute intervals during induction of anaesthesia and during release of vascular clamps, but should not be left to cycle at this frequency for prolonged periods since both nerve and arterial damage have been reported.

The anaesthetic machine should be fitted with an oxygen analyzer to monitor the inspired oxygen concentration and a respirometer should be available to check tidal and minute volumes. A disconnect alarm should be fitted and switched on. Breath sounds may be monitored with a precordial or oesophageal stethoscope (or both). Since both hypercarbia and hypocarbia decrease renal perfusion, monitoring of expired carbon dioxide is valuable. The aim should be normocarbia with an end-tidal concentration at about 5% (5 kPa or approximately 40 mm Hg). Pulse oximetry has become a valuable method of confirming the adequacy of oxygenation. Many patients with renal failure require substantially higher concentrations of inspired oxygen than have been used conventionally to maintain satisfactory arterial oxygen saturation (SaO_2). This may reflect some degree of heart failure or of pulmonary oedema. Measurement of central venous pressure via an internal jugular catheter is becoming popular. Not only will this allow a more accurate assessment of the degree of hydration, but in addition, early function of the graft appears to be improved if venous pressure is maintained at between 10–12 cm of water. The use of pulmonary artery catheters is thought to be undesirable in patients wno are soon to become immuno-compromised and increasingly susceptible to infection.

A nerve stimulator is useful, particularly where a short-acting muscle relaxant such as atracurium is being used. Determination of the train-of-four twitch fade allows for proper titration of subsequent doses. It also gives the anaesthetist an idea of the amount of curarization remaining at the end of surgery.

During prolonged surgery, core temperature will fall and should be measured. Humidification of inspired gases may limit the temperature fall and, where appropriate, a heat and moisture exchanger will conserve heat and water vapour and protect the airway against bacterial and viral contamination. Laboratory facilities for rapid determination of electrolytes, blood gases, haemoglobin or haematocrit and glucose are essential for renal transplantation.

6.7. Choice of anaesthesia

The first patient ever to receive a living related donor kidney transplant had a spinal anaesthetic. Spinal or epidural anaesthesia held certain attractions in the early days of transplantation in America. Patients often came to surgery with heart failure, uncontrolled hypertension and high serum potassium levels. Some developed life-threatening arrhythmias, particularly while being intubated. Regional anaesthesia also avoided the unwanted effects of muscle relaxants and may have reduced the risk of pulmonary aspiration. An epidural catheter could be used for postoperative pain relief although recent heparin dialysis would be a contraindication to its insertion. However, many of the early operations were prolonged and spinal anaesthesia was not well tolerated. The sympathetic block associated with spinal or epidural anaesthesia created difficulty in maintaining an adequate systolic blood pressure. Local anaesthetics have a shorter effect when the circulation is hyperdynamic. The introduction of newer inhalational drugs and muscle relaxants has given the anaesthetist much greater control over the patient having general anaesthesia and this has become the method of choice in most transplant units.

A large-bore intravenous cannula is required. Peripheral venous access may be difficult in the patient who has been receiving haemodialysis for years. The intravenous infusion and blood pressure cuff must not be placed on the arm which has a functioning dialysis fistula or shunt. This arm must be carefully protected during surgery and the presence of a bruit noted before and after operation. Episodes of hypotension and the hypercoagulable state that can occur in the perioperative period may lead to loss of a functioning fistula. Induction of anaesthesia is hazardous for the transplant patient. The majority of deaths and serious arrhythmias have been related to hyperkalaemia and levels over 6.0 mmol/l are dangerous. Pre-oxygenation and correctly applied cricoid pressure should be used in patients at risk of regurgitation and aspiration. An intravenous bolus injection of fentanyl, alfentanil or lignocaine (which may depress the heart) will reduce the cardiovascular response to oral intubation. The uses of beta-adrenergic receptor antagonists (beta-blockers) as bolus injections prior to induction is best avoided. All the currently available beta-blockers are long-acting and some are eliminated by the renal route. Esmolol, a short-acting beta-blocker, may establish a place in this regard when it becomes available, but on no account should this type of drug be given to patients with obstructive pulmonary disease or a history of asthma. Chewing a 10 mg capsule of nifedipine which can then be absorbed through the buccal mucous membrane will often give satisfactory control of high blood pressure during the induction.

6.8. *Induction and maintenance*

Unless the timing of organ availability allows time to curtail oral intake, full-stomach precautions are taken during induction. After pre-oxygenation, a rapid-sequence induction with cricoid pressure and oral intubation is performed. Thiopentone (3–5 mg/kg) is given intravenously. If the pre-operative serum potassium concentration is normal, laryngoscopy and endotracheal intubation are facilitated with suxamethonium (1.0–1.5 mg/kg). If the serum potassium is raised, vecuronium 0.1 mg/kg or atracurium 0.6 mg/kg is used in preference to suxamethonium. Isoflurane, nitrous oxide in 50% oxygen and supplementary doses of non-depolarizing muscle relaxant and fentanyl is the current choice for maintenance. A urinary catheter and, if required, a central venous pressure cannula are inserted. Central venous pressure will be high in well hydrated patients and in those with a good functioning arterio-venous fistula. The electrocardiogram is closely observed for evidence of hyperkalaemia. Washout hyperkalaemia may occur when vascular clamps are released. Blood loss averages 200–400 ml and should be replaced with whole blood (which has been previously ordered). Crystalloid solutions should be potassium free. Compound sodium lactate (Ringer's or Hartmann's solution) is not used. Isotonic sodium chloride, dextrose 5% in 0.45% sodium chloride or dextrose 4% in 0.18% sodium chloride (solution 18) are acceptable. Losses of blood not requiring transfusion can be replaced by plasma or isotonic sodium chloride. Transfusion may be required if excessive bleeding occurs when the vascular clamps are released. Blood should be warmed prior to transfusion to reduce the infused serum potassium level. Intravascular volume is titrated using central venous pressure and systolic arterial pressure measurements rather than making use of any standard formula. Maximum hydration short of precipitating pulmonary oedema encourages early graft function. Intermittent positive pressure ventilation during anaesthesia can mask pulmonary oedema until after resumption of spontaneous breathing and extubation.

Individual transplant teams vary in the pharmacological agents which may be used to encourage graft function. Frusemide (10–20 mg) has been shown to be effective in many animal models of acute renal failure and in clinical studies provided it is given at the time of injury and that the subject is not dehydrated or hypotensive. Mannitol (25–50 g), in addition to its osmotic action on the renal tubules, is a renal vasodilator. It can also cause a rise in serum potassium (0.4–0.7 mmol/l). Upon release of the clamps the kidney should turn from grey to pink. Sometimes hypotension results which should be treated by cautious administration of volume expanders, although use of low dose dopamine (not more than 10 μg/kg/min) has been described. Less commonly, clamp release may result in renin release by the ischaemic kidney, resulting in a transient hypertensive episode.

If significant hyperkalaemia (greater than 6.5 mmol/l) is present at the end of the operation, it may be wise to continue artificial ventilation into the post-operative period to maintain a respiratory alkalosis. Otherwise, the neuromuscular block is reversed with neostigmine (0.035 mg/kg) and glycopyrrolate (0.01 mg/kg) or atropine (0.02 mg/kg) and the patient extubated. Although the slow elimination of anticholinesterase agents in anuric patients may facilitate the reversal of muscle relaxants, there is an increased incidence of delayed unwanted effects such as bradycardia.

For the first 24 hours post-operatively, the patient is nursed in a high dependency area in the transplant ward or in an intensive care environment. Monitoring of heart rate, arterial blood pressure and arterial oxygen saturation should continue during this period, while the patient receives adequate oxygen by disposable face mask. The central venous pressure commonly falls to near zero within a few hours after renal transplantation as the kidney begins to function and adequate fluid replacement is essential. Good oxygenation is important. The medullary thick ascending limb of the loop of Henle has a high oxygen demand and low oxygen supply from the medullary counter current exchange system. The medullary thick ascending limb is thus particularly vulnerable to relatively mild hypoxic insults.

6.9. *Post-operative complications*

In terms of graft function, three scenarios can be imagined. Firstly, there may be good immediate function, and elimination of drugs is undistinguishable from that which occurs in patients with normal renal function. Another common pattern is a high flow of urine but with accumulation of toxic metabolic products resembling the diuretic phase of acute tubular necrosis. Thirdly, there may be delayed graft function requiring haemodialysis but without evidence of rejection.

Cardiac complications remain the most serious cause of post-operative morbidity and mortality. Cardiac death occurs in about 1% of patients, myocardial infarction in 0.5% and serious arrhythmias in 5–10%. Hypertension may require vigorous attention as it threatens both patient and graft survival, especially in diabetic patients. Complications which may lead to other surgical procedures in the early postoperative period include problems with ureteral obstruction or fistulae, vascular problems from haemorrhage, kinking of the renal artery, or thrombosis, and acute rejection (see Chapter 16).

7. Renal transplantation in children

Renal transplantation is now established as the treatment of choice for older children; however, the approach to the infant and young child remains controversial, despite the introduction of dialysis procedures suitable for the very young. The results of transplantation in children under the age of two years were particularly discouraging although there have been recent improvements with greater emphasis on live related donor allografts. Management of anaesthesia for these patients does not differ in detail from that in adults. It should be remembered that children with end-stage renal disease may have severe growth retardation and that due allowance should be made when calculating drug dosage, tracheal tube size and gas requirements for ventilation. Intermittent positive pressure ventilation is used and the intravascular volume maintained steady with a central venous pressure between 10 and 15 cms of water.

Intraoperative volume losses are replaced with a combination of packed cells and plasma, maintaining adequate blood pressure. The immunosuppressive therapy used in Belfast for paediatric recipients is described in Chapter 15. If there is no diuresis within 30–60 min, intravenous frusemide is given over 10–15 min in the dose of 2–5 mg/kg. In the small patient receiving an adult kidney the organ may need to be placed within the abdomen; the renal vessels can be anastomosed directly to the aorta and vena cava. Meticulous attention to peri-operative management and fluid and electrolyte balance is required; intra-transplant sequestration can occur when the vascular clamps are released and a significant proportion of blood volume and cardiac output is diverted to the newly transplanted kidney.

Post-operatively, hourly urine volumes are replaced as 0.45% sodium chloride. Electrolyte measurements are carried out 4 hourly. Insensible loss is replaced by 5% dextrose and other fluid loss by half volume 0.9% sodium chloride and half volume 5% dextrose. If urinary volume is very large potassium loss should be replaced by giving potassium chloride 30 mmol per litre of intravenous fluid.

Organ transplantation in children is fraught with emotional problems. Patients often cope better with their illness than do their parents who may require particularly sensitive and tactful handling.

Acknowledgement

I am grateful to Dr Michelle Brady who provided valuable advice regarding clinical problems and constructive criticism on reading the manuscript.

Further reading

Gallo, J. A., Brown, B. R. R, Newton, D. E. F. Anaesthesia for organ transplantation. In Nunn, J. F., Utting, J. E., Brown, B. R. eds. *General Anaesthesia* 5th edn. London, Butterworth; 1989: 868–871.

Graybar, G. B., Tarpey, M. Kidney transplantation. In Gelman, S. ed. *Anesthesia and Organ Transplantation*. Philadelphia, Saunders; 1987: 61–110.

Linke, C. L. Anaesthesia considerations for renal transplantation. In Brown, B. R. ed. *Anesthesia and Transplantation Surgery; Contemporary Anesthesia Practice* vol 10. Philadelphia, Davis; 1987: 183–231.

Mazze, R. I. Anesthesia and the renal and genitourinary systems. In Miller, R. D. ed. *Anesthesia* 3rd edn. New York, Churchill Livingstone; 1991: 1791–1808.

Sear, J. W., Holland, D. E. Anaesthesia for patients with renal dysfunction. In Nimmo, W. S., Smith G. eds. *Anaesthesia*. Oxford, Blackwell; 1989: 912–932.

CHAPTER 15

Immunosuppression

MARY G. MCGEOWN

In Chapter 1 the story of immunosuppression was left at the stage when it had become clear that whole body irradiation would not become a useful clinical tool. In 1958 Dameshek and Schwartz in the New England Medical Center were attempting to treat aplastic anaemia and leukaemia with bone marrow transplantation. They too tried irradiation of the recipient and found a high mortality. In search of a better method they reasoned that an anti-cancer drug such as 6-mercaptopurine (6 MP) might be used and reported that rabbits treated with this drug showed little response to injection of foreign protein. Their report led Calne in London, and Zukoski in Richmond, Virginia, to use 6 MP for kidney transplants in dogs, with some success, but this too proved to be toxic and some of the animals died.

Between 1960 and 1961 6 MP was used as immunosuppression for renal transplants by Hopewell in London, Murray and his colleagues in Boston and Küss in Paris. None of these transplants were successful but Küss reported prolonged survival of a kidney from an unrelated donor when the recipient received irradiation, 6 MP, and intermittent prednisone – the first successful chemical immunosuppression.

In the meantime Calne had gone to Boston. Working in Murray's laboratory, he tested derivatives of 6 MP produced by Hitchings of Burroughs Wellcome. One of these, azathioprine, later known as Imuran, proved in dogs to be both more immunosuppressive and less toxic than the parent drug for kidney transplants. Murray and Calne began to use azathioprine for transplants in man in 1962. Their third attempt succeeded and despite several rejection episodes the kidney continued to function for about two years. Azathioprine became generally accepted as the main immunosuppressive drug for transplantation for the next two decades. Murray received a Nobel prize in 1990.

The use of azathioprine did not solve the problem of rejection but in 1962 Goodwin reported that steroid injections reversed several rejection episodes in a mother-to-child transplant – the child later died of sepsis. After this the combination of azathioprine and steroid was accepted as the standard immunosuppression for kidney transplantation. The age of drug

Mary G. McGeown (ed.), Clinical Management of Renal Transplantation, 201–229.
© 1992 *Kluwer Academic Publishers, Dordrecht. Printed in the Netherlands.*

Table 32. Immunosuppressant methods used in man

1. Whole body irradiation
2. Azathioprine
3. Corticosteroid
4. Antilymphocyte serum
5. Cyclophosphamide
6. Splenectomy
7. Thymectomy
8. Thoracic duct drainage
9. Bilateral nephrectomy
10. Blood transfusion 1. third party
                              2. donor specific
11. Local irradiation of the graft
12. Subtotal irradiation
13. Cyclosporin A
14. Monoclonal antisera
15. Plasma exchange
16. New immunosuppressive drugs: FK 506; rapamycin

immunosuppression had arrived, but much had still to be learnt. Steroid was a useful adjunct and it was thought the more the better. While the combination of azathioprine and high doses of steroids often permitted long-term survival of kidney grafts, many patients died from infection and numerous other serious side effects often occurred. Indeed many nephrologists preferred the greater safety of dialysis for their patients in spite of the less good quality of life. The combination of azathioprine and steroid continued to be the mainstay of immunosuppression for the next two decades. The results in terms of patient and graft survival remained disappointingly poor and other methods were introduced in the hope of improving graft survival (Table 32). Let us consider the immunosuppressive methods used in man.

1. Total body irradiation

Total body irradiation and the serious toxicity associated with its use has been considered already.

2. Azathioprine

Azathioprine is the imidazole derivative of 6 mercapto-purine (6 MP). It is absorbed very rapidly and completely, significant amounts appearing in the blood within 15 minutes after oral administration. It is partially transformed into 6 MP yet it is a more effective immunosuppressive than is 6 MP in kidney grafts in dogs and skin grafts in mice. Neither azathioprine nor 6 MP have significant intrinsic activity and their activity depends on the formation of their metabolites, so there is a time lag even when they are given intravenously. *In vitro* it alters most T cell markers and functions, inhibiting the mixed lymphocyte reaction and the generation of cytotoxic T cells. It is active against B lymphocytes, though less strongly than against T cells. It inhibits both DNA and RNA synthesis.

2.1. *Side effects of azathioprine*

These are shown in Table 33.

Table 33. Side effects of azathioprine

1. Increased incidence of infection
2. Bone marrow depression
3. Liver toxicity
4. Malignancy

2.1.1. *Infection.* In spite of its immunosuppressive effect, when given on its own azathioprine has little effect on the occurrence of bacterial infections. The incidence and severity of viral infections is increased, herpes simplex, herpes zoster and cytomegalovirus (CMV) being particularly common.

2.1.2. *Bone marrow depression.* Bone marrow depression is not particularly common in normal clinical use (see Dosage of azathioprine). It is heralded by a falling white cell count, when the drug should be discontinued, and recommenced at a lower dose when the white cell count reaches a satisfactory level. The coincidental appearance of a viral infection, especially CMV infection, often leads to a more worrying fall in white cell count, which may persist for weeks after the drug has been withdrawn. The red cell series and platelets are also depleted in severe toxicity especially when associated with CMV infection. Azathioprine depression of the bone marrow most often occurs early after transplantation, but may (rarely) appear after years of good tolerance.

2.1.3. *Liver toxicity.* Liver damage by azathioprine is said to be common in the dog, but in our experience is rare in patients. Most patients who develop jaundice after renal transplantation have viral hepatitis. Cholestatic jaundice is said to be induced directly by azathioprine, but the incidence of this appears to be very low.

2.1.4. *Malignant diseases.* All immunosuppressive agents increase the incidence of malignant tumours. Israel Penn, who established the International Transplant Tumour Registry, estimates that the incidence of tumours in transplanted patients is about 100 times greater than that in the general population of the same age. The incidence is even greater when multiple immunosuppressive agents are used, especially ALG and CYA when used in high dosage. The type of tumours associated with immunosuppression differ in incidence from those in the general population, squamous cell carcinomas and carcinomas of the cervix occurring with considerably greater frequency amongst transplant recipients. The incidence of other common malignancies such as carcinomas of lung, breast, prostate and colon remain the same as in the general population. Lymphomas account for about 21% of tumours in transplant patients, while Kaposi's sarcoma which is very rare in the general population accounts for 6% of tumours. Lip cancers account for 6% of tumours in transplant patients compared with 0.4% in the general population. Cancers of kidney and liver and sarcomas are also more common than in the general population. Exposure of skin to excessive amounts of ultra-violet radiation seems to increase the incidence of skin neoplasia and should be avoided. We advise our patients to use strong sun-screen protection cream when prolonged exposure of skin is necessary and to avoid deliberate sun-bathing and use of sun beds. Female patients should have regular yearly cervical smears because of the increased risk of carcinoma of the cervix.

2.2. *Dosage of azathioprine*

Azathioprine is generally available as yellow 50 mg and orange 25 mg coated tablets which do not readily divide. The coating is intended to reduce skin exposure to azathioprine but it means that many patients require to have supplies of both strengths of tablet. There are also non-proprietary, uncoated 50 mg tablets scored for easy division.

The dose used is very variable. The author carried out a survey of the immunosuppressive therapy being used in transplant centres in UK in 1972 and found that the daily maintenance dose of azathioprine varied from 1.0 to 3.0 mg/k. A more recent Australian study used lower doses. Many of the long established European centres, including Belfast, gave 3 mg/kg as a single daily dose. A higher dose (5 mg/kg/dy) may be given just prior to or early in the course of the operation, or in the first three days after operation. Generally the first dose only is given intravenously. A falling white cell count requires a reduction in dosage or cessation of the drug and careful search for infection, especially CMV. After the white cell count returns to satisfactory levels (e.g. $5000 \times e9/1$) azathioprine should be recommenced at lower dosage.

It is often said that the tolerance of the bone marrow to azathioprine is not affected by the level of renal function. Our own experience is otherwise. The introduction of the maintenance dose of 3 mg/kg/dy before reasonable kidney function is established may lead to leucopenia. We have used 1.5 mg/kg/dy until the creatinine clearance exceeds 30 ml/min. We recommend that the dosage should be reduced if the renal function deteriorates, but there is a danger of using inadequate dosage and the situation should be regularly reassessed. If there are no signs of intolerance the dose of

3 mg/kg/dy of azathioprine is continued as the long term maintenance dose. We have adopted a policy of modest reduction of the dose after 5 years, (to 1.0–1.5 mg/kg/dy) because of the high incidence of skin malignancy.

Allopurinol inhibits the metabolism of azathioprine and should be avoided if possible. If both must be given the dose of azathioprine will probably need to be considerably reduced. Frequent review will be necessary.

3. Corticosteroid

Prednisone was the first corticosteroid (steroid) used for organ transplantation. In the early 1950s it was shown to have immunosuppressive activity but the effect is less in man than in rabbits. It prolongs survival of skin and organ grafts only slightly. It is more effective in combination with other immunosuppressive agents, potentiating their effect. It has a powerful anti-inflammatory effect which may be confused with immunosuppression. It produces biochemical changes in lymphocytes. The target cell has not been precisely defined. The action on T and B lymphocytes is complex, and it also depresses macrophages and polymorphs.

Steroid is never used alone for organ immunosuppression but, since Goodwin reported that it reversed rejection (see Anti-rejection therapy), it has been the main drug used for rejection crises.

Prednisone is rapidly converted into prednisolone by the liver and there is no evidence to indicate which is the better immunosuppressive. In the early days of transplantation prednisolone was the more widely used in UK and we have continued to use it. Methylprednisolone is generally used for intravenous therapy.

There is a wide inter-subject variation in blood concentrations achieved after oral dosage of prednisone or prednisolone, either may be prescribed. On average the bioavailability of prednisone is about 80% of that of prednisolone. The pharmacokinetics of prednisolone are age dependent as well as dose dependent. Liver disease prolongs the half-life of prednisolone.

A by no means exhaustive list of side effects of steroid is given in Table 34.

Table 34. Side effects of steroid

1. Weight gain
2. Cushingoid appearance
3. Acne
4. Increased incidence of infection
5. Gastrointestinal complications
6. Diabetes mellitus
7. Adreno-pituitary suppression
8. Steroid psychosis
9. Avascular necrosis of bone
10. Posterior polar cataracts
11. Hypertension

3.1. Side effects of steroid

These vary in significance from cosmetic changes in appearance, which are merely displeasing to both patient and physician, to those which are life-threatening.

3.1.1.–3.1.4. Cosmetic and skin changes. Most patients gain weight following transplantation, due to increased appetite and delight in self-chosen as opposed to prescribed diet. In the previously malnourished this is salutary but sensible advice about diet is required lest the weight gain gets out of hand. The cushingoid appearance resulting from excessive use of steroid (but also due to the idiosyncratic response of some patients, particularly adolescents) may, in its early stages, be difficult to distinguish from simple obesity. Acne may be troublesome especially in adolescents who are in any event more prone. Skin thinning occasionally occurs in patients past middle age, when large areas of skin purpura may result from trivial injury.

3.1.5. Infection. The excessively high doses of steroid used through the 1960s, and indeed for most of the 1970s in many centres, led to a high incidence of life-threatening infection. Infection was the commonest cause of death in the high dose steroid era accounting for up to 30% of patients. The infection was (and is) often non-bacterial, due to viruses or fungi. Particularly common are CMV, generalized herpes, or unusual infections such as pneumocystis carinii, aspergillosis, and cryptococcus, which are rare in non-immunosuppressed patients. An outbreak of pneumocystis carinii spreading through a renal unit has been described. Tuberculosis is common in parts of the world where this is still endemic and led to the need to give anti-tuberculous drugs after transplantation.

3.1.6. Gastrointestinal complications. Gastrointestinal complications are common in patients given high dose steroid. These range from increase in frequency and severity of dyspepsia, especially at night, to haemetemesis, gastric or duodenal perforation (especially if other gastric irritants are also taken, e.g. alcohol, aspirin, non-steroidal anti-inflammatory drugs), or perforation of diverticular disease.

3.1.7. Diabetes mellitus. Diabetes mellitus may appear for the first time after transplantation and occasionally presents acutely and, if not recognised, can rapidly become life-threatening. As steroids antagonise the effect of anti-diabetic agents, increased doses of these may be needed to control glycaemia in known diabetic patients.

3.1.8. Adrenopituitary suppression. Prolonged daily steroid administration will usually lead to some degree of adrenal suppression, which is dose dependent, and also related to how the medication is given, being most marked when given in divided doses over the day. Adrenopituitary suppression is least when the total daily dose is given in the early morning, before or with breakfast. There is a wide variation in the peak levels attained after a given dose, and the peak levels may occur from half to 4 hours after oral ingestion. The half life does not correlate well with clinical cushingoid changes. In patients who seem to be developing cushingoid signs or excessive weight gain despite low dosage, especially adolescents, the dosage may be changed to double dose on alternate days. This must be done with care, spread over a few weeks as the dosage is gradually adjusted in aliquots from the full dose daily to double the dose on alternate days (instead of 20 mg daily, 30 mg and 10 mg are given on alternate days for one week, then 35 mg and 5 mg on alternate days for a further week, changing to 40 mg on alternate days after three weeks, provided the patient continues to feel well). The patient should be reviewed frequently over this time. There is a slight risk of producing a rejection and the change to double dose/alternate day therapy is probably better done between three to six months after transplantation, before adrenal suppression is established.

Patients who have been on prolonged maintenance steroid therapy are usually given modest doses of hydrocortisone to cover stresses such as surgery or childbirth. Adrenal suppression seems likely to exacerbate the effect of steroid withdrawal in any clinical situation. This may contribute to the increased risk of rejection when steroid is withdrawn to achieve late cyclosporin monotherapy (see Cyclosporin).

3.1.9. *Avascular necrosis of bone.* Avascular necrosis involving the hips, less commonly the shoulders or knee joints, is a painful and disabling complication of steroid therapy. It may sometimes lead to the need for joint replacement.

It seems to be dose related, in that it occurs much less frequently with our low dose therapy. It has occurred in patients given large intravenous doses of methylprednisolone for reasons other that renal transplantation. It may be more common in patients who already have some form of renal osteodystrophy, though evidence for this is sparse.

3.1.10. *Osteoporosis.* There is abundant evidence that prolonged use of steroid may of itself lead to osteoporosis and this may be a reason for choosing a steroid-free method of immunosuppression in elderly female recipients. It is also important to keep the total dose of steroid as low as possible, remembering that many patients, whatever their other immunosuppressive treatment may be, may need to continue to take steroid for the rest of life.

3.1.11. *Posterior polar cataracts.* Posterior polar cataracts are not uncommon and seem to be related to steroid rather than other aspects of the treatment of these patients. They are a serious complication in patients whose life-style has been enhanced by a successful transplant.

3.1.12. *Steroid psychosis*. Steroid psychosis seems to be rare, at any rate when low dose steroid is used, and in Belfast has occurred only in three patients with previous psychiatric history.

3.1.13. *Hypertension*. Steroid therapy may antagonise the effect of hypotensive drugs, making hypertension more difficult to control. This may be of significance in patients receiving cyclosporin which, of itself, predisposes to hypertension.

3.2. *Dosage of steroid*

Although steroid has been used for immunosuppression for transplantation from the earliest days, the dosage of steroid was empirical and could be judged only clinically by the appearance of unwanted side effects. Specific assays were developed only in the late 1970s. Huge doses were used in the mistaken belief that more was better. Table 35 shows the dose used routinely during the later 1970s in four of the largest centres in US, France, and Oxford and Belfast in UK. In Figure 44 the amounts of steroid which the patients received over the first 30 days is shown graphically. The area under the curve is a measure of the amount of steroid the patient received during the early post-operative period in each of the centres, showing the much lower dose used in Belfast. This was maintenance steroid only, patients who developed rejection received much more. Using azathioprine with this low dose of steroid and without other methods of immunosuppression (though almost all recipients received blood transfusion) Belfast was able to achieve a one year graft survival of over 80% and a remarkably low incidence of fatal infection and other side effects.

The standard prednisolone tablets are 25 mg, 5 mg (scored) and 1 mg tablets. In this form prednisolone dissolves in the stomach within a few

Table 35. Steroid treatment given for renal transplantation

Author	Initial treatment
Najarian (US, 1977)	20 mg methylprednisolone/kg/dy for 3 dys; tapered to 0.5 mg/kg/dy at one month
Kountz (US, 1978)	120 mg/dy − 30 mg at one month
Traeger (France, 1978)	1 mg prednisolone/kg/dy tapered
Morris (UK, 1978)	100 mg prednisolone reduced by 5 mg every 5 dys to 20 mg
McGeown (UK, 1968)	20 mg/dy from day following transplantation

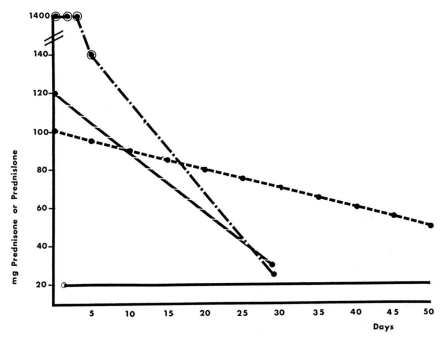

Figure 44. Initial steroid dose used.

minutes leading to peak serum levels within one to two hours. When prednisolone is taken with food there is reduction in gastric irritation and the delay
in absorption is not significant. Enteric coated prednisolone tablets were
introduced to avoid irritation of gastric mucosa, but absorption has been
shown to be less predictable, with lower but more prolonged peak levels.
The enteric coated tablets are available in 2.5 and 5 mg strengths and cannot
be divided.

We advise the standard rather than the enteric coated preparation. The
prescribing doctor must be aware of the difference in pharmacokinetics
between the standard and the enteric coated formulations as the following
case history illustrates:

Mrs. F. complained of indigestion to her general practitioner who then
prescribed enteric coated prednisolone. She did not understand the instructions and changed from taking two 5.0 mg standard formulation tablets to
two 2.5 mg enteric coated tablets. This was discovered at routine review
some months later. She agreed to have tests which showed considerably
delayed absorption of prednisolone (Figure 45) and more marked adrenal
suppression than other patients despite taking only half the dose (Figure 46).
Where duration of therapy and dose are equal the interval between the
doses inversely relates to the degree of adrenal suppression. The delayed
absorption resulting from enteric coating appears to have the same effect as
a frequent dosing regimen.

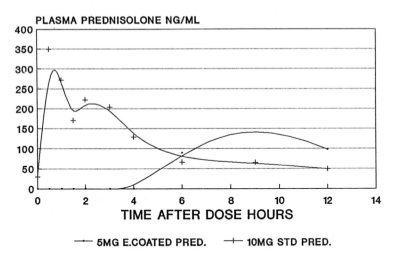

PLASMA PREDNISOLONE
AFTER ORAL PREDNISOLONE

Figure 45. Plasma prednisolone concentrations in two patients following oral prednisolone taken in standard or enteric coated tablets.

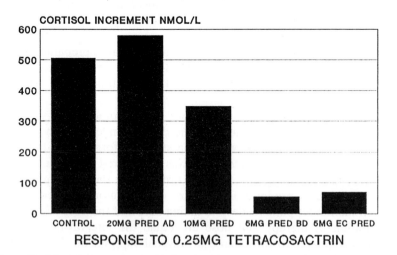

ADRENAL RESPONSE
TO ACTH

Figure 46. Adrenal suppression in relation to maintenance steroid dosing interval: AD = alternate days, BD = twice daily, EC = enteric coated tablets.

3.3. *Anti-rejection therapy*

Large doses of steroid are used, given either orally or intravenously. Some centres give 0.5–1.0 g methylprednisolone intravenously, repeated up to three times at 24 hour intervals. We prefer the oral route and have found that oral administration of prednisolone in dosage commencing at 200 mg/dy in divided doses, repeated for two or three days, depending on response, followed by a reducing dose through 150, 100, 75, 50 back to our usual early maintenance dose of 20 mg/dy (Table 36) will abort the majority of rejection episodes. Patients with any history of dyspepsia are given a course of H_2 antagonist. Many centres give additional anti-rejection therapy in the form of antilymphocyte serum (ALG) or monoclonal antibody (OKT3). ALG has been used recently in Belfast with success for steroid resistant rejection. We gave a single intravenous dose of actinomycin C until 1972 after which it became unobtainable.

Table 36. Anti-rejection therapy used in Belfast

Drug	Dose (mg)	Duration
Prednisolone (oral)	$200 \rightarrow 150 \rightarrow 100 \rightarrow 75 \rightarrow 50 \rightarrow 20$	2 or 3 dys at each dose
Azathioprine (oral)	1968–1974: double dose 1974 onwards: usual dose	5 dys only, continued at usual dose

4. Antilymphocyte serum

By the middle of the sixties attempts to produce a more specific immunosuppressive agent were made by Woodruff in Edinburgh and Starzl in the United States. Many of the cells which infiltrate rejecting grafts are small lymphocytes and they succeeded in producing an antiserum in horses to human peripheral blood lymphocytes. The antiserum (ALG) was effective in transplantation in dogs but was somewhat disappointing in man, where it proved less effective and serious allergic reactions occurred.

Many attempts have been made to produce better antisera. It has been purified to contain only antilymphocyte globulin. The use of splenic, or better, thymic lymphocytes or cultured lymphoblasts led to purer more potent sera. Horse serum often produces reactions in man so smaller animals, such as goats or rabbits, are preferred but their use greatly increases the cost of the serum. Each batch of serum must be standardized and its effectiveness can only be tested in primates.

The best way to use ALG is still unclear, whether to cover the early post-operative period or to use it to treat rejection episodes, and it must be used in combination with other immunosuppressive drugs. It has been widely used in America and in Europe, but relatively less in Britain. The use of ALG may be associated with a high mortality from opportunistic infections such as CMV, pneumocystis carinii and toxoplasmosis. Rubin in Boston, a world expert on infection, attributes the high death rate in transplant patients to ALG rather than steroid and azathioprine. He considers that the addition of ALG greatly enhances the later risk of malignant neoplasms in immunosuppressed patients.

5. Cyclophosphamide

Cyclophosphamide is another cytotoxic agent which was used for transplantation in Leeds early in the 1960s. It is a very toxic drug with many side effects many of which are very unpleasant for the patient, including nausea (often severe), hair loss, and haematuria from bladder irritation. It produces leucopenia and the dose needs very careful control, the main reason why it was soon abandoned. It causes amenorrhoea and depression of spermatogenesis and, finally, it is likely to lead to neoplasia in prolonged usage. More recently it has been used for short periods for treatment of rejection, along with cyclosporin.

Despite the use of azathioprine combined with high dose steroid and sometimes ALG, renal transplant survival remained disappointingly low, one year graft survival rates being less than 50% in many centres even as late as the end of the 1970s. Many attempts were made to improve graft survival by pre-treatment of the recipient before transplantation (Table 32), using protocols of which the aim was to deplete the body store of small lymphocytes.

6. Splenectomy

Rejecting grafts are heavily infiltrated with cells and it was thought that removal of the spleen would reduce lymphoid mass and perhaps also allow greater tolerance to immunosuppressive drugs. Splenectomy was practised in some American centres with varying success, some finding no improvement in graft survival rate in splenectomized patients and others that there was a much lower rejection rate in recipients splenectomized before the transplant than in those not splenectomized or splenectomized later. Some centres claimed that it was particularly helpful in black patients where the results of renal transplantation were usually worse than in white recipients. However, in Newcastle-upon-Tyne, a comparison of the results of transplantation in splenectomized patients with those retaining their spleens did not show any advantage for splenectomy and there was a greater mortality from infection in the splenectomized. Leucopenia was as common in the splenectomized as in the non-splenectomized patients and, when it occurred, was very dangerous – 12 out of 14 such patients died. It was later shown that in non-transplant patients splenectomy increases susceptibility to infection, especially to the pneumococcus, and also predisposes to deep venous thrombosis.

7. Thymectomy

Thymectomy was used by Starzl in Denver during the middle 1960s in the hope that the recipient would become depleted of B lymphocytes. There was a high mortality, it was never widely used and was soon abandoned.

8. Thoracic duct drainage

Another method of depleting the body of small lymphocyles was thoracic duct drainage. The thoracic duct was cannulated and the effluent collected, and after the cellular content was removed the fluid was re-infused into the patient. This certainly depleted the patients of lymphocytes but the effect was short lived. It could only be used when the date for transplantation was already fixed (for a living related donor transplant or when a poorly matched graft was acceptable). There were technical difficulties in keeping the drainage tube patent, and there was a high risk of serious infection. This treatment was always combined with azathioprine, high dose steroid and usually ALG. Traeger and his colleagues in Lyon seem to have used it extensively but it was never widely used. Fish reported in 1983 that in spite of six weeks of thoracic drainage, 14 of 21 grafts developed hyperacute or acute rejection.

9. Bilateral nephrectomy

Bilateral nephrectomy was used as a preparation for renal transplantation almost routinely in many centres, including Belfast up to the end of the 1970s. It was thought that removal of the recipient's own kidneys might help in preventing post-operative infection in patients whose renal tract was infected or potentially the site of infection. It was thought that it might prevent recurrence of the original renal disease, which it does not. It does, however, reduce the incidence of hypertension requiring therapy after successful transplantation. It also removes a potential site of neoplasia, especially if the kidneys are cystic. Michielsen (1992) continues to advocate bilateral nephrectomy for patients whose blood pressure is not controlled by volume depletion and ACE inhibitor. Bilateral nephrectomy is discussed in more detail in Chapter 6.

10. Blood transfusion

Since 1968 when Dossetor showed that graft survival was improved in transfused dogs compared to non-transfused animals, blood transfusion has played an interesting and changing role in renal transplantation. In 1969, several centres found cytotoxic antibodies in patients who had been transfused. Since it is much more difficult to find donors for recipients with antibodies, especially if present in high titre to common HLA antigens, many renal units adopted a non-transfusion policy for their patients on haemodialysis awaiting transplantation. Over the next few years the results of renal transplantation, far from improving, grew worse.

In 1973 Opelz and Terasaki published the results of a large study in the United States in which they found improved graft survival in recipients who had previously been transfused. There was criticism of their study, which was multicentre and lacked validation of the transfusion history of the patients. However, it was noted that the survival of grafts had become less good since the introduction of the non-transfusion policy in renal units. Improved graft survival was demonstrated in transfused dogs and rhesus monkeys (1976–1978). Gradually studies appeared with well-documented transfusion histories some of which, but not all, showed that graft survival was better in the transfused recipients.

There was no evidence to show how blood transfusion worked, but it was suggested that it produced "enhancing" antibodies. There has been no convincing demonstration of these. It was not clear at first which component of blood was responsible for the beneficial effect, but eventually the evidence pointed to the white cells, which were absent from frozen blood and blood freed of the buffy coat. Persijn in Leiden found that even one unit of blood transfused many years previously was sufficient for benefit, but most of the centres which adopted a deliberate policy of transfusing patients before transplantation gave several units of blood. Opelz produced evidence that very large numbers of transfusions (over 20) were more helpful than a few.

The question of when the transfusion should be given was investigated. Obviously when the recipient was awaiting a cadaver graft the interval between transfusion and operation could not be determined in advance, but a time between three months and about three weeks came to be thought optimum. It was then suggested that blood given during surgery was sufficient to produce the benefit, but the evidence for this was not strong.

Undoubtedly in some patients blood transfusion was followed by the formation of cytotoxic antibodies (Chapter 9). It was only after many epidemiological studies that it was accepted that the formation of antibodies was more likely to occur in female recipients who had borne children, especially if multiparous, in previously transfused males or in patients of both sexes who had previously had a graft which had failed. It was shown that about 15 to 18% of patients developed antibodies after their first transfusion and that, in these patients, the titre increased with further transfusion. However, in some patients the titre fell again as the interval after the last transfusion increased.

It should be remembered at this point, in view of the controversy which arose later about the value of blood transfusion in cyclosporin A (CYA) treated recipients, that the evidence cited for benefit from blood transfusion in human transplantation came from recipients treated with azathioprine and steroid as their main immunosuppression. However, a comprehensive study of the effect of transfusion on graft survival (in 1990), which included more recent patients treated with CYA, concluded that one-year graft survival rates were 5–8% higher for transfused patients transplanted for each year between 1982 and 1987. Transplants performed in 1988 and 1989 showed 3% improvement with transfusions. Transfusions decreased the risk and apparent severity of early rejection episodes. Moreover, this effect was more marked in recipients who received mismatched grafts. It was more marked in Asians (7%) than in Blacks (6%) and least in Whites (4%). However there has been a change in transfusion policy in some units and a recent UK survey (1991) reported that 59% of units did not give elective transfusions before transplantation. Of those which still give elective transfusions 62% restrict them to non-sensitized men and non-parous women awaiting first grafts. All the above investigations related to random third party transfusions, i.e. blood not HLA typed.

10.1. *Donor specific transfusion*

In the late 1970s in San Francisco, Salviterria reported a test that appeared to be of value in predicting the results of living related kidney donation. He reported that, when the patient had shown a positive response in the mixed lymphocyte test (MLT), it was possible to predict whether the kidney would be rejected by testing the response to repeated small transfusions of the proposed donor's blood, donor specific transfusion (DST). If the patient did not form antibodies, graft survival was almost 100% and about two-thirds of patients did not form antibodies. In the remainder of patients who did form antibodies, if the transplant was carried out almost all rejected. However, the sensitization was "specific" in the sense that these patients could have a successful graft from another donor. DST became the vogue for living related donation over the next few years, but not all centres found it useful.

11. Local irradiation of the graft

Local irradiation of the graft was used both for early immunosuppression and for the treatment of rejection, especially in America. It was used with azathioprine, large doses of steroid, and often with ALG. There was no convincing evidence of its value. It was well recognised that in the non-transplanted situation the kidney responds to local irradiation by interstitial fibrosis.

12. Subtotal irradiation

Irradiation of the trunk of the recipient, using the inverted Y-shaped field used for treatment of Hodgkin's disease, shortly before transplantation, was introduced by Myerburgh in Johannesburg. This method was piloted in baboons and used at first with azathioprine and steroids, later as part of a pre-treatment protocol with CYA. Many of the patients died of infection and the protocol has not had widespread acceptance in spite of enthusiastic reports from South Africa.

13. Cyclosporin A

Borel in 1970 working in Sandoz Laboratories in Basle, noticed that the effluent of a previously unknown fungus had immunosuppressive properties *in vitro* and in rodents. He eventually reported this in 1978 at a scientific meeting attended by White who works with Calne in Cambridge. They used it for kidney grafts in dogs and heart and liver grafts in pigs and found it to be a very effective immunosuppressive agent in organ transplants. It seemed to have few side effects.

Calne commenced to use CYA for kidney grafts in man in 1978. The doses are now considered huge (first 25 mg/kg/dy, later reduced to 17 mg/kg/dy). He immediately encountered serious side effects. The most unexpected was the nephrotoxicity of CYA. There were many other side effects (Table 37), and Calne reported that CYA is toxic to all cells and is oncogenic.

Table 37. Side effects of cyclosporin A

1. Nephrotoxicity
2. Hypertension
3. Anorexia, nausea
4. Hirsutism
5. Coarsening of features
6. Gum hypertrophy
7. Leucopenia
8. Neurological side effects
9. Infection
10. Breast adenomata
11. Lymphoma
12. Metabolic effects: hyperkalaemia, hyperglycaemia

13.1. *Side effects of CYA*

13.1.1. *Nephrotoxicity.* Calne found that graft function deteriorated when CYA was used even when the graft came from a well matched living related donor. Indeed in some living donor grafts function was very delayed and only commenced after CYA was discontinued. The biopsies of deteriorating grafts did not show the usual appearances of rejection. Vacuoles in tubules and other minor changes were eventually described in the renal biopsies, but these are not now considered characteristic of CYA damage to the kidneys.

The one thing characteristic of CYA nephrotoxicity was that graft function improved when CYA was withdrawn or the dose reduced. It was first thought that the damage was completely reversible, but biopsies taken after only three months of CYA treatment showed interstitial fibrosis, and vascular changes were described in later reports (Chapter 18). CYA was used for immunosuppression for heart transplants (where it proved very effective) and it was found that renal function deteriorated in these patients whose kidneys had been normal or nearly so. On longer follow-up some of the CYA treated heart transplant patients developed end-stage renal failure and required maintenance dialysis.

The dosage of CYA was considerably reduced and it was found that it was better to delay its use until urine was being produced. While the more generalized use of CYA greatly improved the one year graft survival rate in many centres, there were fears that the longer term graft survival might be less good than had been obtained in the best centres using azathioprine and steroid (now called "conventional therapy"). While the development of reliable methods for assay have been useful, toxicity does not always run parallel with blood level. Nephrotoxicity remains a serious problem as it is difficult to distinguish from other causes of early delay or deterioration in graft function (Chapters 17 and 18) and the diagnosis of CYA toxicity is one of exclusion. The longer term follow-up of CYA treated patients already suggests that early toxicity may prejudice the graft's future.

At first CYA was used without other immunosuppressive agents and Calne thought that its great virtue was that patients would be spared the numerous side effects of steroid. However, as the side effects of CYA itself, and the need to reduce the dose were recognized, CYA began to be used with steroid and other agents. Monotherapy, double, triple, quadruple and even quintuple therapy will be described later (Dosage of CYA).

13.1.2. *Hypertension.* All patients treated with CYA develop some elevation of blood pressure. This may be slight and not significant but in many the rise is sufficient to require hypotensive drugs, in some it may be severe. This is the clinical response to the vascular changes found on biopsy of CYA treated grafts (Chapter 18), and may be responsible for the rather disappointing long term results.

13.1.3. *Anorexia and nausea.* When first commenced on CYA almost all patients complain of nausea and lack of appetite. This is ameliorated by giving the drug with milk and it tends to become less with time.

13.1.4. *Hirsutism.* This is very common, occurring in at least 50% of patients, and affects both males and females. The growth of hair may be copious over the limbs and face. It causes great distress to female patients who may need to shave daily.

13.1.5. *Coarsening of features.* While less obvious than overgrowth of facial and limb hair, coarsening of features is fairly common in CYA treated patients and may be very disfiguring in young women. It may lead them to discontinue the treatment or demand that it should be changed.

13.1.6. *Gum hypertrophy.* Hypertrophy of the gums occurs in about 30% of patients taking CYA. This annoying complication has not been abolished by the lower dosage now generally used. It is to some extent related to poor mouth hygiene. Neoplastic change in gum hypertrophy has recently been reported.

13.1.7. *Leucopenia.* A significant fall in white cell count is much less common with CYA treatment than with conventional therapy.

13.1.8. *Infection.* About 30% of patients treated with CYA develop infection during their operative admission. There is a reduced incidence of bacterial and fungal, but not viral infection. With conventional therapy using low dose steroid most of the lethal infections were in the chest. It was recently reported from Manchester which adopted CYA therapy early and has treated a large number of patients, that they have not lost a patient from pneumonitis who had not received steroid during the past eight years. This is a great improvement.

13.1.9. *Neurological side effects.* Neurological side effects occur in about 20% of patients. The commonest are tremor, burning paresthesia of palms and feet, headache, flushing, depression and confusion. Seizures may occur, especially in children.

13.1.10. *Breast adenomata.* One of the side effects noted in Calne's early patients treated with CYA was the occurrence of lumps in the breasts. These patients received much higher doses than would be given to-day. They were not receiving steroid. On biopsy the lumps were found to be benign adenomata. This condition has not been mentioned in recent reports.

13.1.11. *Lymphoma and other malignancies.* Four of Calne's first 32 patients developed lymphoma within the first year and this aroused fear that patients receiving CYA were at high risk of developing malignancy. At the 1990 meeting of the International Transplantation Society, Penn reported for the International Tumour Registry that tumours are developing earlier in transplant patients and that there is a disproportionate rise in the incidence of lymphoma and Kaposi's sarcoma. He suggested that the changing pattern of malignancy may be due to over-immunosuppression, implicating the triple, quadruple and quintuple regimens.

13.1.12. *Metabolic effects.* Hyperkalaemia is fairly common and requires vigilance during early treatment. Hyperglycaemia without ketosis occurs occasionally, which may be due to impaired hepatic synthesis of glycogen.

13.2. *Assay of CYA*

When CYA was first used an assay was not available. When one was devised there was considerable uncertainty as to whether it should be carried out on serum, separated red cells or whole blood. It is now accepted that the whole blood level should be measured and that it is best to use the trough level, i.e. blood withdrawn before the morning dose is given.

At first it was thought that the therapeutic range lay between 400 and 800 ng/ml, but the desirable level has been reduced progressively and is now considered to be between 150 and 250 ng/ml. The target level differs if the assay method measures metabolites as well as parent compound.

13.3. *CYA protocols*

At first CYA was used alone in high dosage and this led to the discovery of the toxic side effects already described. As attempts were made to use lower doses, it was found that rejection frequently occurred and other immunosuppressive agents were added, in the hope of retaining the improved graft survival (obtained by most centres with CYA after the "learning curve") while reducing the undesirable side effects. CYA is used in different ways in different centres and may be used either alone or in combination with other immunosuppressive regimens. The main treatment combinations are shown in Table 38, but within these there are a considerable number of variables. Many centres have changed their protocols repeatedly and comparisons were made between small groups of patients. The protocols shown in Table 38 all have been used for prophylaxis, but sometimes first steroid and then other agents are added after rejection occurs and fails to be controlled.

It is common practice to reduce the dose of CYA after 6 to 12 months after transplantation. Borel believes that this may allow chronic rejection to occur.

Table 38. CYA protocols

---

1. CYA monotherapy from transplantation
2. CYA monotherapy after graft functions (sequential therapy)
3. CYA with steroid   1. *ab initio*
                      2. for rejection
4. CYA with/without steroid, converted to conventional therapy
5. CYA with steroid and azathioprine (triple therapy)
6. CYA with steroid, azathioprine and ALG (quadruple therapy)
7. CYA with steroid, azathioprine, ALG and monoclonal antibody (quintuple therapy)

13.3.1. & 2. *CYA monotherapy.* One great difference between CYA and conventional therapy is the importance of early function of the graft. Using azathioprine and low dose steroid, we obtained one year graft function of over 80% in spite of the fact that graft function was delayed for a week or more in almost 100%. When CYA is given before the graft is producing urine the graft may not begin to function for a prolonged period and this early toxicity seems to be prejudicial to its longer term welfare. For this reason many centres do not commence CYA until the graft produces urine and give azathioprine and steroid for the initial immunosuppression. Some centres, particularly in the US give ALG as well as azathioprine and steroid, replacing the ALG with CYA once good graft function is established. Both of these protocols are sometimes described as sequential therapy.

When rejection occurs in a patient receiving CYA monotherapy, steroid is given, either as a short course intravenously or more often continued indefinitely. Such a patient may still be counted as receiving CYA monotherapy, as it was the intention to treat by monotherapy.

13.3.3. *CYA with steroid.* A great advantage of CYA is that some patients can be spared steroid therapy, which is particularly helpful for children, diabetics and older patients. There have been several randomised trials (containing relatively small numbers of patients) which have not shown advantage for steroid treatment unless rejection occurs. However, many centres give steroid from the beginning, sometimes in quite high dosage especially for the first week, while others add steroid for control of rejection, which may or may not be discontinued later. At least 25% of patients for whom CYA monotherapy was planned end up taking steroid. Some believe that steroid has some protective effect against nephrotoxicity, while others think that the immunosuppression is better with steroid and it is possible to use less CYA.

13.3.4. *CYA with/without steroid, converted to conventional therapy.* Conversion from CYA to conventional therapy may be carried out for a variety of reasons. It is done most often for nephrotoxicity, but sometimes because patients find other side effects intolerable. The high cost of CYA may make it necessary when the patient must pay for it. Conversion may be carried out when the need arises, but some centres change the treatment electively. The time at which this is done varies. It probably should not be before three months and is better done after six to 12 months. There is risk of rejection while the change is being made and the conversion should be gradual with overlap between the protocols.

13.3.5. *Triple therapy*. Relatively small doses of CYA, azathioprine and steroid are combined in triple therapy. The CYA is not given until after the graft has begun to produce urine. Typical doses may be CYA 8–10 mg/kg with azathioprine 1 mg/kg and prednisolone 15–20 mg.

Triple therapy has been used most in North America. Morris reports that while triple therapy is simple to use and other side effects are minimal, nephrotoxicity still occurs and graft survival is not better.

13.3.6. & 7. *Quadruple therapy and quintuple therapy*. The addition of ALG to CYA, steroid and azathioprine has been described by Morris as using a sledge-hammer to crack a nut. A high incidence of serious infection has been reported. The high risk to the patient from infection and later malignancy seem good reasons for avoiding this blunderbuss therapy. The addition of monoclonal antibody to this cocktail does not seem to have anything to recommend it. Those who are prepared to use such potent immunosuppression seem to have lost sight of the fact the survival of the recipient is more important than that of the graft.

13.4. *Treatment of rejection during CYA therapy*

Although the introduction of CYA therapy has led to improved graft survival in most centres, about 75% of grafts have at least one rejection. Rejection occurring while on CYA therapy may be treated in different ways (Table 39).

Table 39. Treatment of rejection while on CYA

1. Steroid
2. Steroid and azathioprine
3. Steroid and ALG
4. Steroid and monoclonal antibody

13.4.1. *Steroid*. Many centres begin with a short course of intravenous methylprednisolone, e.g., 0.5–1.0 g daily for up to three days. If graft function improves oral prednisolone in doses of 15–20 mg daily are continued along with CYA.

13.4.2. *Steroid and azathioprine.* If the addition of steroid alone fails to abort the rejection, in many centres the next option is to add a small dose of azathioprine. The patient is now receiving triple therapy.

13.4.3. *Change to conventional therapy.* When triple therapy fails to abort rejection the dose of azathioprine may be increased and CYA gradually withdrawn. This sometimes succeeds when the first two measures have failed. Usually the patient would then remain on conventional therapy.

13.4.4. *Steroid and ALG.* Some centres, especially in America, give both steroid and ALG for treatment of rejection. Since many rejections respond to steroid alone, the addition of ALG may be just another hazard for the patient, but the case for giving it is better if steroid alone has been tried already. In other centres ATG (or OKT3) is given after failure to respond to steroid, without further additional steroid.

13.4.5. *Steroid and monoclonal antibody.* A monoclonal antibody, such as OKT3, is given usually only after ALG has been tried and failed. The risk of infection becomes much greater when ALG and OKT3 or other monoclonal is given, and one needs to be very certain that the condition being treated is rejection and not nephrotoxicity. However, Morris claims that 80% of steroid resistant rejections are reversed by OKT3 treatment.

13.4.6. The use of CYA has led to a worthwhile increase in early graft survival. This is due mainly to improved patient survival which can be attributed to reduction in infection. The reduction in the amount of steroid given contributes importantly to the reduction in infection. The advantages of low dosage of steroid, including improved patient survival, were reported from Belfast before the introduction of CYA.

14. Monoclonal antibodies

Monoclonal antibodies are essentially more specific forms of antilymphocyte globulin. Those most used have been OKT8, OKT3 and very recently OKT4 and Campath 1. In a small number of patients treated with conventional therapy OKT8 and OKT3 were used for treatment of steroid and, usually, ALG resistant rejection. The early patients had severe generalized reactions. Rejection was sometimes reversed but life-threatening infection and even death was common.

OKT3 is sometimes used in patients treated with CYA where other methods of antirejection treatment have failed. It may succeed after failure with ALG. It is claimed that there is a higher rate of re-rejection after OKT3 than after ALG. This may simply reflect the fact that only the most resistant rejection episodes are treated with OKT3. Good early results with OKT4 have been reported from Lyon.

15. Plasma exchange

Plasma exchange has been used for treatment of steroid resistant rejection, especially if the graft biopsy shows vascular involvement. We have had modest success with this treatment. It has been used occasionally when an ABO incompatible graft has been transplanted inadvertently, and also in preparation of highly sensitized patients for transplantation.

16. FK 506; rapamycin

It is claimed that FK 506 and rapamycin are 50 to 100 times more potent immunosuppressive agents than CYA. They have been found to be highly toxic in primates and in dogs, but do not seem to be nephrotoxic. They have been tested for organ transplants in animals in Cambridge, Pittsburgh and Japan. At the time of writing they have been used for liver transplantation in man, with success, but not yet for renal transplantation.

FK 506 acts similarly to CYA and should not be combined with it. Rapamycin shares the same binding protein as FK 506, but acts differently. It can be combined with FK 506 but steroid should not be given with it.

17. Immunosuppression in Belfast

When renal transplantation was commenced in Belfast in 1968 much thought was devoted to the immunosuppression regimen to be used. At that period azathioprine with high dose steroid was used universally. It was sometimes combined with ALG and one or other of the methods already described. None of the patients from Belfast who had received successful grafts in London or Cambridge had received ALG, showing that it was not essential. We therefore decided to use azathioprine with steroid.

The dose of azathioprine chosen was that used in St. Mary's Hospital in London – I had already used this without encountering any serious problems. The dose of steroid to be used was more difficult. I had of course experience with the use of steroids in the treatment of the nephrotic syndrome and other diseases. I became impressed by their side effects.

It should be borne in mind that as well as receiving azathioprine and steroid, the patients were transfused. Before 1975 almost all underwent bilateral nephrectomy. Thereafter, only selected patients with severe uncontrolled hypertension, polycystic disease, reflux nephropathy or stone disease as the cause of their renal failure had bilateral nephrectomy.

17.1. *Initial immunosuppression*

The first dose of the immunosuppressive drugs is given intravenously in theatre, as soon as possible after the intravenous infusion is set up. It consists of hydrocortisone 200 mg and azathioprine 5 mg/kg body weight. During the first 24 hours after surgery three further doses of hydrocortisone 200 mg are given intravenously at intervals of six hours, the second dose being given six hours after the dose in theatre.

On the day following transplantation the drugs can almost always be given by the oral route. The dose of azathioprine is 1.5 mg/kg body weight, which is continued until graft function is established and the creatinine clearance reaches 30 ml/min.

The dose of prednisolone is 20 mg daily, except for small recipients (below 35 kg) when the dose is reduced to 15 mg. Prednisolone is increased if rejection is diagnosed. The diagnosis of rejection is discussed in Chapters 16 and 17.

17.2. *Anti-rejection therapy*

Prednisolone for treatment of rejection is often given intravenously as methylprednisolone 0.5 or 1.0 gm, repeated two or three times at intervals of 24 hrs. There have been occasional reports of sudden death, thus the drug must be given very slowly. Controlled trials have not shown advantage from the higher dose. In Belfast only a small number of patients have received intravenous methylprednisolone because we observed that rejection often recurred and then responded to a more protracted course of oral prednisolone. The oral course of prednisolone for anti-rejection is shown in Table 5.

17.3. *Maintenance therapy*

Azathioprine is continued at 3.0 mg/kg unless the white count falls to $4000 \times e9/1$, when it is withheld for a few days, then commenced at a lower dose depending on the trough white cell count. The majority of patients tolerate 2.5–3.0 mg/kg, but occasional patients can sustain a satisfactory white cell level only on very low doses. One such patient was changed to CYA 10 days after transplantation, during which he received only prednisolone 20 mg daily following the initial single dose of azathioprine. He has never had a rejection episode and the graft continues to function well more than six years later. Other similar patients with intolerance to azathioprine have been changed to CYA.

The dose of 20 mg of prednisolone is gradually reduced after three months of stable function, after some 15 months to 10 mg daily. In patients with excessive weight gain uncontrolled by diet, severe acne, a florid appearance or difficult to control hypertension, it is often helpful to change the steroid to double the daily dose, given on alternate days. The importance of doing this with care has been emphasised already.

17.4. *CYA protocol used in Belfast*

When it was decided to use CYA as routine immunosuppressive therapy it was recognised that CYA monotherapy was unlikely to be suitable for all patients. Patients are classified in advance of transplantation into three categories, for each of which there are detailed protocols. It is hoped that this will avoid haphazard changes of drugs.

17.4.1. *Standard patients*. This group excludes recipients with increased immunological risk and patients who have been selected for CYA monotherapy. A form of "sequential therapy" is used.

17.4.2. *Patients at increased immunological risk*. This group includes patients who are highly sensitized with over 50% antibodies (Chapter 9) and patients awaiting a second or later graft. Patients for whom it is particularly difficult to find a well-matched kidney because of rare tissue type might also be included. Triple therapy is used.

17.4.3. *Patients selected for monotherapy*. This group includes children under the age of 15, patients older than 60 years, patients with osteoporosis and some diabetics. These patients receive sequential therapy followed by withdrawal of steroid.

17.4.4. *Sequential therapy as used in Belfast*. Treatment commences as described already as initial therapy for conventional immunosuppression (methylprednisolone 800 mg intravenously as four doses of 200 mg at six hour intervals and a single dose of azathioprine 5 mg/kg). From the day following operation azathioprine 1.5 mg/kg and prednisolone 20 mg are given orally. This is continued until the creatinine clearance exceeds 30 ml/min, and azathioprine has been increased to 3.0 mg/kg (unless the white cell count falls to less than $4000 \times e9/1$). When graft function is judged to be good (i.e. falling serum and creatinine clearance) CYA is added at 10 mg/kg. The daily dose of CYA is given divided into two doses, in milk in a ceramic cup (CYA is inactivated by plasticizers in plastic). The aim is to achieve a CYA blood level of between 150 and 250 ng/ml. When this is attained the azathioprine is reduced progressively at the rate of 1 mg/kg per week, and then discontinued.

17.4.5. *Monotherapy as used in Belfast*. Treatment is commenced as for sequential therapy. When graft function is judged to be stable, usually at about one month after surgery, the dose of prednisolone is reduced by 2.5 mg every two weeks to 10 mg daily at about three months. During this time the prednisolone may be changed to double dose on alternate days. The prednisolone is then withdrawn by 2.5 mg decrements at monthly intervals until the dose reaches zero. There is an increased risk of rejection during steroid withdrawal and the patient should be seen at least once weekly.

17.4.6. *Triple therapy as used in Belfast.* Intravenous azathioprine and hydrocortisone followed by oral azathioprine and prednisolone are given as usual. CYA is given either orally as 3 mg/kg before operation followed by 3 mg/kg 12 hours later (6 mg/kg over first 24 hours) *or* intravenously as 2.5 mg/kg in 100 ml normal saline commenced in theatre and given over four hours. A second similar infusion of 2.5 mg/kg is commenced 12 hours later (total dose over first 24 hours 5 mg/kg).

Maintenance triple therapy continues with prednisolone 20 mg daily, azathioprine 1.5 mg/kg daily and CYA 5 mg/kg, all given orally. When renal function seems established and improving the dose of CYA is gradually increased to achieve a blood level of 150–250 ng/ml.

17.5. *Treatment of acute rejection when on CYA therapy*

Rejection is treated as described for rejection on conventional therapy, by increase of the oral dose of prednisolone to 200 mg (divided into four doses) daily, and reducing the dose stepwise back to the maintenance dose of 20 mg daily (Table 5). Patients with a history of dyspepsia, proven duodenal ulcer or hiatus hernia are given prophylactic ranitidine or cimetidine during anti-rejection therapy. Recently in a few patients severe steroid resistant rejection has been treated successfully with ALG.

17.6. *Maintenance prednisolone*

Whichever CYA protocol is chosen for the individual recipient, the original maintenance dose of prednisolone is gradually reduced by 2.5 mg daily to reach a dose of 10 mg daily at three months. In patients selected to have CYA monotherapy, steroid is withdrawn as already described under Monotherapy.

18. Immunosuppressive therapy for children as used in Belfast

Paediatric recipients are given an immunosuppressive regime, suitably scaled down, similar to that given to adults. Until 1990 they received azathioprine and steroid only, following the protocol for adults already described. Since 1990 azathioprine and steroid have been used as before for induction and during the early post-transplant period, until stable graft function is established. CYA is then added, and azathioprine is withdrawn, with an overlap period, and the dose of steroid is progressively reduced. The aim is to use CYA monotherapy, but this is usually achieved only in children without rejection episodes. The dose of CYA given is tailored for the individual child to give blood levels within the therapeutic range. The protocol for immunosuppressive therapy used for children is given in the Appendix to this Chapter.

Blood levels of CYA tend to fluctuate more in children than in adults. It has been found helpful to give the daily dose divided into three aliquots. Fluctuating blood levels tend to be more troublesome in those children who do not have regular once or twice daily bowel motions (Savage, personal communication).

19. Appendix. Immunosuppressive therapy for children as used in Belfast

19.1. *Admission protocol*

19.1.1. On admission for a possible kidney transplant information on the following points must be recorded in the case notes:
1. 24 hour urinary output; residual renal function
2. presence of recent infections, e.g. peritonitis, urinary tract infection
3. any recent contact with children or adults with infectious disease
4. type of dialysis therapy and usual protocol
5. drug therapy – antihypertensive, anti-epileptic drugs
6. height and weight
7. state of nutrition and hydration
8. blood pressure
9. condition of catheter exit site, or arterio-venous fistula

19.1.2. Investigations required on admission:
1. 10 ml clotted blood required by Tissue Typing Laboratory
2. full blood count including platelets
3. serum urea, electrolytes and total protein
4. repeat blood group and four units of blood to be cross-matched
5. if treated by CAPD, culture peritoneal fluid
6. chest X-ray

19.2. Consent for operation must be obtained in writing from a parent or guardian. If they do not have it already the parents should be given the booklet on kidney transplantation.

19.3.1. Haemodialysis may be required before operation.

19.3.2. The anaesthetist should be consulted about any anti-hypertensive or anti-epileptic drug doses due.

19.3.3. An intravenous infusion of 5% dextrose should be set up to run at minimum rate, before sending the patient to theatre. If the initial examination suggests that the child is hypovolaemic or hypo-albuminaemic the appropriate fluid should be given instead of 5% dextrose.

19.4. *Immunosuppression*

19.4.1. *Intra-operative*: hydrocortisone 5 mg/kg is given intravenously as a stat dose; azathioprine 5 gm/kg intravenously as a stat dose.

19.4.2. *Post-operative 24 hours*: hydrocortisone 5 mg/kg is given intravenously at six hour intervals for four doses. No further azathioprine is given over this period.

19.4.3. *Early post-operative immunosuppression*: provided the white cell count is above $4,000 \times e9/l$, azathioprine is given at a dose of 3 mg/kg/dy until the creatinine clearance has reached 1/3 normal for age, after which it is increased to 3 mg/kg/dy.

From the end of the first 24 hours prednisolone is given orally in a dose of 1 mg/kg/dy (or the equivalent dose of hydrocortisone – 4 mg/kg divided into two doses intravenously). This continued for five days. The dose of prednisolone is then reduced to 0.5 mg/kg given as a single morning dose.

After one month the dose of prednisolone is changed to 1 mg/kg on alternate mornings.

19.4.4. Once graft function is stable, CYA is added orally at 9 mg/kg/dy, divided into three doses. The dose will require to be adjusted according to blood levels, the therapeutic (trough, i.e. before the morning dose) level being 100–200 ng/ml. When the level of CYA is stable azathioprine is gradually withdrawn.

19.5. In the early post-operative period the child will have the following tubes *in situ*:
  1. multiple lumen central venous catheter, to be used for measurement of central venous pressure, intravenous fluids and analgesia
  2. arterial catheter for recording of blood pressure
  3. urethral catheter.

19.6. *Analgesia*

A morphine infusion at 10–20 mg/hr is given at a rate sufficient to control pain, but care must be taken to avoid causing respiratory depression.

19.7. *Common problems of the post-operative period*

19.7.1. *Hypertension* is common during the immediate post-operative period and is best managed by the appropriate dose of hydralazine or labetalol given intravenously. Check for volume expansion.

19.7.2. *Low urinary output* necessitates checking the vital signs, and correcting fluid intake, *etc.*, as necessary. One dose of frusemide (2 mg/kg) may be given intravenously. Haematuria associated with a low urinary output suggests renal vein thrombosis.

19.7.3. *Hypotension* may require volume expansion (check the CVP and urinary output). Check for blood loss, and its source. Check whether hydralazine or frusemide has been given recently; if so omit the next planned dose. If dopamine is being given the rate may need to be increased, or it may be commenced.

Conclusion

CYA is undoubtedly a good immunosuppression agent but needs to be used with caution. There are many possible combinations of CYA and other immunosuppressive agents. Ideally the treatment should be chosen to suit the individual patient, with the objective of minimizing immunosuppression, especially the amount of steroids given. The logistics of tailoring immunosuppression for each patient in a busy unit are formidable. The method of triage already described is one way of addressing this problem.

All potent methods of immunosuppression have numerous and often dangerous side effects. It is important to remember that the patient is more important than the graft. The patient should live to have another transplant. There should be very careful investigation of declining graft function, before giving additional potent immunosuppressive therapy for what may prove to be a mistaken diagnosis of rejection.

Further reading

Kahan, B. D. Cyclosporine. *New Engl. J. Med.* 1989; 321: 1725–1738.

McGeown, M. G. *Clinical renal transplantation and immunosuppression.* In Salaman, J. R. ed. Lancaster, MTP Press; 1981: 143–176.

Salaman, J. R. Cyclosporin monotherapy – who needs it? *Clin and Experiment. Perspectives in Sandimmun Therapy* 1991; 1: 1–3.

CHAPTER 16

Nursing care of the patient with a renal transplant

MARY G. McGEOWN

The nurse plays an important part in the management of all stages of chronic renal failure.

Chronic renal failure, once established persists for the remainder of the patient's life and may need to be treated in different ways at different times. In the early stages control of diet, and treatment of hypertension if needed, may be sufficient to keep the patient feeling reasonably well and at work, but as renal function continues to decline a plan for the future needs to be made. This plan may include a renal transplant at some time, usually after a period of some form of dialysis treatment. The patient must be made aware that the transplant may not succeed, or may fail after months or years of good function and dialysis may become necessary again (Figure 47). The patient needs to be informed that there are different types of dialysis and understand the reasons why one type may be suitable for the present but another may be better as circumstances change over a longer period of time. In planning it is important to preserve blood vessels which may be needed in the future for haemodialysis. The object is to restore reasonable health with as little disturbance to ordinary existence as possible and the initial choice of treatment may need to be changed with time in pursuit of this goal.

The renal team includes doctors, nurses, technicians, artificial kidney assistants, the pharmacist and the social worker as well as secretaries and transplant co-ordinators all working together for the treatment and support of the patient. Ideally the same staff should continue to look after the patients as they progress through different modalities of treatment, but this is often not possible.

The role of the nurse is not confined to the physical care of the patient. It includes psychological support, counselling and education about the nature of the illness and its treatment.

1. Nursing care in the immediate post-operative period

In the Belfast Unit after transplantation patients are nursed in protective isolation until sutures, drains and catheter are removed. The patient has a single room and toilet with positive pressure ventilation. All nursing and

Mary G. McGeown (ed.), Clinical Management of Renal Transplantation, 231–241.
© 1992 *Kluwer Academic Publishers, Dordrecht. Printed in the Netherlands.*

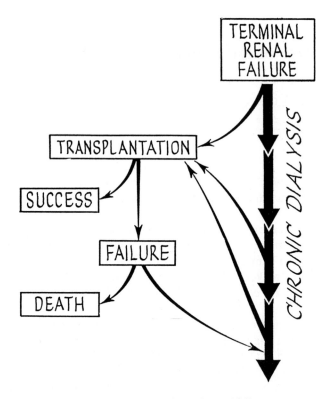

Figure 47. Treatment of chronic renal failure.

medical care comes to the patient from the inner clean corridor and used materials of every sort are discharged through a pass-through to the outer corridor (Chapter 1). If dialysis is required it is carried out in the patient's room. Visitors are not admitted to the room until the period of isolation is ended. They are able to see and talk to the patient through a plastic panel in the outer door. An exception is made for young children, whose parents are admitted wearing gown and overshoes. Protective isolation and its purpose of prevention of infection has been fully explained before going "on-call" for a kidney, and again before admission for operation. The period of isolation may be difficult for some patients to accept, but very frequent visits from the nurses and the instruction given about all aspects of the treatment helps it to be accepted, usually quite willingly.

Nursing care is very similar to that following any major operation. Important points are summarized in Table 40.

1.1. *Vital signs*

On return from theatre monitoring and recording of pulse, blood pressure, temperature and respiration rate are commenced at intervals of 15 minutes

Table 40. Immediate post-operative care

1. Vital signs and CVP monitoring
2. Fluid and electrolyte balance and prevention of uraemia
3. Management of the wound and post-operative pain
4. Administration of immunosupppressive drugs and monitoring side effects
5. Observing and monitoring for early signs of rejection
6. Nursing the patient in isolation
7. Advice on discharge

for the first hour, 30 minutes for the next two hours, then hourly for four hours and two hourly for six hours, the interval continuing to be lengthened provided the patient's condition does not give cause for special concern.

1.1.1. *Blood pressure.* The blood pressure is often mildly elevated in the immediate post-operative period, probably because replacement of blood and fluid losses during operation tend to be generous. If the blood pressure falls significantly the grafted kidney may be at risk of acute tubular necrosis, or vascular thrombosis. The significance of any fall in blood pressure obviously depends on the previous level but a fall of more than 10 mm Hg may be significant, and a cause should be sought, remedied if found, and if none is found the frequency of recording should be increased until it becomes stable at a satisfactory level. One potent cause of hypotension apart from haemorrhage and hypovolaemia, is excessive administration of analgesia.

1.1.2. *Pulse.* A fast pulse rate needs an explanation, and may indicate haemorrhage, shock or pain. An irregular pulse should be reported to the medical staff. Many older patients, and those suffering from diabetes mellitus, may have ischaemic heart disease.

1.1.3. *Respiration.* Any change in respiration rate or quality may be a response to shock or pain, which needs to be dealt with. The patient is receiving oxygen by face mask and the nurse is responsible for ensuring that the mask is applied correctly, and that the flow rate and concentration are as prescribed by the doctor.

The patient who is still drowsy and confused will not understand the need for the mask and this must be explained repeatedly to gain co-operation. In patients receiving morphine-based analgesia respiration may become shallow, especially when the analgesia is self-administered by infusion pump. If this happens the dose of analgesia should be reduced.

As soon as the patient is conscious enough to co-operate, breathing exercises are commenced. These are particularly important if the patient has been a smoker. Ideally the patient should have stopped smoking some time ago and been instructed in breathing exercises prior to operation, but this is not always possible.

1.1.4. *Temperature*. A modest pyrexia is common during the first 48 hours after transplantation. It may be an early sign of rejection, but is often present in patients who do not develop other signs of rejection. If the temperature reaches 38°C medical staff should be informed and blood cultures taken. Meantime the patient is made more comfortable by tepid sponging and giving paracetamol.

1.1.5. *Central venous pressure monitor*. This may be used for the first 24–48 hours after transplantation, as an indicator of the hydration status. It is often not necessary but it is particularly helpful in small children. It is not an accurate guide to the need for fluid replacement, and should be used in conjunction with the vital signs as recorded above and the records of urinary output.

When the patient returns to the ward after surgery a chest x-ray is taken to check that the CVP catheter is in the correct position.

The CVP is recorded hourly. The normal range for the CVP is 2–6 mm Hg or 6–10 cm H_2O. If the reading looks inconsistent with previous readings it should be repeated before giving any additional fluids.

The CVP should be measured with the patient in the prone position without pillows. If this is not possible, it is important to ensure that the patient is placed in the same position for each recording. A reference point is marked, using an indelible pencil, on the patient's chest at the mid-axillary line in the 4th/5th intercostal space. The zero point on the manometer scale is aligned with this mark at each reading, which is taken with the observer's eye level with the scale. Before each recording the equipment should be checked for kinks and leaks. The 3-way tap is primed to allow fluid from the intravenous infusion to enter the manometer, and the reading is taken – the figure at which the column of fluid becomes stable, measuring from the zero point. The 3-way tap is then adjusted to allow the fluid in the manometer to flow back into the patient, checking that the intravenous infusion continues to run at the correct rate. The CVP infusion line is usually reserved for this purpose only, being adjusted to run at a rate just sufficient to keep the line patent, but it may be used also to give extra boluses of fluid if needed. At each use the dressing should be checked for bleeding, or discharge, and should be renewed with full aseptic ritual if necessary. If the patient complains of discomfort or pain related to the catheter the dressing should be removed and the wound inspected for discharge and reddening.

The most serious hazard associated with the presence of the CVP catheter is the risk of infection, which in the immunosuppressed patient can rapidly become life threatening. The catheter should be removed as early as possible and is seldom needed longer than 24 hours. Complications other than this are therefore rare.

2. Fluid and electrolyte balance

On return from theatre the patient has a urethral catheter attached to a urinometer bag. The urinary output is recorded hourly. The urine is usually heavily blood-stained and occasionally, especially if the output is low, the catheter may become blocked with clot in which case the patient will usually complain of pain (bladder spasm). A bladder lavage may be needed, with full aseptic technique using sterile water for flushing. This is uncomfortable and the patient needs reassurance that the bladder spasm will be relieved as soon as the catheter is unblocked.

The initial prescription for intravenous fluids assumes that the urinary output may be modest in amount, but it should take into account any output from the patient's own kidneys prior to operation. If substantial quantities of urine are produced the intravenous fluid prescription must be increased accordingly, tailoring it to the previous 12, later 24 hour output. The intravenous fluids are given through a peripheral line, if possible ensuring that the fistula arm is not used for this purpose. Intravenous fluids are usually not necessary after bowel sounds become audible, unless the new kidney produces so much urine that the patient is unable to drink sufficient fluids to keep up with the output.

The patient is always very concerned if the urinary output is low, especially if this continues for more than a day or two. The situation should be discussed frankly with the patient, explaining that it is not unusual for function of the new kidney to be delayed, and that there is good reason to hope that it will do well.

Blood samples are taken each morning for monitoring urea, creatinine, electrolytes, full blood picture and 24 hour creatinine clearance. The laboratory treats as urgent specimens from recently transplanted patients, which enables early decisions about treatment to be made.

A rising serum potassium concentration is particularly important, and if above 6.5 mmol/l requires urgent action. If this occurs during the first 48 hours after surgery an intravenous "cocktail" of dextrose and insulin, sometimes with sodium bicarbonate or calcium chloride, is given to delay the need for dialysis for a short period, during which the urinary output may be improving. If this does not happen quickly enough dialysis, either haemodialysis or CAPD according to the patient's previous method of treatment, will become necessary.

The patient may become very anxious if dialysis should be necessary and may think that the graft has failed. Reassurance is needed that this is a common occurrence at this stage and does not mean that the kidney has failed.

NAME   AGE   WARD   DIET

DRUGS

MEDICAL HISTORY

	Initial Assessment	Date	Comments Concerning Wound Progress	Treatment	Signature
1 Type of wound	Surgical Pressure Other				
2 Location					
3 Area	Reddened Skinned Open				
4 Exudate	None Amount Colour				
5 Pain	Continuous Occasional @ Dressing None				
6 Dimensions	Breadth Length Depth				
7 Tissue	Healthy Sloughing Necrotic				

Figure 48. Wound assessment chart.

3. Care of the wound

It is helpful to use a "Wound assessment chart" on which to assess the progress of wound healing (Figure 48). The findings at the initial assessment are recorded and the type of suture used should be noted under "Comments". The wound is dressed on the day following operation (Day 1) using full aseptic no-touch technique. Provided the dressing appears clean and dry, it is left untouched on succeeding days, but if there is any discharge this should be swabbed, and the specimen marked "urgent", redness or swelling noted and reported. Provided there are no open areas the wound is left exposed from Day 6–7.

Elderly, obese, diabetic or poorly nourished patients are particularly susceptible to wound infections. Patients who receive additional steroid for treatment of rejection are especially vulnerable.

4. Control of post-operative pain

Failure to relieve post-operative pain is not only inhumane, but may delay recovery. Pain is difficult to define and tolerance to it is very variable.

Table 41. Patient control administration of opoid (PCAS)

Recommended drug and concentration	Morphine 1 mg/ml
Recommenced bolus	0.5–2 mg
Recommended lock out interval	20 minutes
Recommended background infusion	Not more than 0.5 mg/hour

Frequent physiotherapy to the chest and limbs is very important for prevention of infection and deep venous thrombosis but pain must be controlled to allow the patient to co-operate fully. Pain control permits better physiotherapy and therefore less lung collapse occurs (some degree of pulmonary collapse follows almost every abdominal surgical procedure – a collapsed area may become infected by inhaled or blood-borne organisms).

The standard management of pain following surgery is the intermittent administration of a fixed dose of an opiate 4–6 hourly intramuscularly. This does not take into account the different responses of different patients to analgesia, nor their different responses to pain.

Recently a method has been introduced of tailoring analgesia to the needs of the individual patient. The patient control administration system (PCAS) allows the patient to titrate the delivery of opiate to achieve the desired degree of analgesia.

The system consists of a syringe containing a dilute solution of analgesic, usually morphine or a derivative of morphine. The syringe is locked into a computerized pump which delivers a pre-set bolus of analgesia when triggered by the patient. The bolus is a small dose of, usually, morphine (0.5–2.0 mg morphine). A "lock-out time" is programmed to prevent too frequent use of the analgesic. This should be sufficiently long to allow the effect of the dose to be appreciated, but short enough to allow the patient to obtain sufficient analgesic for adequate pain relief. There is a continuous background infusion set to deliver not more than 0.5 mg morphine per hour. It is important that the patient does not receive so much opiate that respiration is depressed (Tables 41 and 42). The intravenous cannula used for the PCAS must be reserved for this purpose only and the settings for dose and lock-out time must be prescribed by the anaesthetist.

5. General management

Patients are encouraged to become mobile as early as possible following transplantation. The risks associated with remaining immobile are

Table 42. Observations while receiving analgesia via PCAS

Respiratory rate, sedation level and pain score
  1/2 hourly for first hour
  Hourly for 2 hours
  Every 2 hours for following 8 hours; then every 4 hours
  Syringe volume checked and recorded by the nurse every 2 hours

explained – stasis of peripheral circulation with increased risk of deep venous thrombosis. The importance of deep breathing to guard against chest infection is stressed. They are shown how the wound may be supported while moving around.

Some patients have an altered body image following surgery. This is usually not a problem after transplantation – the incision for a renal transplant is unobtrusive in a low position close to the inguinal ligament. Most of our patients are elated at receiving a new kidney and the scar seems unimportant in comparison to the gain.

The diet is important. During the first few days, especially if urine production is low, potassium and sodium intake must be kept low – usually the diet given to patients suffering from acute renal failure is adequate. Intake of protein and vitamins should be increased to normal as soon as the need to restrict potassium and sodium is over.

Patients who are treated with steroid usually experience increased appetite. If they are poorly nourished this is beneficial up to a point, but it is important that a habit of over-eating does not develop and lead to excessive weight gain. The dietician discusses this potential problem with the patient before it arises, and provides a booklet giving sensible advice about choice of diet.

6. Drugs

The drugs used for immunosuppression are described in Chapter 15. Their prescription for the patient takes into account to some extent the individual situation. Consideration is given to special need to avoid altogether or to reduce steroid dosage rapidly (the elderly or those with severe bone disease), and to those at increased hazard of rejection (second and later grafts where a previous graft has failed from rejection).

During the first 24 hours the immunosuppression is given intravenously, after this they can usually be given orally. From this stage onwards the patient is familiarized with the appearance of the drugs, their names and how they should be taken. The patient records the drugs as taken on a treatment card (as well as the nurse's record on the Drug Kardex). CYA should be given mixed in milk in a ceramic cup as plastic vessels inactivate CYA. Recently it has become available in tablet form. Despite the fact that the tablets are rather large even children can swallow them. CYA may be with-held until the kidney is producing urine. The drugs should be taken at the time prescribed – the total daily dose of steroid should always be taken about half an hour before breakfast because divided dosage spread over the day increases adreno-pituitary suppression.

There will be several changes of drugs over the early period after operation and each change needs to be explained to the patient, indicating that most of the changes are part of a planned programme of drug administration, and that the change from one drug or set of drugs to another must be gradual with overlap between the two regimes. Once the immunosuppression regime becomes fairly stable from day to day, the patients are given packs of drugs containing the day's supply, which they take and record on the treatment card at the times prescribed.

The patient often requires drugs other than those used for immunosuppression. These may include nifedipine (given for protection of the new kidney against the nephrotoxic effect of CYA and/or for control of hypertension), acyclovir for prophylaxis against CMV, and other drugs. The patient learns to recognize each drug required, why it is given, how it should be taken and to record it on the chart. When at home the routine of recording each drug as taken is soon abandoned, but the drugs should be taken in the amounts and at the times prescribed. This education on the drugs and how they should be taken will help prevent mistakes and omissions later.

All drugs have side effects and patients should be told about the commoner ones. CYA often produces increase in body and facial hair, which is distressing for women, the worst afflicted of whom may need to shave the upper lip and chin area. Cosmetic advice should be given, as the patient may omit the drug with disastrous results for the graft. Somewhat less common is gum hypertrophy, which can be reduced by good mouth hygiene. The tendency for steroid to cause increase in weight, and rounding of the face with increase in ruddiness is lessened by taking the total dose in the morning as prescribed. If necessary the dosage schedule can be changed (gradually) to double dosage on alternate days.

7. Early symptoms and signs of rejection

Rejection can often be suspected before there is clear evidence to support its presence (Table 43). The patient may seem less cheerful or slightly depressed. The appetite often becomes less and there may be slight elevation of the temperature. The first firm indication of rejection is often a reduction in urinary volume after a continuing increase. As a urethral catheter is in place during the first week any fall in output should be readily detected by inspection of the fluid intake/output chart at least twice daily. If the urine continues to be blood-stained a blocked catheter must first be excluded

Table 43. Signs of rejection

1. Tenderness and enlargement of graft
2. General malaise
3. Failure to regain appetite
4. Pyrexia
5. Hypertension
6. Drop in urinary output and rise in serum creatinine
7. Unusual anxiety

before diagnosing rejection. The diagnosis of rejection is described in Chapter 17, and its treatment in Chapter 15.

8. Advice before discharge

Over the whole period of the stay in hospital the patient has been given gradually the information which will be needed when he is discharged. As recovery occurs and the patient feels increasingly well the programme of education helps to combat boredom as well as being useful for the future. There is opportunity to bring up the fact that sexual intercourse can take place as soon as the individual patient feels ready for it. Women of reproductive age need to be warned that they can become pregnant even before periods return, and that it is important to follow the contraceptive advice given by their doctor. It is advisable to wait for a year or more before planning a pregnancy, and this should be fully discussed in advance with their doctor.

The future should include return to employment, whether full-time or part-time, or housework or studies. The younger patients with return to health may wish to take up new interests such as sport or improve their achievement at some activity previously enjoyed. We suggest that for the first month after surgery, even if the whole procedure has gone smoothly and discharge from hospital has been at about 14 days, the patient should live quietly at home and avoid crowded places, and ask friends who have colds or who may appear to have infection to stay away. The patient who has recently commenced relatively high dosage of immunosuppression has an increased susceptibility to infection.

Table 44. Aspects of home care

1. Signs and symptoms of rejection
2. Measuring and recording urinary output
3. Collecting 24 hour urine collections and MSSU samples
4. Attending out-patient clinics
5. Advice on diet control
6. Advice on "crowd" control for 6–8 weeks post discharge
7. Discharge Booklet and formal discharge talk

Finally, the day before discharge from hospital the patient is given a short concise booklet which contains all the necessary information including how to obtain help if needed. This should be read and fully understood before leaving hospital.

It must be appreciated that good nursing plays a very important role in all transplant programmes. In Belfast we have had the good fortune to have from the very beginning highly motivated and intelligent nurses whose contribution to all stages of development has been immense.

Two very useful recent developments were due to nursing initiatives. All patients about to be discharged after transplantation are invited to join a Patient Support Group. General advice reinforces that given during convalescence, and help is available for individual problems as may be needed. Ex-patients are available on request to discuss with the patient difficulties they have encountered.

An Education Unit has been set up, with the support of the Northern Ireland Kidney Research Fund. Patients are made aware of the Fund which has as one of its aims the furtherance of knowledge about kidney donation in the general population, as well as raising funds for research. There is a very informative set of slides covering the transplant operation and its aftermath, accompanied by an oral commentary spoken by a well known TV personality. Patients are encouraged to join a physical fitness programme tailored to individual needs. Advice about nutrition, diet and the importance of weight control is stressed. If necessary psychiatric advice can be obtained. The room shows photographs of local patients taking part in the national and international Transplant Games, being awarded medals and cups. Many become aware for the first time through this Unit that they can become fit enough to take part in serious competitive sport. Training and coaching can be arranged if desired. One patient whose transplant took place 17 years ago learnt to swim after his transplant and has regularly won medals for swimming over many years. He has also completed the Belfast Marathon five times.

Acknowledgement

This chapter is dedicated to the memory of Kay Maguire who contributed greatly to the development of the renal service and whose vision of the renal nurse inspired so many others.

Mrs Rosemary Wilson, S.R.N., and Sister Laura Johnston, S.R.N., gave much advice about the preparation of this Chapter and generously permitted quotation from as yet unpublished written material.

CHAPTER 17

Graft dysfunction and its differential diagnosis

C. C. DOHERTY

The quality of clinical management in the early post-operative phase has an important influence on the outcome of renal transplantation. This chapter deals mainly with graft dysfunction as manifested by deteriorating renal function, but also examines post-transplant proteinuria. Some problems special to renal transplantation in children and the elderly are discussed.

It is convenient and practical to consider renal transplant dysfunction in two main clinical settings – firstly, the early post-operative phase prior to discharge from hospital and secondly, the patient who is re-admitted from the outpatient clinic because of later transplant dysfunction. The point of this distinction is that there are certain causes of graft failure which occur in the first but not the second of these two settings. The initial approach to graft dysfunction in all cases requires a careful assessment of the clinical background, the symptoms and physical signs, and preliminary laboratory investigations. The differential diagnosis requires a knowledge of the general principles of renal failure and of the urological and infectious complications of renal transplantation. Where the diagnosis remains uncertain, ultrasound, isotope renography and graft biopsy are the most valuable investigations.

1. Early post-transplant graft dysfunction

Some transplanted kidneys function immediately, graft dysfunction does not occur and clinical management is straightforward. This is exceptional and it is more common for one or more episodes of graft dysfunction to occur. Thus the kidney may (1) never function, (2) function for a short period and then lose function or (3) show delayed onset of function. Important clues may be found in the antemortem history of the kidney (e.g. cardiac arrest in the donor, prolonged total or operative ischaemia), the peri-operative events (e.g. intra-operative hypotension, sub-optimal perfusion on removal of clamps) or the early post-operative pattern of vital signs and fluid balance charts (a good diuresis of heavily bloodstained urine followed by sudden anuria not attributable to hypotension suggests clot obstruction).

Mary G. McGeown (ed.), Clinical Management of Renal Transplantation, 243–262.

Table 45. Causes of early post-transplant graft dysfunction

1. Hypovolaemia
2. Obstruction
3. Acute tubular necrosis
4. Urinary leak
5. Vascular complications
6. Infection
7. Cyclosporin nephrotoxicity
8. Nephrotoxicity due to other drugs
9. Rejection

The common causes of abnormal renal function in the early post-transplant period (defined here as the first 3 weeks) are listed in Table 45. The clinical presentation may be a rising serum creatinine in an otherwise well patient, or there may be additional features which aid the differential diagnosis.

1.1. *Hypovolaemia*

Assessment the volume status of the dialysis patient admitted for renal transplantation is critically important. The patient's target 'dry weight' must be compared with body weight on admission. If the patient has been kept fasting for a significant period awaiting the transplant procedure and continues CAPD during this time, negative balances must be assessed. The average 24 hour volume of urine produced by the patient's own kidneys, if any, must be taken into consideration. This is particularly important in children who may have salt-wasting and polyuria (often 1.5–3 litres) as a feature of their primary renal disease. Central venous pressure monitoring is essential in children and the elderly and should also be used in cases where clinical assessment of volume status is difficult. Blood loss in theatre should be replaced volume for volume with blood and in patients in whom the CVP is monitored, adequate isotonic saline should be given to ensure a CVP of at least 10–12 cm of water at the time the arterial clamps are released. For the first 12–24 hours post-operatively the CVP should be maintained above 5 cm of water and during this initial period when urinary volume may vary from zero to torrential diuresis (which may be 1 litre or more per hour) hourly urinometer readings should be kept and the fluid prescription revised every 3–6 hours if necessary. For those patients with immediate allograft function, adequate fluid balance can usually be maintained by replacing hourly urine volumes plus 30 ml, using alternative dextrose 5% and normal saline. Intravenous fluids can usually be discontinued by 24–48 hours. The cardiovascular response to hypovolaemia can be masked by beta-blockade and this may contribute to dangerous delay in diagnosis of post-operative haemorrhage. Therefore beta-blockers should be omitted prior to renal transplantation and alternative agents used to control hypertension. In the Belfast

Unit, pre-operative and post-operative fluid is prescribed by the consultant nephrologist in charge. Approximately one third of cadaver renal allografts do not function initially. If obstruction of the urinary catheter by blood clot is excluded, the approach to fluid and electrolyte balance should be as for acute renal failure. Particular attention is paid to control of serum potassium. If ion exchange resins such as calcium resonium or sodium polystyrene are used to control hyperkalaemia, a laxative such as lactulose 10–20 ml must be given concurrently to prevent formation of concretions in the colon which might precipitate diverticulitis or colonic perforation. The likelihood of this adverse event is enhanced by post-operative constipation secondary to general inactivty and ileus following the operation.

1.2. Obstruction

The commonest cause of obstruction in the early post-operative stage is blood clot from the bladder cystotomy blocking the Foley catheter. The occurrence of clot obstruction may be suggested by abrupt alteration in the recorded urinary flow rate per hour, or the complaint of supra-pubic discomfort and desire to void urine (even though some urine drainage is occurring). If clot obstruction is suspected, bladder lavage should be carried out. The catheter should be changed if any question of inadequate drainage persists. Other causes of obstruction include compression of the pelvis or ureter by haematoma, urinoma, seroma or lymphocele, ureteric narrowing due to ischaemic necrosis, kinking and ureteric involvement in the rejection process. Ultrasound is the most helpful investigation in suspected obstruction (a small degree of dilatation of the renal pelvis is a normal finding in a transplanted kidney). Ultrasound may indicate the level of obstruction and the cause if it is extrinsic fluid collection.

1.3. Acute tubular necrosis (ATN)

This diagnosis is usually reached by exclusion of the other causes of early post-transplant graft failure. ATN may result from hypotension/hypovolaemia in the donor, prolonged warm ischaemia (greater than 1 hour) in removing the kidneys, difficult nephrectomy with induced cortical spasm, and prolonged ischaemia during transplantation. Identification of such factors may predict ATN and aid diagnosis. ATN may manifest two different patterns of graft dysfunction; most commonly, the kidney produces urine for 1 or 2 hours to a few days followed by progressive oliguria. Isotope renography at this stage may show an excellent vascular phase or may be totally flat depending on the severity of the damage. In most cases, urinary output recovers in 1 or 2 weeks but particularly in elderly patients may take as long as 4–6 weeks. A second clinical pattern of ATN is that of adequate urine volume without satisfactory renal function, daily creatinine levels remaining static or rising only slightly. This resembles the diuretic phase of ATN and should be followed by improvement in renal function unless further complications develop or there is co-existent rejection. To prevent leucopenia and marrow toxicity it is important to keep the dose of azathioprine low (1.5 mg/kg body weight) during functional renal failure.

1.4. *Urinary leak and other urological complications*

Urine leak at the vesico-ureteric anastamosis or mechanical obstruction of the ureter are common complications which may occur early or late in the post-operative period. It is important to note that although urine output may diminish abruptly, dramatic changes in urine volume do not necessarily occur and a necrosing ureter may function for several days before a leak develops. Urinary leak is a serious complication and is usually caused by damage to the arterial supply of the transplant ureter or rarely by dehiscence at the cystotomy site. It may cause fever, graft tenderness, oedema of the scrotum or labia and increased wound drainage. If sufficient fluid oozes from the wound or via a wound drain, biochemical analysis of such fluid will distinguish lymph or serum from urine (the creatinine levels of lymph and serum are identical) and is a valuable diagnostic test. Prompt surgical repair is the usual management.

1.4.1. *Lymph leak and lymphoceles.* A lymphocele may cause progressive decline in renal function by local compression of the graft and its adjacent structures. Ultrasound is usually diagnostic and small collections may resolve without decompression or drainage. Large collections can be aspirated with a needle or catheter under ultrasound guidance.

1.4.2. *Rupture.* Life-threatening haemorrhage can occur from spontaneous graft rupture and is usually associated with rapid parenchymal swelling during an acute rejection episode. This is a rare event and is probably even less common when CYA is used in primary immunosuppression. There is severe graft pain with circulatory shock and emergency nephrectomy is usually required.

1.5. *Vascular complications*

1.5.1. *Haemorrhage.* Acute haemorrhage due to dehiscence of a vascular suture line may occur within a few hours after transplantation. There may be excruciating pain in the region of the graft, the back or flank, with radiation toward the rectum. Hypovolaemic shock may ensue and emergency graft exploration is indicated.

Later haemorrhage may occur associated with perinephric abscess or mycotic aneurysm. Iliac artery involvement may produce catastrophic bleeding. Occasionally, significant post-operative bleeding arises in the retroperitoneal space with acute flank pain, and a drop in haemoglobin. A large haematoma extending up the psoas gutter may be visible on ultrasound. This type of bleeding is often self limited but can be a potential site of sepsis.

1.5.2. *Arterial thrombosis.* This event may produce complete or segmental infarction of the kidney and may result from multiple renal arteries, technical difficulties or atherosclerosis of recipient or donor vessels. Complete infarction of the graft is suggested by absence of renal function and continued need for post-operative dialysis. There may be significant urine production from the patient's native kidneys and surprisingly little systemic disturbance. The kidney may appear small in size on ultrasound with increased echogenicity and reduced cortical thickness. There may be a sensation of little resistance on needle graft biopsy and the tissue core may be a pale muddy colour on naked eye inspection. Concern has been expressed that CYA may increase the risk of primary graft non-function due to arterial thrombosis (especially in children). This increased risk may be due to the significant renal vasoconstriction and decrease in renal blood flow induced by CYA. I^{131} hippuran renography will aid assessment of blood flow to the kidney. If there is a normal vascular phase one can assume that the arterial supply is intact. Duplex doppler scan and arteriography may also be used to confirm the diagnosis. Operative salvage of such kidneys is unlikely and nephrectomy is indicated.

1.5.3. *Venous thrombosis.* This may occur as a primary event or in association with severe acute rejection. It causes graft swelling and tenderness and is usually – but not always – associated with signs of iliac vein thrombosis in the form of marked swelling of the leg on the side of the transplant. Lesser degrees of ipsilateral leg swelling are not uncommon post-transplant and are probably due to extrinsic pressure of the kidney on the iliac veins. Diagnosis may be aided by absence of uptake of isotope on renography (suggesting graft infarction) and duplex doppler ultrasound scanning can also be useful to assess blood flow in the renal vein. Selective contrast venography to image the renal vein is often technically difficult and carries a risk of damage to the venous anastomosis if carried out in the early post-operative period. Arteriography with venous phase films may be preferred. Salvage of the kidney by operative intervention is rare. However, a Belfast patient developed venous thrombosis three weeks after transplantation. The thrombus was removed, and the kidney continued to function until death from myocardial infarction over 21 years later.

1.6. *Bacterial infection*

Systemic bacterial infections in the post-operative period may cause significant graft dysfunction and ATN. Infections with this potential include klebsiella pneumonia, severe wound or urinary infection, or staphylococcus aureus bacteraemia from central venous lines. It is of critical importance to distinguish fever due to serious bacterial infection from that due to rejection, as inappropriate increase in immunosuppression in this setting could have disastrous consequences. This principle is illustrated by the following case history.

A 59 year old man with a history of chronic obstructive airways disease received a cadaver kidney transplant and experienced graft dysfunction in the first week post-operatively with fever, rising creatinine and abdominal pain in the region of the graft in the left iliac fossa. Physical examination, graft ultrasound and renography were unremarkable and the provisional diagnosis was probable rejection. Over the next 24 hours he developed grossly purulent sputum and was noted to have marked faecal loading on abdominal X-ray. The diagnosis of 'rejection' was revised to 'pneumonia plus constipation' and improvement followed treatment with antibiotics and laxatives rather than increased immunosuppression.

In the transplant patient with early post-operative dysfunction and fever, it is therefore essential to seek symptoms, signs and radiological/laboratory evidence of bacterial infection. Fever which responds promptly to antibiotic therapy is unlikely to be immunological in origin.

1.7. *Cyclosporin nephrotoxicity*

There are both acute and chronic forms of CYA nephrotoxicity. CYA administration is associated with a variety of changes in the renal vasculature, predominantly affecting the arterioles; these changes may be (1) a reversible dose-dependent arteriolar vaso-constriction (renal vascular resistance may increase by 50%) with substantial reduction in blood flow to the transplanted kidney, (2) an arteriolopathy characterised by luminal narrowing due to intimal proliferation (note these same features may occur due to chronic rejection) and (3) arteriolar and capillary thrombi probably due to increased platelet aggregation secondary to CYA induced inhibition of endothelial prostacyclin synthetase. This latter form of CYA nephrotoxicity may be associated with thrombocytopenia and microangiopathic haemolytic anaemia resembling the haemolytic uraemic syndrome.

CYA nephrotoxicity may therefore occur as an acute early effect producing renal vasoconstriction with reversible decreases in GFR and renal blood flow, or as later irreversible injury associated with chronic renal failure. CYA can also affect proximal and distal tubular function and may cause hyperkalaemic hyperchloraemic metabolic acidosis.

Prevention of early CYA nephrotoxicity involves either reduction of the dose of the drug or avoidance of its use entirely during the initial period following transplantation before graft function has become established. An alternative approach is concurrent administration of drugs to ameliorate the adverse effect on renal blood flow. Frusemide, misoprostol and calcium antagonists have been used, at present the most convincing evidence favours the calcium antagonists. In the Belfast Unit, the induction immunosuppressive therapy is tailored to the individual patient and early use of CYA is influenced by whether or not there is immediate graft function. Exceptions to this are all highly sensitised patients (cytotoxic antibody titre greater than 0.50 or previous transplants) who receive CYA from the time of transplantation with concurrent administration of nifedipine to counteract renal vasoconstriction (see Chapter 15). CYA is either given *orally* as a dose of 5 mg/kg body weight pre-operatively and a dose of 5 mg/kg 12 hours post-operatively (equivalent to 10 mg/kg daily dose) or *intravenously* as 2.5 mg/kg pre-operatively followed by a second i.v. dose of 2.5 mg/kg 12 hours later (equivalent to 5 mg/kg daily dose); nifedipine 10–20 mg orally is administered concurrently. In non-sensitised recipients, initial immunosuppression is with intravenous hydrocortisone and azathioprine; CYA is introduced at an oral dose of 10 mg/kg body weight when graft function is established (as judged by significantly increasing urinary output and falling creatinine), and again with concurrent administration of nifedipine. In all cases subsequent CYA dosage is adjusted according to serum levels, triple therapy continues until CYA levels are stable within the therapeutic range, and azathioprine is then gradually reduced and withdrawn.

An important aspect of CYA therapy is knowledge of drug interactions which may result in enhanced nephrotoxicity (aminoglycosides, amphotericin B, co-trimoxazole, ciprofloxacin, acyclovir, colchicine); marked elevations of CYA concentration (erythromycin, ketoconazole, diltiazem); or aggregation of adverse effects on glomerular haemodynamics (ACE inhibitors). Clinical clues which may suggest the presence of CYA nephrotoxicity are tremor, hypertension, renal tubular acidosis and hyperkalaemia. Drugs which decrease CYA levels include isoniazid, phenytoin and rifampicin.

1.8. *Nephrotoxicity due to other drugs*

The list of drugs with nephrotoxic potential is lengthy and the possibility of the implication of a drug should always be considered in the differential diagnosis of early graft dysfunction. Obvious candidates for drug nephrotoxicity in the early post-transplant setting are CYA and aminoglycosides. Acyclovir (given for treatment or prophylaxis of CMV) may cause significant decrease in renal function. Thus its dose must be adjusted according to the level of renal function.

1.9. *Rejection*

There are 3 main forms of clinical rejection pattern – hyperacute, acute and chronic.

1.9.1. *Hyperacute rejection.* Hyperacute rejection involves interaction between preformed cytotoxic antibodies and antigenic determinants on the graft vascular endothelium. Characteristically it occurs in patients with high titres of cytotoxic antibodies, usually multiparous women, recipients who have had multiple transfusions and recipients who have rejected previous transplants. A small number of patients have hyperacute rejection without demonstrable cytotoxic antibody. Hyperacute rejection may be apparent in the operating theatre when the kidney fails to assume the typical pink colour and healthy firm turgor immediately after the renal artery and vein are unclamped. The kidney is a dull blue with a soft spongy feel and occlusion of the renal vein with the surgeon's fingers fails to cause the kidney to swell as is the case with normally perfused transplants. If this occurs on the operating table, immediate nephrectomy is indicated otherwise severe disseminated intravascular coagulation and bleeding diathesis will ensue. In other instances only mild changes occur at operation but anuria, hyperkalaemia and a catabolic state rapidly become apparent in the first 24–48 hours.

1.9.2. *Acute rejection.* Classic acute rejection is characterised by fever, graft swelling, rising creatinine, oliguria and frequently hypertension. Patients often complain of vague malaise, feeling 'not quite right'. A good appetite is uncommon in the presence of acute rejection. The clinical manifestations of acute rejection tend to be less marked in CYA treated patients. Isotope renography may show diminished uptake of varying degree. Clinically the most reliable signs are moderate decreases (200–500 ml) in urinary output, oedema, weight gain and rise in blood pressure. Acute rejection episodes can occur at any time but are most common in the first 3 months after transplantation. The diagnosis may be based on the clinical features combined with exclusion of other causes of graft dysfunction. Rapid reduction in serum creatinine following anti-rejection therapy (usually apparent within 2–4 days) confirms the diagnosis. If the clinical picture is atypical or response to anti-rejection therapy is unsatisfactory, graft biopsy is indicated. In cases of steroid resistant rejection, the biopsy may show both cellular and humoral components of host responsiveness, including necrotising vasculitis and interstitial haemorrhage; such features indicate a need to consider aggressive immunosuppression with antithymocyte globulin (ATG).

1.9.3. *Chronic rejection.* This is associated with a clinical picture of very slow progressive rise in serum creatinine, often accompanied by hypertension and proteinuria of variable amount. In some patients there may have been previous bouts of acute rejection, while others will never have shown signs of acute rejection. Careful study of the transplant clinic flow chart may reveal that the onset of rising creatinine coincided with alterations in immunosuppressive therapy (withdrawal of azathioprine, reduction in prednisolone, etc.) or rapid weight gain with resulting reduction in azathioprine dose in mg/kg body weight. In patients where azathioprine has been reduced or withdrawn

Table 46. Causes of late post-transplant graft dysfunction

1. Obstruction
2. Cyclosporin nephrotoxicity
3. Nephrotoxicity due to other drugs
4. CMV Infection
5. Transplant artery stenosis
6. Recurrent prnary disease
7. Hypertension
8. Graft pyelonephritis
9. Graft athero-embolism
10. Rejection

for temporary leucopenia, failure to return azathioprine dosage back to the maximum tolerated may be observed in the period prior to onset of slowly progressive rise in serum creatinine. Whatever the precipitating factor progression to end-stage uraemia usually involves a time frame of some years and treatment seldom appears to be effective once the serum creatinine has risen above 200 μmol/l. In some patients where study of the preceding clinical course identifies a potentially culpable alteration in immunosuppressive regime, reversal of this combined with a course of conventional anti-rejection treatment may stabilise graft function if the serum creatinine has not yet risen above 200 μmol/l. Graft biopsy may be helpful in this situation; if histologic changes of acute as well as chronic rejection are present, rejection therapy is likely to be of benefit.

2. Late post-transplant graft dysfunction

Common causes of late graft dysfunction are listed in Table 46.

2.1 & 2. *Obstruction & CYA nephrotoxicity*

When they occur later after transplantation these do not differ from when they occur in the early stage.

2.3. *Drug nephrotoxicity*

There are three drugs which may cause a rise in serum creatinine in the late post-transplant phase. Trimethoprim, frequently prescribed for urinary tract infection, affects tubular creatinine re-absorption and may produce an elevation in serum creatinine of the order of 50–80 μmol/l. This effect is reversed immediately on stopping the drug. ACE inhibitors may cause reversible renal failure in transplant patients by causing hypotension, interstitial nephritis or 'functional' renal failure due to graft artery stenosis or the combination of ACE inhibition of efferent arteriolar vasoconstriction and CYA induced constriction of the pre-glomerular arteriole. Irreversible anuric transplant failure after ACE inhibition treatment has been reported in patients with graft artery stenosis, due to superimposed occlusive thrombosis. Plasma creatinine levels should therefore be measured daily for several days after introducing or substantially increasing the dose of an ACE inhibitor (ACE1) in a renal transplant patient. Conversely, any transplant patient who is taking an ACE1 and who develops a rising creatinine, should have the ACE1 discontinued and alternative hypotensive therapy given while the effect of ACE1 withdrawal on creatinine is determined. The third drug which (less commonly) may adversely affect graft function is vitamin D. This may be contained in a multiple vitamin preparation prescribed by the patient's general practitioner or as 'cod liver oil' taken by the patient on their own initiative; in the recently transplanted patient with parathyroid hyperplasia resulting from their previous chronic uraemia, even small doses of vitamin D may induce hypercalcaemia and mild elevation of serum creatinine.

2.4. CMV infection

The clinical syndromes caused by CMV in immunosuppressed patients include fever, pneumonia, hepatitis, chorioretinitis, and renal allograft dysfunction. Virtually all post-transplant CMV infections occur 1–4 months after transplantation (with a peak occurrence at 6–8 weeks). A infected donor kidney is the major source of primary CMV infection but post-operative blood transfusion containing leucocytes may also cause primary infection. Prevention of CMV infection after transplantation can be achieved by administration of prophylactic acyclovir to sero-negative recipients who receive a CMV positive donor kidney, and by use – when blood transfusion is required – of packed red cells free of viable leucocytes. Clinical CMV disease begins insidiously with constitutional symptoms of anorexia, malaise, fever and occasionally myalgia. The peripheral blood film may shown 5–10% atypical lymphocytes. Approximately one-third of patients develop a non-productive cough and some progress to respiratory distress, pulmonary infiltrates and hypoxaemia on arterial blood gas determination. Laboratory investigations may reveal leucopenia, thrombocytopenia and hepato-cellular dysfunction. CMV infection may also adversely affect renal function under certain circumstances and produces a distinctive glomerular lesion on biopsy. The corresponding clinical picture is of variable graft swelling and tenderness and rise in creatinine of the order of 100–150 μmol/l.

2.5. Transplant artery stenosis

This may arise as a result of atherosclerosis, faulty surgical technique, arterial injury during donor nephrectomy or chronic rejection. The antecedent clinical picture usually includes severe hypertension refractory to treatment and progressively rising creatinine. Operative repair may be technically difficult and hazardous due to intense scarring around the vessels; it should only be undertaken if there is unmanageable hypertension or progressive renal dysfunction. Percutaneous transluminal angioplasty is not recommended.

2.6. Recurrent primary disease

Several types of glomerulonephritis (especially type 2 membrano-proliferative GN, IgA nephropathy, focal segmental glomerulosclerosis, anti-GBM nephritis, and haemolytic uraemic syndrome) and metabolic disorders (type 1 diabetes, amyloidosis, cystinosis, oxalosis) may recur in the transplanted kidney and cause graft dysfunction. The clinical picture may show the same variable pattern seen when the primary disease occurs in native kidneys; IgA nephropathy for example may produce graft dysfunction ranging from asymptomatic microhaematuria to frank haematuria with exacerbations of renal failure, or rapidly progressive renal failure with crescentic changes on biopsy.

2.7. Hypertension

The incidence of hypertension after transplantation is about 50% in patients one year after operation. Hypertension after transplantation may arise from retention of native kidneys, graft rejection (acute and chronic), recurrent primary disease, obstruction, transplant artery stenosis, hypercalcaemia, corticosteroid and/or CYA therapy. Uncontrolled hypertension may be a primary cause of graft dysfunction or a secondary factor in patients with chronic rejection. In renal transplant patients not on CYA, captopril challenge has been advocated as a means of distinguishing hypertension due to native kidneys from that due to transplant artery stenosis; in the latter situation captopril causes a marked decline in GFR whereas in transplant patients whose hypertension is induced by their native kidneys, there is instead a dramatic increase in effective renal blood flow.

2.8. Graft pyelonephritis

As in the normal population, the incidence of asymptomatic bacteriuria is greatest in the older transplant patient group. In patients with symptomatic urinary tract infection following renal transplantation, the majority are mild in degree with symptoms of cystitis only and there is no effect on graft function (with the exception of artefactual rise in creatinine if trimethoprim is prescribed). Occasional patients however develop malaise, fever, graft pain and a rise in creatinine associated with urinary tract infection. This represents graft pyelonephritis and should be treated promptly with appropriate antibiotic and copious fluid intake. Recurrent severe urinary tract infection should raise suspicion of obstruction or stone formation. In some patients bladder dysfunction (e.g. megacystis/megaureter, neurogenic bladder) or the native kidneys may be a source of recurrent infection. Young female patients may have vaginal warts or other gynaecological pathology. In older male patients prostatic enlargement should be considered.

2.9. Rejection

Precipitating factors can sometimes be identified in events prior to the onset when acute rejection occurs in the late post-transplant period. Rejection is likely to occur during conversion from CYA to conventional immunosuppression (azathioprine/prednisone) especially if this is implemented over a short time and without adequate drug overlap. It may similarly occur during gradual withdrawal of prednisolone while attempting to convert patients to CYA monotherapy. Attempts at steroid withdrawal in patients on azathioprine/prednisone suggested there was a critical threshold of prednisolone dosage of approximately 7.5 mg daily. Recent studies have shown that about one-third of CYA treated patients cannot be managed on CYA monotherapy and require concurrent steroid. In some patients, errors in immunosuppressive drug dosage may precede rejection and non-compliance with treatment may be elicited from some adolescent transplant recipients. Recorded CYA serum levels prior to and at the onset of acute rejection may be in the subtherapeutic range. Serum drug level monitoring has never been available to assist azathioprine therapy in similar fashion; this drug is most often commenced at a dosage which varies in different centres from 2–3 mg/kg body weight. This dosage is frequently lowered subsequently either due to leucopenia or in the longer term because of concern about malignancy. There is however evidence that prolonged reduction of azathioprine below 100 mg/day for more than 1 year when implemented for reasons other than leucopenia, is associated with a high incidence of rejection. Transplant patients who develop excessive weight gain in the early (first 12 months) post-transplant period form another potentially important group which receive sub-optimal azathioprine dosage. Body weight in some transplant patients who neglect dietary advice concerning calorie intake may increase by as much as 40% in the first year. If azathioprine dosage is not adjusted accordingly, the azathioprine dosage in mg/kg terms is effectively reduced during the period of greatest rejection risk.

Clinical clues to rejection as the cause of graft dysfunction may therefore be found from careful scrutiny of the outpatient clinic flow chart, from details of CYA levels, body weight change, recent alterations in blood pressure, proteinuria, immunosuppression, etc. As with acute rejection occurring in the early post-transplant phase, diagnosis may be based on the clinical picture and exclusion of other causes of graft dysfunction. If however the diagnosis is unclear following preliminary investigations (urine culture, quantitation of proteinuria, serum calcium, graft ultrasound) percutaneous graft biopsy may be indicated to distingish rejection from recurrent disease or CYA nephrotoxicity.

3. Renal transplantation in older patients

Older patients (over 50 years old) are generally considered to be at risk in renal transplantation, with a higher mortality rate in the early post-operative period due to infection, cardiovascular complications and malignancy. However results in recent years have improved due to growing experience with immunosuppression. Transplantation is the preferred treatment for end-stage renal disease in patients aged 50–64 years in the absence of contraindications. Diverticulitis, atherosclerotic vascular disease and steroid induced diabetes have been reported more frequently in older patients after renal transplantation, and this should be kept in mind when evaluating graft dysfunction in the elderly transplant patient. Renal allograft athero-embolism should for example be considered in the differential diagnosis when graft dysfunction occurs in elderly patients with angina or intermittent claudication. Graft biopsy in this situation may show diagnostic cholesterol clefts and CT scan of the abdomen may show atheromatous plaques in the aorta. It should also be noted that elderly patients show age-related decline in kidney function and this tends to be reflected in the creatinine clearance values of the older renal transplant patient.

Donor age may also affect the level of renal function achieved after transplantation. Ageing is associated with alterations in renal structure, the most striking change being glomerular hyalinisation and changes in the intra-renal vasculature. Donor age is therefore a relevant consideration when interpreting appearanoes on graft biopsy. Use of paediatric cadaver kidneys from donors under 6 years of age may result in decreased graft survival rates and an increased incidence of technical complications including vascular thrombosis.

4. Post-transplant proteinuria

Nephrotic range proteinuria in renal allograft recipients is usually secondary to recurrent or *de novo* glomerulonephritis or the glomerulopathy associated with chronic rejection. Proteinuria may also increase with and may precede acute rejection episodes. Nephrotic range proteinuria with minimal change glomerulopathy on graft biopsy has been reported in the first year post-transplant, but in contrast to the natural history of this disorder when it occurs in native kidneys, the majority of such patients have developed progressive uraemia with subsequent histological features of chronic rejection.

4.1. *De novo glomerulopathy*

The commonest form of *de novo* glomerulopathy in renal allografts is membranous glomerulonephritis which has a reported incidence varying from 2–9%. It usually presents as asymptomatic proteinuria or nephrotic syndrome, and the later usually indicates a poor graft prognosis. Morphologically, some pathologists consider that *de novo* membranous GN in most instances has distinct differences from idiopathic membranous GN in native kidneys; the presence of varying features of rejection may point to *de novo* GN. About 50% of grafts which develop *de novo* membranous GN eventually fail and this may represent the consequences of the associated chronic rejection.

Some cases of so called *de novo* membranous GN may be a complication of transplant glomerulopathy rather than the results of mechanisms totally independent from rejection.

4.2. *Recurrent renal disease*

The diagnosis of recurrent renal disease after transplantation requires an accurate diagnosis of the initial cause of renal failure and a determination of the cause of graft failure. The overall incidence of recurrent disease may be as high as 10–20% but it accounts for less than 2% of graft failure. Probably all types of glomerulonephritis recur, but with great variation in frequency and severity. In some forms of glomerulonephritis, recurrence may be frequent and definite on histopathological criteria, but may have only a minor clinical expression (e.g. IgA nephropathy, anti-GBM antibody glomerulonephritis) while in others, recurrence is less predictable yet is clearly associated with premature graft failure (e.g. focal glomerulosclerosis, membranous GN). Where the initial glomerulonephritis was aggressive and caused kidney failure over a short time, recurrence is more likely and, when present, will lead to graft failure with an increased frequency. It is relatively rare for disseminated lupus erythematosis to affect a transplanted kidney. Diabetic nephropathy appears to follow a remarkably similar time course in the transplanted patient to that seen in native kidneys in type 1 diabetic patients. Amyloidosis usually does not recur when the causative inflammatory disease has 'burnt out'. Oxalosis, cystinosis and Fabry's disease are other metabolic disorders which may recur in the graft. It has been suggested that the likelihood of recurrence of haemolytic uraemic syndrome affecting the transplanted kidney may be increased by the use of CYA and that this drug should not be used in patients with this primary diagnosis. Anti-GBM nephritis has been reported to occur in the transplant kidney of a minority of patients with Alport's syndrome. This may represent a sensitisation phenomenon to the antigens which are deficient in the glomerular basement membrane of patients with Alport's syndrome, resulting in anti-GBM antibody-mediated GN affecting the graft. Severe acute deterioration of graft function with gross haematuria has been reported with recurrence to IgA nephropathy; in this setting, graft biopsy may show only mild glomerular lesions but acute tubular cell injury (in relation to phagocytosis of erythrocytes or pigments and/or tubular obstruction).

5. Graft biopsy

5.1. Indications and timing of biopsy

It often proves relatively easier to biopsy a transplant kidney in the early rather than the later post-transplant phase, as with time the graft may become encased in a dense layer of fibrous tissue. This fibrous capsule must first be punctured before the graft biopsy can be taken.

Biopsy before the seventh day following transplantation is exceptional as biopsies during the first week are technically more difficult, and likely to be associated with higher risk as tenderness and swelling make localisation difficult and the kidney may be more friable. The main indications for graft biopsy in the first week post-operatively, are signs of hypercatabolism (rapidly rising urea and potassium) in the absence of infection, or a 'flat' isotope renogram; such features suggest a non-viable graft due to severe rejection or vascular occlusion.

Graft biopsy should in general be carried out when the result seems likely to influence management. The commonest indications are to assist differential diagnosis of both early and late graft dysfunction (especially in differentiating ischaemic damage, rejection and CYA nephrotoxicity), and to assess the success of anti-rejection therapy, in order to help decide whether such potentially dangerous therapy should be continued. Percutaneous needle biopsy should not be attempted in cases (usually paediatric) where the kidney has been implanted in the peritoneal cavity.

5.2. Technique

Prior to carrying out graft biopsy the nature of the procedure should be explained to the patient as the word 'biopsy' often invokes patient anxiety. Essential steps to minimise complications are control of hypertension (diastolic blood pressure less than 100 mm Hg), assessment of coagulation screen (followed by administration of vitamin K, fresh frozen plasma etc. if indicated) and prior dialysis if the patient has uraemia of a degree likely to contribute a bleeding tendency (blood urea greater than 30 mmol/l) or to

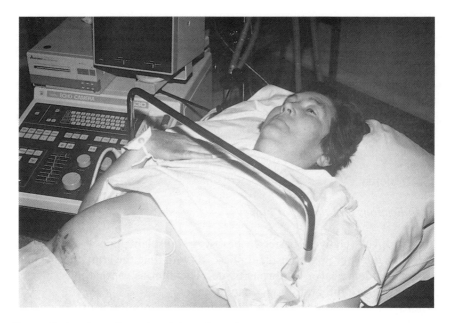

Figure 49. An elevated metal cross-bar allows the sterile drapes to shield the operative site from the patient's view.

require dialysis soon after the biopsy (at the first dialysis after a biopsy, minimal or no heparin must be used). Pre-medication with diazepam 10 mg orally should be given 15 minutes before biopsy. If possible the procedure should be carried out in the operating theatre with full aseptic technique and on an operating table whose height can be varied. It is helpful to have a nurse to assist and reassure the patient. An elevated metal cross-bar across the patient's chest over which the sterile drapes may be placed is useful to shield the lower abdomen from the patient's view (the sight of a Trucut needle disappearing into the abdomen may be distressing for the patient). Each step should be explained to the patient as the operator proceeds.

Abdominal ultrasound using a sector scanning probe should be used to locate the upper pole of the graft, to measure the distance in centimetres from skin to capsule and to define the angle of approach shortly to be followed by the biopsy needle. Ideally scanning should be carried out by the nephrologist as this affords the best 'feel' for the subsequent needle pass. This done, the skin site should be marked (firm pressure using a one penny piece is convenient), the ultrasound gel wiped off and the site re-marked with an indelible fibre tip pen. Care during this part of the procedure will reward the operator by increasing the likelihood of obtaining diagnostic tissue, and of avoiding damage to hilar structures or calyces. The patient should be instructed not to move after the preliminary ultrasound localisation and marking is carried out. Following skin preparation, 15–20 ml of ligno-

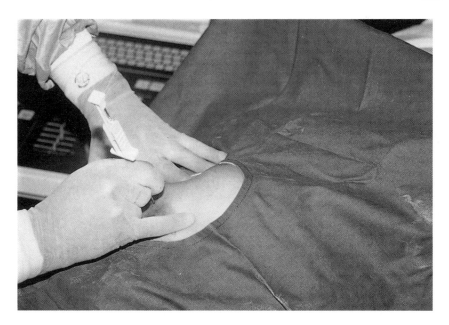

Figure 50. The index finger and thumb are used to steady the upper pole of the kidney as the needle is advanced.

caine 1% as local anaesthetic are infiltrated into the skin and tissues overlying the kidney. As the distance of skin to kidney may vary from 2–7 cm in individual patients, use of a long spinal needle (19–22 gauge is best) is necessary to infiltrate adequate local anaesthetic close to the kidney. This is facilitated by having a sterilised centimetre ruler on the instrument tray which allows the spinal needle to be inserted to the depth of the skin to kidney distance previously measured by the ultrasound scanner. As the spinal needle reaches the kidney, a change in resistance may be felt (or a 'pop' if the needle enters the kidney) and this allows, on removal of the spinal needle, a check on the depth of the kidney which can be read off on the sterile ruler. After opening the skin with a scalpel blade just (Figure 50) enough to admit the biopsy needle, 2 cores of tissue should then be taken with either a Trucut or modified Menghini needle. This should be relatively painless provided adequate local anaesthetic has been properly infiltrated beforehand. It can be disappointing to obtain apparently good cores of renal tissue only to later find that they consist of medulla, contain no glomeruli and are therefore non diagnostic. It is useful to change the angle of the needle slightly before taking the second core so that a different area of kidney is sampled.

The most significant recent advance in graft biopsy technique is the automated, spring-fired biopsy device known as the Biopty Gun (Radiplast, Uppsala, Sweden). With the aid of a needle guide attached to the ultrasound scanner probe, the biopsy needle can be visualized throughout the procedure.

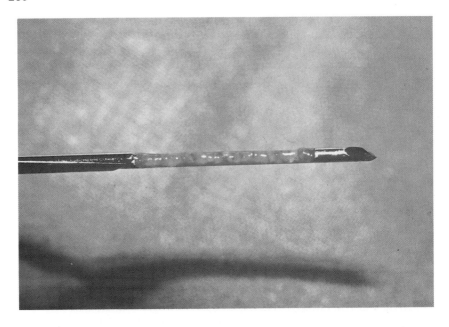

Figure 51. Examination of tissue cores in the operating theatre under a low power microscope may permit identification of glomeruli.

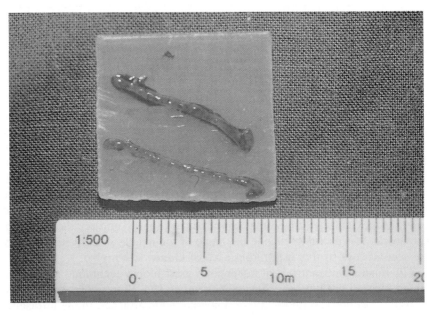

Figure 52. Two cores of tissue are taken.

Table 47. Key points in evaluation of graft dysfunction

1. Exclude easily reversible causes (drugs, obstruction, infection)
2. Beware of conditions which may mimic rejection (CMV infection, diverticulitis, urine leak, obstruction, graft pyelonephritis).
3. Make every effort to distinguish fever of infection from that of immunological origin.
4. Employ graft biopsy at an early stage
5. Exercise vigilance after any changes in immunosuppressive therapy at the outpatient clinic.
6. Rapid weight gain in the early post-transplant phase may result in sub-optimal azathioprine dosage.
7. The clinical course preceding transplantation may hold valuable clues as to the causation of graft dysfunction.
8. The most reliable signs of acute rejection are moderate decrease in urinary volume, oedema and progressive rise in creatinine.
9. Meticulous flow sheets are invaluable in assessing graft dysfunction.

This allows the gun to be "fired" when the needle is seen to touch the renal capsule, and results in a high success rate. Complications are minimised especially the likelihood of obtaining a non-diagnostic deep sample consisting of only medullary tissue. The method offers distinct practical advantages and is now the technique of choice in the Belfast Unit.

Examination of the cores in the operating theatre under a low power microscope may permit identification of glomeruli and assessment of adequacy of the core. The material is subsequently prepared for light microscopy, electron microscopy and immunoflourescent staining (see Chapter 18). After obtaining the tissue cores, manual pressure is applied to the biopsy site for 3–5 minutes, a pressure dressing should then be strapped over the biopsy site and the patient confined to bed for the next 24 hours.

5.3. Biopsy complications

The patient should be informed that transient haematuria may follow the procedure and that mild discomfort may be experienced when the local anaesthetic wears off. Severe post-biopsy pain is rare if the procedure is carried out as described here. If it occurs it is usually due to retroperitoneal haematoma or clot colic. This latter complication should be treated with adequate analgesia and bladder catheterisation if there are sufficient clots to cause urinary retention. Pulse and blood pressure are recorded every 15 minutes for 2 hours and then hourly. All urine samples are inspected for haematuria and nursing staff are instructed to call the medical staff if there is pain, bleeding, swelling or any change in vital signs. Occasionally haemorrhage after biopsy may be severe enough to fill the renal pelvis with clot and cause acute anuria; large clots may also induce distressing bladder spasms. Anuria due to obstruction clot may require a percutaneous nephrostomy or ureteral stent placed under ultrasound guidance. Large bladder clots may be difficult to evacuate and it may be necessary to use a 3-way irrigation catheter.

Further reading

Donovan, K. L., Thomas, D. M., Wheeler, D. C. *et al.* Experience with a new method for percutaneous renal biopsy. *Nephrol. Dial. Transplant.* 1991; 6: 731–733.

Fine, R. N. Renal transplantation in the infant and young child and the use of paediatric cadaver kidneys for transplantation in adult recipients. *Amer. J. Kidney Dis.* 1988; 12: 1–10.

Huraib, S., Goldberg, H., Ktaz, A. *et al.* Percutaneous needle biopsy of the transplanted kidney: technique and complications. *Amer. J. Kidney Dis.* 1989; 14: 13–17.

Kahan, B. D. Drug therapy – cyclosporine. *New Engl. J. Med.* 1989; 321: 1725–1737.

Matis, A. J., Sibley, R., Mauer, M. D. *et al.* A retrospective study of biopsies performed during putative rejection episodes. *Ann. Surg.* 1983; 197: 226–237.

Mathew, T. H. Recurrence of disease following renal transplantation. *Amer. J. Kidney. Dis.* 1988; 12: 85–96.

Peterson, P. K., Anderson, R. C. Infection in renal transplant recipients. Current approaches to diagnosis, therapy and prevention. *Amer. J. Med.* 1986; 81, Suppl. 1A: 2–10.

CHAPTER 18

The pathology of renal transplantation

CLAIRE M. HILL

The pathological findings in a transplanted kidney are influenced by many factors relating to the donor, the vascular and ureteric anastomoses, by the presence of rejection, *de novo* or recurrent disease and by the effect of drugs such as cyclosporin (CYA) on the kidney. The accurate recognition of rejection in biopsy specimens is of considerable practical importance. Equally important is the identification of other abnormalities such as tubular necrosis or pyelonephritis which would alter the clinical management and influence the dose of immunosuppressive drugs required by the patient at that time.

1. Historical background

The first descriptions of renal transplant pathology were made during experimental animal studies in the early 20th century. In these non-immunosuppressed animals the main findings were interstitial oedema and mononuclear cell infiltration but relatively normal glomeruli. It was shown later that rejection was accelerated if the donor had already given skin or a kidney to the recipient. In these animals there was interstitial haemorrhage and necrosis of blood vessels and glomeruli in the transplanted kidney. Further understanding of the rejection process came from experimental observations on skin grafting and tumour transfer by Medawar who described the features of first and second set rejection. First set rejection was shown to be cell mediated whereas second set was due to circulating antibody against the grafted tissue. These studies provided a very basic understanding of rejection and its histological appearances.

Following the extension of renal transplantation to human patients Hume and his co-workers in Boston described the pathological findings in a series of nine transplants some of which were from unrelated donors. As in the animals the main abnormalities in the kidneys were interstitial oedema and a "round cell" infiltrate. However, if there was a major blood group incompatibility between donor and recipient, the intrarenal arteries in the transplanted kidney had thrombosed.

Mary G. McGeown (ed.), Clinical Management of Renal Transplantation, 263–275.

The introduction of azathioprine and prednisone as immunosuppressive agents in the early sixties was a major advance and prolonged survival after renal transplantation became possible. Immunosuppressive treatment meant that the lesions in the transplanted kidneys were less florid in these "modified" recipients. The pathological changes due to rejection were described by Porter. Much of the diagnostic pathology of renal transplant biopsies is based upon his careful observations. The introduction of CYA almost two decades later has complicated the pathological scene. CYA, as well as being a powerful immunosuppressive drug, is nephrotoxic and transplant biopsies are often performed in order to try and distinguish between rejection and CYA toxicity, since the management of the two conditions is very different.

2. Technical aspects

As described in Chapter 17 renal transplant biopsies are usually obtained percutaneously using a Tru-cut needle. It is helpful if details of the case are discussed with the pathologist in advance as this may influence the allocation of the tissue to the various forms of investigation. In some centres a specially trained medical laboratory scientific officer attends the biopsy and deals with the tissue "on the spot". This is particularly helpful if the renal unit and the transplant pathologist are in different hospitals as in several U.K. centres. Other laboratories send out a "biopsy box" with appropriate instructions. Needle biopsy produces small precious specimens and it is important that an experienced person handles them immediately after they are taken so that the optimum yield of diagnostic information is obtained. If possible two cores of tissue should be taken, ideally with the needle at different angles. This reduces the problem of sampling error if localised lesions such as small polar infarcts are present.

The mainstay of biopsy assessment is light microscopy usually of paraffin sections. As soon as it is taken from the patient one of the biopsy cores is placed on a small piece of dental wax or firm paper to which it will adhere slightly and thus remain flat. The tissue and its support are placed into freshly prepared fixative which has been provided by the laboratory. Ten per cent formalin or a similar solution is widely used. However, in Belfast a modified Bouin fixative, Duboscq Brasil, has been used for many years for renal biopsies. This gives excellent, crisp fixation for light microscopy but does not permit reliable demonstration of immunoglobulins and complement by immunoperoxidase methods.

Since 1972 immunofluorescence has been performed in Belfast on transplant biopsies. For this purpose one tissue core is snap frozen using isopentane pre-cooled by liquid nitrogen. On return to the laboratory a preliminary frozen section is examined by light microscopy. This can be helpful in deciding if a non-functioning kidney is necrotic. Dense cellular infiltrates are observed in untreated rejection episodes. However, caution is needed in interpreting lesser degrees of abnormality. In these circumstances it is more prudent to await the paraffin histology rather than over-interpret a frozen section. Direct immunofluorescence takes less than two hours and can give information about blood vessel staining and glomerular deposits which is helpful in differential diagnosis.

Electron microscopy is most useful in biopsies taken months or years after transplantation, particularly if there is any suspicion of *de novo* or recurrent glomerulonephritis. It is less important in early samples where the diagnostic questions are concerned with viability and the distinction between rejection and acute tubular necrosis. When electron microscopy is planned, a small piece of tissue is taken immediately from each end of a biopsy core, fixed in buffered gluteraldehyde and processed into resin. This normally takes at least one day but can be speeded up in exceptional circumstances. The recent introduction of microwave ovens into pathology laboratories is a useful development and may shorten the fixation times without loss of quality.

A biopsy taken from the donor kidney at the time of harvesting or after completion of the anastomoses can be used for comparison with later samples from the same kidney. This is not routine practice in Belfast unless some abnormality is suspected by the surgeon. Diagnostic transplant biopsies are used in Belfast for the investigation of transplant dysfunction or proteinuria. This means that some recipients have no biopsies, whereas others have several. It has not been our policy to examine regular biopsies at pre-arranged time intervals. This avoids unnecessary biopsy trauma to the transplant.

The nephrologist should give as much information as possible on the biopsy request form. This must include the transplant date and type of immunosuppression as well as the clinical indications for the biopsy. The pathologist's records should contain details of any previous biopsies.

In some centres fine needle aspiration cytology is used to study cells within a transplanted kidney. This procedure is more valuable if immunoperoxidase staining is performed on the aspirate to identify the T cell subtypes present within it. The preparations should be assessed by a cytopathologist in order to gain maximum information, particularly if conditions other than rejection are present.

3. Rejection

Rejection is classified as hyperacute, acute or chronic.

3.1. *Hyperacute rejection*

Hyperacute rejection is thought to be due to preformed antibodies and results in a reaction beginning immediately the kidney is revascularised. It is analogous to experimental xenograft rejection (between different species) and was observed in early human renal transplants with ABO incompatibility between donor and recipient. Preformed cytotoxic antibody can cause hyperacute rejection and a number of patients are now described in whom hyperacute rejection is thought to be due to antibody against the vascular endothelial cells. Perfusion injury to the endothelium may occasionally have a similar appearance. In practical terms the kidney with hyperacute rejection goes blue on the table shortly after removal of the vascular clamps. It becomes progressively infarcted. If it is removed within a few hours the main pathological finding is a deeply cyanosed kidney with patent major vessels. Histological examination reveals early thrombosis of glomerular capillaries and cortical arterioles. If the non-functioning kidney is not removed a biopsy some days later will show necrotic non-viable tissue. The nephrectomy specimen is infarcted and there is secondary thrombosis of the hilar vessels. It may be very difficult to determine the precise cause of infarction at this stage and the distinction between hyperacute rejection and primary venous thrombosis may be impossible.

3.2. Acute rejection

Acute rejection is initially predominantly cellular as in first set animal rejection. Later there is prominent vascular involvement as was observed in second set rejection in animals. This is probably due to antibody formed after transplantation. These are the changes most commonly encountered in biopsies from rejecting renal transplants.

Cellular rejection is characterised by infiltration of the interstitium by mononuclear cells of the lymphoid series, particularly T lymphocytes (Figure 53). The interstitium is frequently very oedematous during rejection, particularly in azathioprine treated cases but less so when the patient is receiving CYA. The infiltrate is most dense in the deeper part of the cortex and tends to aggregate around the arcuate arteries at the corticomedullary junction, which should be included in a biopsy sample to permit this assessment. In acute cellular rejection the cells also infiltrate the walls of tubules and blood vessels (Figure 54). Involvement of these structures indicates activity of the process. Neutrophil polymorphs are not a feature of cellular rejection. Their presence in a transplant biopsy suggests either infection or necrosis, probably associated with more severe changes in the adjacent tissues.

Cellular rejection is potentially reversible but episodes which do not resolve completely are followed by further injury to peritubular capillaries, arterioles and arteries. The early cellular infiltration and intimal oedema are followed by fibrinoid necrosis and thrombosis. Secondary changes are found in the surrounding tissues. A reliable hallmark of severe rejection is interstitial haemorrhage. If this is seen in a needle biopsy it usually indicates vascular rejection even if the affected vessels are not present in the tissue sample. Fibrinoid necrosis may extend from the afferent arterioles into the glomeruli

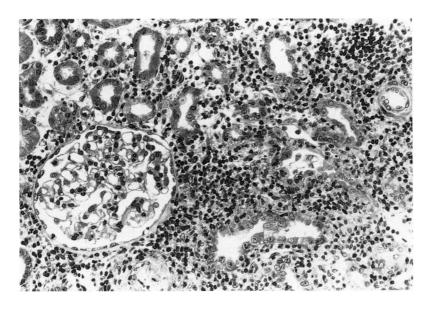

Figure 53. Acute cellular rejection. A dense lymphocytic infiltrate in the interstitium separates the tubules widely. Masson trichrome ×200.

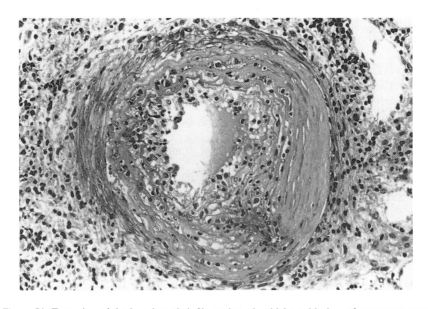

Figure 54. Extension of the lymphocytic infiltrate into the thickened intima of an arcuate artery in acute rejection. Periodic acid Schiff ×200.

and this change does not reverse completely even with aggressive therapy. When advanced lesions such as these are seen in transplant biopsies from a patient who has already been maximally immunosuppressed, a transplant nephrectomy may be advisable. The kidney will be enlarged, congested and mottled often with multiple small infarcts. The renal artery appears narrowed because the wall is swollen by the rejection process.

3.3. *Chronic rejection*

The main histological finding in chronic rejection is marked narrowing of the lumen of arteries and arterioles by fibrous intimal thickening. Although known as chronic, the lesion can be present as early as a few weeks after transplantation. The progressive reduction in blood flow leads to secondary ischaemic changes, with tubular atrophy, interstitial fibrosis and scattered lymphocytes in the interstitium. Antibody mediated endothelial damage, particularly to arcuate and interlobular arteries, is the probable cause of this lesion. Patients with chronic rejection have often had previous acute rejection episodes. As outlined in Chapter 17 it is an important cause of failing function in later transplants.

Interstitial and vascular lesions tend to be the most prominent abnormalities in rejection but some cases with allograft dysfunction have very abnormal glomeruli. The glomerular capillary loops are blocked by swollen endothelial cells. Infiltrating mononuclear cells in the glomeruli add to the hypercellular appearance which resembles post infectious proliferative glomerulonephritis. This lesion is known as acute allograft glomerulopathy. Recent studies indicate that it is a distinct form of allograft rejection in which the glomerular endothelium is the target for injury by cytotoxic T cells. There is an association with cytomegalovirus (CMV) infection in some of the patients. The relationship between viral infection and rejection is complex and not clearly understood. The prognosis of acute allograft glomerulopathy is said to be poor, though the rate of progression is very variable since many factors are involved.

In chronic rejection with proliferative vascular lesions the glomeruli become progressively ischaemic. In a biopsy they may appear shrunken due to wrinkling and collapse of the capillary loops. The spectrum of glomerular lesions in rejection also includes changes which resemble membranoproliferative glomerulonephritis. The subendothelial space is widened by deposited material which is very pale on electron microscopy and stains positively for IgM and fibrin. Similar deposit is found in cases of haemolytic uraemic syndrome and it has been suggested that they result from laying down of incompletely polymerised fibrin. This lesion results in proteinuria and is found in biopsies from patients who develop proteinuria and renal impairment months or years after transplantation. Increasing the dose of immunosuppressive therapy has little effect on these glomerular changes and the reduction in renal function is likely to be progressive.

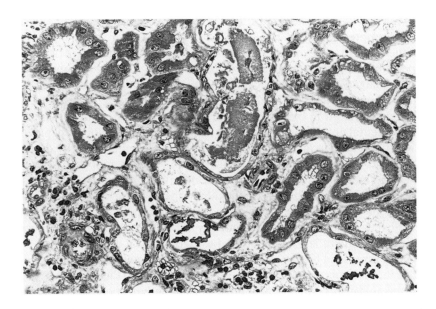

Figure 55. Acute tubular necrosis with flattening of the epithelium of some but not all of the tubules. Cellular debris and casts are present in the lumen. Masson trichrome ×250.

4. Differential diagnosis

One of the main questions to be answered by an early biopsy from a kidney which has not yet functioned is whether or not the tissue is infarcted either following hyperacute rejection or arterial or venous thrombosis. The other common diagnosis to be considered in the early post-transplant period is acute tubular necrosis. The histological evidence for this may be relatively sparse and does not correlate well with the clinical severity. Suggestive features are flattening and necrosis of the epithelium of some of the tubules which appear dilated (Figure 55). Interstitial oedema and scattered inflammatory cells are observed in cases of acute tubular necrosis but since these may be also part of cellular rejection the situation is quite complicated in the transplanted kidney.

There has been considerable debate as to what pathological alterations are diagnostic of CYA toxicity and several of the lesions originally thought to be important are now regarded as non-specific. A transplant biopsy from a CYA treated patient with renal impairment has to be assessed for evidence of rejection, tubular necrosis and other lesions in the usual way. A peculiar histological pattern known as striped interstitial fibrosis may be a pointer to CYA toxicity but it is difficult to recognise this pattern in small biopsy cores. Fibrin deposition in the walls of arterioles is also described in CYA toxicity but must be distinguished from the arteriolar lesions of rejection. Isometric vacuolation of tubular epithelium is not specific to CYA toxicity. Confirmation of the diagnosis of CYA toxicity is provided if renal function improves following reduction of the CYA dose without increasing any other immunosuppressive agent.

Patients with a fever and reducing transplant function are sometimes suspected of having cytomegalovirus (CMV) infection and a biopsy may be taken to diagnose rejection or CMV infection of the kidney. However, CMV inclusions are only found in the kidney in overwhelming infection and are rarely encountered in biopsy material. A few years ago a glomerular lesion with segmental necrosis was attributed to CMV. However, there is an overlap between this change and so-called acute allograft glomerulopathy described in an earlier section of this chapter. The main value of a biopsy under these clinical circumstances is the exclusion or otherwise of active rejection.

Pyelonephritis in a transplanted kidney may be the cause of functional impairment. It may arise from blood-borne infection in an immunosuppressed recipient but is more commonly the result of ascending infection, particularly if there is some degree of ureteric obstruction (see below). The diagnosis is made in biopsy material when there are collections of polymorphs in the interstitium and within the lumen of tubules (Figure 56). We have seen this in several patients who have subsequently responded to antibiotics and relief of partial ureteric obstruction. Difficulty arises if the biopsy also shows evidence of cellular rejection, which can certainly co-exist with infection and both should be treated. Polycystic kidneys are a potential source of infection and this is one of the arguments in favour of their removal prior to transplantation. Many of the earlier patients in this series have had bilateral nephroureterectomy for end-stage reflux nephropathy to avoid the risk of infected urine from the refluxing ureters reaching the transplant. More recently only a few such patients have been nephrectomised.

5. Recurrent disease

An interesting question which arose in human renal transplantation was whether or not the recipient's original disease would recur and, if so, would it cause the new kidney to fail. The answer is that quite a number of conditions do recur in the transplant but do not invariably lead to its failure.

Several types of glomerulonephritis have been shown to recur in transplants. The diagnosis should be established from positive histological features, comparing them with previous biopsies from the patient's own kidneys.

5.1. Dense deposit disease

Type II membranoproliferative glomerulonephritis is very prone to recur and has caused the failure of several transplants in our series, particularly when the initial clinical presentation was rapidly progressive and histologically characterised by multiple crescents superimposed on the basic pattern of

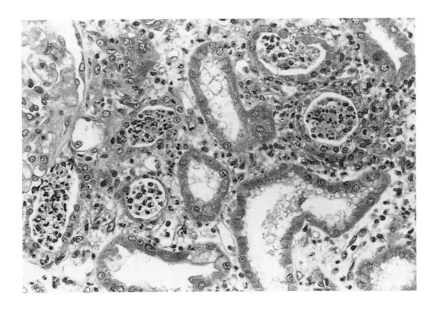

Figure 56. Acute pyelonephritis. Numerous neutrophil polymorphs are seen in the tubules and the adjacent interstitium. Masson trichrome ×250.

dense deposit disease. The first patient in whom we observed this presented with an acute nephritic syndrome when aged 16. He became dialysis dependent within two weeks and several months later his kidneys were removed because of uncontrollable hypertension. The glomeruli showed numerous epithelial crescents and advanced type II membranoproliferative GN with widespread ribbon-like electron dense deposits in the glomeruli and the basement membranes of Bowman's capsules and proximal tubules. This material stained positively for C'3 on immunofluorescence. C'3 was virtually undetectable in the patient's serum which contained C'3 nephritic factor. He was dialysed for almost three years before a suitably matched kidney was obtained. He achieved good graft function but at 18 months proteinuria recurred. The lower ureter had become stenosed after having a urinary leak in the the early post transplant period. At the time of surgery to his stenosed ureter his kidney was noted to be pale and a biopsy was taken. This showed definite dense deposit disease with early crescents. There was no evidence of rejection. A subsequent biopsy showed more severe glomerular disease and within six months he was in advanced renal failure. The kidney was removed because of the very heavy urinary loss of protein and he was also having life threatening infections. It was a large pale kidney typical of this type of glomerulonephritis. A small number of other patients in this series have lost their transplants from dense deposit disease. Others with recurrent disease have had a more benign course.

5.2. *Type I membranoproliferative glomerulonephritis*

Recurrence of type I membranoproliferative glomerulonephritis is much more difficult to prove as the lesion closely resembles glomerular rejection. However, we observed recurrence in one well documented case in whom the pattern of fluorescence in his own kidneys (which had been removed) was reproduced exactly in his transplant, biopsied after the onset of nephrotic syndrome. The kidney functioned for two more years, before he required dialysis.

5.3. *IgA nephropathy*

Another glomerular lesion which recurs is IgA nephropathy a complication seldom seen in our series despite the frequency of this lesion in patients requiring a transplant.

5.4. *Anti-glomerular basement membrane (GBM) nephritis*

Recurrence of anti-GBM nephritis is usually prevented by waiting several months after the serum antibody level has become negative before carrying out a transplant. Recently we observed a florid recrudescence of anti-GBM nephritis after a 'flu like' illness in a man transplanted four years earlier. Anti-GBM antibody has been reported in patients transplanted for Alport's syndrome whose native glomerular basement membranes are biochemically and antigenically different from the transplant.

5.5. *Focal segmental glomerulosclerosis (FSGS)*

FSGS is said to recur early in transplants leading to nephrotic range protein-uria but this has been rare in the Belfast series. Transplant biopsies may show sclerotic segments arising as part of glomerular scarring for a variety of reasons and the diagnosis of recurrent FSGS should be made with caution.

5.6. *Haemolytic uraemic syndrome (HUS)*

HUS may also recur and cause renal damage. It has to be distinguished from the spectrum of vascular changes attributed to CYA toxicity. It is probably better to avoid this drug in patients whose original disease was HUS.

5.7. *Diabetes mellitus*

The glomerular and vascular lesions of diabetes mellitus may reappear in a transplant.

5.8. *Other metabolic diseases*

Metabolic diseases such as xanthinosis and oxalosis may cause considerable damage. Cystinosis affecting a transplant is a less severe lesion with the characteristic hexagonal crystals mainly within interstitial macrophages. We have observed this in one patient.

5.9. *Amyloid*

Amyloid is said to recur in approximately one third of cases, occasionally leading to renal failure. This complication has not been seen in our series.

The identification of recurrent disease is of great importance. It may alter the immunosuppressive management if something other than rejection is causing the transplant to fail. In conditions such as dense deposit disease which frequently recur and progress to cause serious damage, the use of live donors may be unwise.

The protracted course of several of these recurrent lesions has been attributed to the immunosuppressive treatment which modifies their natural history even if it does not prevent them.

6. Donor disease

A lesion in a renal transplant may have been present in the donor kidney.

On one occasion several years ago, a young male with severe head injury was being considered as a potential donor. His name however, identified him as a patient with steroid-resistant nephrotic syndrome who attended Nephrology Outpatients. Clinical investigation following his injury had not yet revealed this problem which made him quite unsuitable to be a donor. Another donor's kidneys were noted by the surgeon to be an unusual colour when they were being harvested. Urgent frozen section examination of a biopsy revealed heavy accumulation of iron in the renal tissue. This made the kidneys unsuitable for transplantation. The donor had apparently had haemolysis from a prosthetic aortic valve. These anecdotes illustrate the necessity for careful evaluation of donors whose earlier clinical records may not be immediately available during an acute and final admission and whose unconscious state prevents them giving their own medical history. There are several reports in the literature of inadvertent transplantation of metastatic tumours within the kidneys. A small primary may not have been apparent until detected at donor necropsy. Such tumours have led to the death of the recipient.

7. *De novo* glomerulonephritis

Any form of renal disease can develop in a transplant. However, one which has received particular attention is *de novo* membranous glomerulonephritis. It has distinct pathological features and several grades which can be clearly demonstrated by electron microscopy. We have occasionally observed this lesion in our series. One interesting patient whose polycystic kidneys were removed a year before transplantation developed increasing proteinuria 18 months later, rising to a level of 16 g/24 h. Transplant biopsy revealed membranous glomerulonephritis with finely granular capillary wall deposits of IgG and silver positive spikes on the epithelial aspect of the glomerular basement membranes. The findings were confirmed on electron microscopy. The patient was further investigated to exclude an underlying malignancy, HBs antigenaemia and renal vein thrombosis as underlying causes for proteinuria but none of these lesions was found. He continued to have nephrotic range proteinuria with slowly progressive renal impairment over a period of several years. His biopsy showed no other histological features of rejection and therefore he was diagnosed as having *de novo* idiopathic membranous glomerulonephritis. The kidney functioned for two more years before he required dialysis. In other cases the membranous pattern may be part of chronic rejection in which anti-HLA antibody-antigen complexes have lodged subepithelially. However, as described in an earlier section subendothelial deposits in transplants biopsied after the onset of nephrotic syndrome are much more typical of chronic rejection.

8. Pathology of the transplanted ureter

It is only logical to assume that the ureter is involved in the rejection process as it is part of the allografted tissue. This is shown to be true when ureters from rejected transplants are examined in the laboratory after nephrectomy. Lesions such as mononuclear cell infiltration and vascular necrosis or narrowing also occur in the ureter. There is often a considerable degree of submucosal oedema. The ureter is a thin walled tube and its lumen is easily compromised when the wall is swollen by accumulating fluid and cells of the immune system. This can be sufficient to cause an isotope renogram to have an obstructive pattern, which resolves after antirejection treatment.

The arterial supply to the lower ureter is delicate. During harvesting the periureteric fatty tissue should be left undisturbed to avoid damaging the vessels within it. In a few patients however the lower end of the ureter becomes ischaemic in the region of the anastomosis which breaks down, resulting in a urinary leak. Under these circumstances a transplant biopsy would show very little abnormality despite a reduction in the urinary output to the exterior. This discrepancy would raise the possibility of obstruction. Lesser degrees of damage to the ureter cause ischaemic narrowing later. The back pressure changes affect the kidney, seen histologically as tubular dilatation and progressive interstitial fibrosis with deposits of Tamm Horsfall protein in the interstitium. Polymorphs in the lumen of tubules are the commonest pointer to the presence of impaired urinary drainage with ascending infection. Reimplantation of the ureter may be necessary.

9. Concluding remarks

Renal transplant biopsies provide the pathologist with very interesting material to study. Rejection is the commonest finding in samples taken during episodes of functional instability particularly in the first few months. This chapter has endeavoured to outline the alternative diagnostic possibilities in transplanted kidneys and their potential relevance to the management of transplant patients.

Frequent discussions about patients requiring biopsies are useful and follow up information should be provided to the pathologist who is part of the transplant team. This type of close collaboration helps increase the understanding of the significance of the complex changes found in transplanted kidneys.

Further reading

Häyry, P. J. Fine needle aspiration biopsy in renal transplanation. *Kidney Int.* 1989; 36: 130–141.

Hume, D. M., Merrill, J. P., Miller, B. F., Thorn, G. W. Experiences with renal homotransplantation in the human: report of nine cases. *J. Clin. Invest.* 1955; 34: 327–382.

Mihatsch, M. J., Thiel, G. Basler, V. *et al.* Morphological patterns in cyclosporine treated renal transplant recipients. *Transpl. Proc.* 1985; 17 (Suppl 1): 101–116.

Porter, K. A., Thomson, W. B., Owen, K. *et al.* Obliterative vascular changes in four human kidney homotransplants. *Br. Med. J.* 1963; 3: 639–645.

Walker, R. G., Kincaid-Smith, P. Recurrence of glomerulonephritis after renal transplantation. In *International Yearbook of Nephrology.* Andreucci, V., Fine, R. N., Kjellstrand, C.-M., Sugino, N. (eds). Boston: Kluwer Academic Publishers, 1990; 37–51.

CHAPTER 19

Surgical complications of renal transplantation

R. A. DONALDSON

Surgical complications following renal transplantation may be defined as those which require operative intervention for alleviation. Non specific surgical complications such as wound sepsis, peptic ulceration and gastro-intestinal haemorrhage to which the immunosuppressed recipient may be more susceptible than normal are not described in this chapter. The surgical complications are usually technical in origin. Since the early days of renal transplantation their incidence has fallen dramatically. This is in part due to better technique and a fuller understanding of the anatomy, both normal and anomalous, of the kidney and excretory tract. The introduction of synthetic suture materials for vascular anastomoses has reduced the incidence of complications. The vast worldwide experience of renal transplantation shared at conferences and through publications has been most helpful in managing surgical complications. The number of surgical complications has been dwindling and as a result they may now seem to be more complicated, but with the help of a shared experience, a remarkable number of innovative techniques have been used to salvage allografts which would otherwise have been lost. Nevertheless, life threatening and graft threatening situations still arise and an awareness of these situations is still essential. Apart from haemorrhage and wound sepsis, the surgical complications of renal transplantation usually come to light during the investigation of early anuria or graft failure. A combined medical and surgical approach to the investigation of anuria and early and late renal failure, using minimally invasive techniques is essential.

The surgical complications of renal transplantation may be conveniently described under the following headings:

1. excretory tract
2. vascular
3. fluid collections
4. miscellaneous

Mary G. McGeown (ed.), Clinical Management of Renal Transplantation, 277–290.
© 1992 *Kluwer Academic Publishers, Dordrecht. Printed in the Netherlands.*

1. Excretory tract complications

Excretory tract complications are those related to the calyces, renal pelvis, ureter and bladder. It should be re-emphasised (Chapter 11) that avoidance of excretory tract complications depends largely upon the care with which retrieval of the kidneys has been carried out. It should be remembered that the blood supply to the ureter is through one or two para-ureteric arteries running within the peri-ureteric sheath supplied by branches from the renal artery, from vessels in peri-renal fat and, as the ureter descends into the pelvis, from branches of the aorta, external iliac artery and internal iliac artery. As branches from the aorta and below obviously cannot be preserved, the ureteric arteries will depend upon the supply from the renal artery and peri-renal fat. This means that, at the time of retrieval, the peri-renal fat between the lower pole of the kidney and ureter should be carefully preserved, as well as that of the tissues in the hilum of the kidney and around the ureter. The ureter should be kept as short as possible, without tension at the uretero-vesical anastomosis, in order that the blood supply via the ureteric arteries to the terminal ureter should not be extended excessively. Minor damage to the ureteric arteries at the time of retrieval may result in early thrombosis of these vessels, resulting in various degrees of ischaemia. At the time of renal transplantation when the blood flow has been restored to the kidney, the blood flow to the ureter should be carefully assessed, ensuring that there is adequate oozing of blood at the tip of the ureter, prior to implantation.

1.1. *Urine leakage*

Urine leakage from the wound usually occurs within the first few days of transplantation. This leakage may be from the cystotomy or from the uretero-vesical anastomosis.

Early leakage of urine should lead one to suspect that the urethral catheter may be blocked, stretching and opening up an inadequate suture line at the cystotomy wound or uretero-vesical anastomosis. In the early hours after renal transplantation, with early renal function, if it is found that the catheter is not draining adequately, gentle washouts of the bladder should be attempted. If this fails the catheter should be changed and careful observations carried out to see if catheter drainage is restored, with cessation of urine leakage through the wound. If the leakage continues, early exploration is advised to re-suture the cystotomy or revise the uretero-vesical anastomosis. It is best to treat these situations aggressively otherwise there is a high risk of infection. Delayed exploration is much more difficult with a high risk of loss of the graft. If the lower end becomes necrotic and sloughs due to poor vascularisation from thrombosis or surgical ablation of the ureteric arteries, the kidney having functioned immediately after transplantation, the urine flow from the urethra will switch to flow through the wound within a few days following transplantation. In these circumstances after a few days all the urinary output will be excreted through the wound. Early exploration is advisable.

Exploration will reveal the amount of remaining viable ureter or renal pelvis and depending upon these findings surgical correction can be initiated. The ureter may be re-implanted into the bladder or the renal pelvis anastomosed to the bladder or ipsilateral ureter if it is still present. The renal pelvis can also be anastomosed to the contralateral ureter if the ipsilateral ureter is not present. If the recipient's kidneys are still *in situ* the ureters can be ligated proximaly with impunity but at some later stage it is advisable to remove the recipient's kidney as there is a risk of hydronephrosis and resultant pyonephrosis. This of course can be carried out at a later stage if the patient's progress is satisfactory.

At a later stage, usually after two weeks, leakage of urine may occur through the wound but at the same time urine is coming from the bladder. Under these circumstances, a leakage of urine from a calyx should be suspected. This is a very rare condition and is due to leakage of urine from an upper or lower pole calyx as a result of de-vascularisation at the time of renal retrieval when a polar artery has been missed, damaged or unsuccessfully re-anastomosed to the main renal artery. When this happens it is most important to have a pre-operative diagnosis, since this condition may easily be missed at surgical exploration. It is best diagnosed by retrograde pyelography. Treatment consists of excision of the ischaemic pole of the kidney and suture of the healthy remaining excretory tract and kidney.

1.2. *Ureteric obstruction*

1.2.1. *Ureteric stenosis.* The most common cause of ureteric obstruction following renal transplantation is ureteric stenosis due to vascular insufficiency. Ureteric stenosis may appear weeks, months or even years after transplantation. The time at which ureteric stenosis appears depends on the degree of vascular insufficiency. Complete vascular insufficiency leads to early sloughing of the ureter, whereas the more minor degrees of vascular insufficiency lead to slow and progressive fibrosis and stenosis of the ureter. The aetiology of vascular insufficiency is mainly technical and due to damage to the ureteric arteries at the time of renal retrieval and transplantation. It should be emphasised that careful handling of the ureter with preservation of a complete peri-ureteric sheath and minimal minipulation with blunt dissecting forceps of the tip of the ureter at the time of transplantation, are the keys to preservation of a good ureteric blood supply.

Complete stripping of the peri-vesical tissues at the time of retrieval usually results in sloughing of the ureter following transplantation but lesser degrees of damage due to careless handling of the ureter can result in thrombosis of the ureteric arteries.

Fresh bleeding from the end of the ureter at the time of transplantation is a most reassuring sign. If fresh bleeding does not occur, the ureter should be cut back in length until fresh bleeding is seen. However, a ureter should be left of such length as is compatible with a ureter-vesical anastomosis which is not under tension. If the blood supply to the entire ureter is suspect at the time of transplantation, it is advisable to utilise the recipient's ureter, anastomosing it to the renal pelvis as a primary procedure or performing a direct anastomosis of the renal pelvis to the bladder.

Thrombosis of the ureteric arteries due to the rejection process is not thought to be a significant cause of ischaemia and ureteric stenosis. Careful histological examination of those ureters which have been stenosed have shown signs of rejection in the ureter only in those cases where there has been overwhelming rejection of the kidney as well as of the ureter.

Ureteric stenosis commences at the tip of the ureter and the degree of proximal extension of the stenosis depends upon the degree of vascular insufficiency. Stenosis at the anastomosis is probably due to a constricting anastomosis usually caused by continuous suturing of the uretero-vesical mucosa. This can be prevented by using interrupted sutures rather than a continuous stitch. As ureteric stenosis develops slowly, progressively and silently after transplantation, with initially only partial obstruction of the excretory tract, decline in renal function tends to be the late and only presentation of this condition. As the transplanted kidney is devoid of nerve supply ureteric colic or pain is not a feature of ureteric obstruction in allograft recipients. If the condition is undiagnosed, it may progress to complete ureteric obstruction and hydronephrosis with eventual graft failure and the risk of pyonephrosis.

Whilst renal function is declining but still adequate, excretion urography will reveal evidence of obstruction of the excretory tract. Dilatation proximal to the stenosis will also be revealed by ultrasound scanning. Retrograde pyelography usually has little to offer in the investigation of ureteric stenosis as the ureteric orifice is on many occasions inaccessible to catheterisation. Furthermore, if the distal end of the ureter is stenosed, it is virtually impossible to pass a ureteric catheter. On the other hand it is important to know the exact site and extent of stenosis pre-operatively so that operative correction can be carefully planned. The most useful pre-operative investigation is antegrade pyelography with percutaneous puncture of the excretory tract under ultrasound control.

At the time of antegrade pyelography, some surgeons recommend the insertion of a stent between renal pelvis and bladder, leaving the stent *in situ* for three months. This could be considered only as a temporary procedure as the ureter is already ischaemic and, following removal of the stent, further fibrosis of the ureter will be inevitable. Definitive excision of the stenosed segment of the ureter should be carried out and followed by reconstruction of the excretory tract.

Although retrograde pyelography is usually unhelpful, it is well worthwhile carrying out a preliminary cystoscopy as the stenosis may be restricted to the tip of the ureter. If a submucosal tunnel has been constructed, the appearances will resemble a conventional ureterocele; and at the time of cystoscopy, the condition can be dealt with adequately by simple incision of the ureterocele.

1.2.2. Reconstruction of the excretory tract. There are numerous methods of reconstruction of the excretory tract and the approach used depends upon the tissues available. After excision of the stenosed segment of ureter, if there is sufficient length of viable ureter remaining to carry out a re-implantation without tension at the uretero-vesical junction, this procedure should be carried out. If there is insufficient length of ureter to reach the bladder and the patient's ipsilateral or contralateral ureters are present then pelvi-ureteric anastomosis should be considered. Ligation of the recipient's proximal ureter usually has no longterm ill effect but there is a potential risk of hydronephrosis of the recipient's kidney with the further risk of pyonephrosis. Under ideal circumstances at some later date, it is probably advisable to remove the recipient's own kidney. If the recipient's ureters are not present and there is insufficient length of ureter to reach the bladder, then the renal pelvis should be anastomosed to the bladder with the assistance of a psoas hitch or Boari flap if necessary. Obviously direct pelvi-vesical anastomosis leads to overt vesico-renal reflux but experience has shown that vesico-ureteric reflux in renal allograft recipients seems to have no deleterious effect on the graft.

Very few surgeons use ureteric stents at the time of initial renal transplantation. However, at any secondary procedure for reconstruction of the excretory tract, stenting is advisable because of the extended handling of tissues at the time of operation causing moderate to severe ischaemia with a high risk of leakage of urine and recurrent stenosis.

Occasionally one may find a pelvi-ureteric junction obstruction resembling a conventional pelvi-ureteric junction obstruction. This is most likely due to a *forme fruste* of pelvi-ureteric obstruction in the donor organ which has not been recognised at the time of retrieval. A conventional pyeloplasty is not advisable as the distal ureteric blood supply may be insufficient to support such a procedure. Pyelo-ureterostomy or pyelo-vesicostomy should be considered.

1.2.3. Other causes of ureteric obstruction. Other causes of ureteric obstruction include external compression of the excretory tract and intraluminal obstruction. External compression of the excretory tract may be caused by fluid collections around the kidney and ureter and this subject will be discussed later. In the early days after transplantation, the lower end of the ureter may be compressed by blood or blood clot within the uretero-vesical tunnel. Oedema within the tunnel may also compress the lower end of the ureter to cause ureteric obstruction. Anuria and oliguria are common after transplantation and other causes such as acute tubular necrosis and rejection receive priority in investigation. If rejection is not present and DTPA renography shows that the kidney is functioning well with a good blood supply, ureteric obstruction will be suspected. Uretero-vesical tunnel compression due to oedema or blood clot may be seen on IVU. This condition requires no operative intervention as it will settle spontaneously with renal dialysis. Tunnel oedema and bleeding within the tunnel can be prevented by careful attention to technique with respect to haemostasis and tissue handling. The ureter will retract from its tunnel if the uretero-vesical anastomosis is under tension and this retraction may result in ureteric obstruction. The findings are much the same as with tunnel oedema and blood clot but exploration and re-implantation are required. The condition may be prevented by an adequate intravesical tunnel at the time of transplantation and a retaining stitch between the ureter and peri-vesical tissues thus preventing retraction of the ureter.

There have been case reports of external compression of the ureter by the spermatic cord. There is a potential risk of obstruction of the ureter by the round ligament of the uterus but invariably this structure is ligated and divided at the time of transplantation. Sometimes the spermatic cord is ligated and divided but one usually attempts to preserve it at the time of transplantation when a space for the kidney is being prepared within the extra-renal portion of the pelvis. When the space is being prepared, the cord tends to sag into the depths of the wound and when carrying out the uretero-vesical anastomosis it is very easy inadvertently to place the ureter anterior to the cord. If this happens, the cord tends to proceed to its normal anatomical position after operation and may kink the ureter sufficiently to cause complete obstruction. When ureteric obstruction has been diagnosed, exploration of the wound will reveal the cause and can be remedied by division and ligation of the cord. This is easier than re-doing the uretero-vesical anastomosis posterior to the cord, which however is appropriate if the opposite cord has been ligated and divided at some previous transplantation operation and sterility is considered of importance.

Following transplantation and especially after re-exploration, fibrous tissue may build up around the ureter. This can cause extrinsic ureteric compression resembling retroperitoneal fibrosis. This condition may be amenable to antegrade stenting of the ureter. If exploration is carried out then ureterolysis in the usual manner as for retroperitoneal fibrosis is not usually feasible and some form of reconstruction should be carried out.

Intraluminal obstruction of the ureter is usually caused by blood clot or clots. Clots may form within the renal pelvis and pass down the ureter causing temporary obstruction only and no special treatment is required. If the clot becomes lodged at the suture line of uretero-vesical junction, it may become organised and very adherent to the ureteric orifice sufficient to cause complete obstruction for days or weeks. Eventually it will be dislodged spontaneously if renal replacement therapy by dialysis has been maintained. It can be diagnosed earlier if ureteric obstruction is suspected and cystoscopy is carried out, at which time the clot can be dislodged easily with small biopsy forceps.

2. Vascular complications

2.1. *Haemorrhage*

During operation serious and uncontrollable haemorrhage may occur when the vascular clamps are released. Haemorrhage from the arterial anastomosis is more frequent but may also occur from the venous anastomosis or from small veins in the hilum of the kidney which have been inadvertently damaged or over-looked at the time of renal retrieval. Carefully constructed anastomoses will reduce the incidence of haemorrhage. Continuous suturing of the arterial anastomosis has been facilitated by the use of a Carrel patch without risk of subsequent stenosis of the renal arteries. If a patch is not available for anastomosis, as is usual in the case of living related donors, then end to end anastomosis of the internal iliac artery to the renal artery is recommended, using interrupted sutures rather than a continuous suture with risk of subsequent stenosis at the suture line. The technique of suturing and the suture material used is very important. Suture should be from within the lumen of the recipient artery (which may be somewhat atheromatous) passing the needle through the media and adventitia. In this way, small atheromatous plaques are tacked down to the media and produce a smooth suture line. In the early days of renal transplantation silk was used, but the introduction of synthetic suture materials has vastly improved the results. Modern sutures ensure that the suture material is wider than the needle used and this means that the needle holes are completely plugged by the suture and needle hole bleeding is completely avoided. Some surgeons advocate wrapping the anastomotic line with synthetic haemostatic material such as Surgicel or Haemocel prior to removal of the clamps. When haemostasis is secured, the material can be picked off from the suture line.

It is very rare to have completely uncontrollable haemorrhage requiring re-clamping of the main recipient vessels and removal of the donor organ. Smaller bleeding points can be oversewn. Small veins within the hilum of the kidney which have been overlooked can be ligated and, as long as one main renal vein remains intact, this can be carried out without detriment to the venous drainage of the kidney.

When the wound is closed, significant haemorrhage may occur in the first few hours after operation and is usually reactionary in nature occurring in those recipients who have been hypotensive during surgery, as the blood pressure rises post-operatively. A drain, if used, may not reveal the full extent of blood loss. In such situations immediate exploration is mandatory. Bleeding tends to be from the anastomoses, especially the arterial anastomosis, or from damaged veins within the hilum of the kidney. The donor organ can usually be salvaged by oversewing the anastomosis if necessary and ligation or oversewing of open veins within the hilum of the kidney.

2.2. *Arterial complications*

2.2.1. *Renal artery thrombosis.* The arterial complication which occurs earliest is thrombosis at the site of anastomosis. This is usually technical in origin as a result of an irregular suture line predisposing to clot. Rarely conditions such as protein C or protein S deficiency predispose to early arterial thrombosis. Intrarenal thrombosis may occur in acute rejection and is not considered to be one of the surgical complications. If arterial thrombosis occurs it is rarely possible to make the diagnosis in time to salvage the kidney by exploration and thrombotomy. If the kidney is anuric or oliguric from the beginning, then the diagnosis will not be suspected. If early function occurs and it is noticed that urine output is declining, then by the time catheter drainage is fully investigated and DTPA renography and arteriography carried out, the ischaemic time has been far exceeded for exploration and remedial surgery to be carried out. A few cases of renal artery thrombosis have been described after the administration of antilymphocyte globulin and after the administration of CYA in the immediate post-operative period. The precise reason why CYA therapy should be implicated in renal artery thrombosis is still a mystery and requires further observation and research. Arterial thrombosis is more common in those kidneys which have multiple vessels requiring bench surgery prior to implantation. If multiple renal arteries arising from the aorta are present, best results are achieved by using several Carrel patches rather than trying to anastomose smaller vessels to the main renal artery.

2.2.2. *Renal artery stenosis.* Renal artery stenosis occurring months to years after transplantation is very uncommon and is usually detected on the investigation of hypertension. This condition is investigated by the use of intra-arterial digital subtraction angiography and by conventional angiography. Stenosis of the arterial supply to the kidney may occur at various sites. The most common site of stenosis is at the suture line where a short segment of stenosis can be identified. There may be stenosis in the common iliac artery proximal to the anastomosis or if the internal iliac artery has been used there may be stenosis within this vessel. The aetiology of stenosis within these vessels may be dense peri-arterial fibrosis or atheromatous plaques within the vessels. Treatment of common iliac internal iliac and suture line stenosis is bypass grafting or venous patch grafting after the vessels have been dissected free of scar tissue. Stenosis of small branches of the main renal artery may be single or multiple and are much more difficult to diagnose and manage. Since the introduction of CYA therapy there appears to have been an increased incidence of clinically significant transplant arterial stenosis. With the increase in the use of donor kidneys harvested from children younger than six years, the incidence of stenosis of the donor artery unrelated to the surgical anastomosis has increased (without evidence of the stenosis being related to vascular rejection). Overall, regardless of the immunosuppressive regime used, the use of small donor kidneys appears to be the most significant factor associated with transplant arterial stenosis. Histological evidence tends to suggest that the stenoses are due to medial fibroplasia which of course may have been present prior to transplantation. Small vessel stenoses are difficult to manage by open surgical procedures and most clinicians agree that as long as the hypertension can be controlled by drugs alone, operative intervention should be avoided. With the introduction of endoluminal angioplasty for the treatment of arterial stenosis this method of management has been universally adopted for transplanted kidneys. The procedure can be easily repeated if necessary and results in minimal renal damage. Results of endoluminal angioplasty will of course depend on the condition of the distal vascular bed and best results are achieved in those patients with a post-stenotic dilation and the fewest arterial lesions. Angioplasty is usually carried out under general anaesthesia using balloon catheters appropriate for the size of vessels involved. Prevention of spasm and heparin therapy are essential adjuncts to this treatment.

2.3. Venous complications

The only significant venous complication is renal vein thrombosis which tends to occur within a few days after operation. The thrombosis probably commences at the anastomotic suture line and propagates along the renal vein and into the common iliac and femoral veins. This results in a grossly swollen kidney and ipsilateral leg. There will be a marked decline in urine output if the kidney has functioned immediately after transplantation. The diagnosis is usually easy and confirmed by DTPA renography, ultrasound of the kidney and exploration. The kidney can usually be salvaged by embolectomy as ischaemia of the organ is incomplete due to the nature of the condition, as the renal artery lumen is patent and there is sufficient blood flow to provide oxygen compatible with viability.

2.4. Arterio-venous fistulae and false aneurysms

These complications tend to occur following percutaneous renal biopsy during the investigation of declining renal function. The condition presents clinically with marked haematuria following biopsy. The diagnosis is usually confirmed by angiography and treatment may include observation or selective intra-arterial embolisation. If the arterio-venous fistula is associated with a pseudo-aneurysm, when intra-arterial embolisation is technically impossible, treatment may be attempted by percapsular embolisation of the pseudo-aneurysm using intra-operative ultrasound guidance. Following embolisation with coils the presence of the coils within the pseudo-aneurysm may act as a guide for subsequent percutaneous embolisation of the arterio-venous fistula.

3. Fluid collections associated with renal allografts

Accumulations of lymph, blood, serum or pus near renal allografts have been held responsible for a variety of complications such as obstruction of the excretory tract, ipsilateral leg oedema and proteinuria. The main clinical signs are suprapubic abdominal swelling, ipsilateral leg oedema, oedema over the allograft and lymph drainage from the wound. Deterioration in renal function with proteinuria and elevated serum creatinine concentrations are frequently encountered in patients with lymphocoeles. Concurrent rejection and urinary tract infection are also common features. Urinary retention is a rare complication of a fluid collection such as lymphocoele. Cases of ureteric obstruction due to collections of pus or peri-pelvic haematoma causing kinking of the ureter have been reported. A collection of pus is probably the most lethal of all these fluid collections but it should be remembered that diffuse pulmonary micro-emboli can occur from localised liquefying haematoma with necrotic tissue within the retroperitoneal space around the kidney.

3.1. *Lymphocoele*

Although a peri-ureteric fluid collection may produce a distortion of excretory tract anatomy, the extent to which it may compromise renal function or cause ureteric obstruction is uncertain.

Theoretically it might produce ureteric occlusion by kinking of the ureter by compression or by the effects of associated adhesions. It is also conceivable that a relatively mild compression might have a greater obstructive effect in a transplanted ureter than in an entirely normal ureter. Cine-radiological studies have demonstrated normal peristaltic activity in the unobstructed transplanted ureter, but the technique, without additional urodynamic information, gives no real estimate of the propulsive strength of the observed contraction or of the extent which they could overcome varying degrees of obstruction. Despite these uncertainties, it is clear that lymphocoeles may be present without causing ureteric obstruction or deterioration in renal function and operative treatment may not be required. If clinical and other circumstances are such that specific therapy is required, open surgical drainage is the treatment of choice. This procedure carries less risk of recurrence or of introducing infection than does repeated aspirations under ultrasound control. Where lymphocoeles or other fluid collections are associated with deterioration in renal function, the graft failure may be attributed to the mechanical effects of the fluid collection and lead to failure to diagnose other serious causes such as infection. This is particularly likely when the incidental fluid collection is large or when there is radiological evidence of ureteric obstruction. Optimal surgical intervention involves the transperitoneal approach with marsupialisation of the lymphocoele and placement of a tail of omentum through the window created. In less fit patients one might consider using drainage and installation of Povidone-iodide. Since the lymph in lymphocoeles appears to come from the lymphatics of the recipient, it might be possible to demonstrate these swellings by lymph-angiography but in most cases the diagnosis may be made on clinical grounds and with the aid of more usual radiological procedures and ultrasonic techniques. Graft recipients tend to be overloaded with fluid with the result that the peri-vascular lymphatics are more prominent in these patients than they are in patients with normal renal function. Ligation of dilated lymphatics that are divided during the course of vascular mobilisation at the time of transplantation would seem to be important for the prevention of lymphocoeles.

3.2. Haematoma/seroma

When this diagnosis is made, simple aspiration under ultrasound control is usually adequate for treatment. Recurrence is most unlikely.

3.3. Abscess

If the patient's condition is poor, it may be necessary to stop immunosuppressive therapy and drain the wound. On the other hand it is sometimes possible with a patient in good condition to continue immunosuppressive therapy with antibiotics and wound drainage.

4. Miscellaneous surgical complications

There are a number of surgical complications directly related to the operation of renal transplantation and these include: spontaneous rupture of the kidney, femoral neuropathy, hydrocoele, renal stones and gastro-intestinal complications.

4.2. *Spontaneous rupture of the kidney*

The aetiology of spontaneous rupture of the kidney is uncertain but it is a most dramatic condition. A number of factors have been incriminated such as renal vein thrombosis, acute tubular necrosis and acute rejection. The condition usually presents within the first 10 days of operation as gross swelling at the site of transplantation and sometimes very severe haemorrhage. Immediate exploration is indicated. If haemorrhage is not severe, it may be possible to salvage the kidney provided that acute rejection does not appear to be a significant feature. The large fissures which are usually present on the surface of the kidney can be covered by synthetic haemostatic material such as Haemocel or Surgicel. Despite the gross swelling in the kidney, the wound can usually be closed with drainage.

4.2. *Femoral neuropathy*

Numerous factors are involved in the aetiology of neuropathy in patients with chronic renal failure and those on haemodialysis. These include diabetes, uremia, abnormalities of uric acid, calcium and phosphate metabolism. Nevertheless, there seems to be a form of femoral neuropathy involving the ipsilateral femoral nerve following transplantation which is of technical origin. It is probably due to compression of the femoral nerve and its blood supply by a retractor at the time of operation. Diabetes may be a cause of spontaneous isolated femoral neuropathy but this condition can occur in non-diabetic patients following transplantation, usually in older patients who already have some degree of vascular insufficiency which is exacerbated by wound retraction. Although the femoral nerve is not exposed during a renal transplant operation, damage may result from cutting, stretching, compression, diathermy or devascularisation of the nerve. The mechanism of neuropathy caused by compression is probably anoxia as the femoral nerve has a relatively poor blood supply and is susceptible to compression anoxia. This is particularly the case when the main blood supply to the nerve is interrupted by ligation of the ileo-lumbar artery during mobilisation of the internal iliac artery. The co-lateral supply to the pelvic portion of the nerve is poor and thus the nerve may be rendered ischaemic. The lateral cutaneous nerve of the thigh may also be damaged during a renal transplant operation and because of the minor degree of disability, these lesions may be overlooked. Femoral nerve palsy, however, is dramatically obvious and incapacitating, with loss of motor power in the quadriceps and sensory loss in the distribution of the femoral nerve immediately following operation. As the injury is a neuropraxia, spontaneous improvement, which may take months to years, may nevertheless occur.

4.2. *Hydrocoele*

A hydrocoele on the side of the renal transplant is common if the cord has been ligated and divided. Prevention of this complication is by preservation of the cord which also preserves fertility. The ureter must be placed posterior to the cord to avoid obstruction of the ureter. Surgical correction of the hydrocoele should be carried out where possible and repeated tapping avoided as there is a risk of introducing infection.

4.3. *Renal calculi*

Hereditary cystinuria is a rare cause of renal failure resulting in renal transplantation. The condition will recur in the transplanted organ often necessitating removal and repeated transplantation. Very rarely a phosphate or oxalate calculus may be discovered in the investigation of haematuria or proteinurea with or without recurrent infections in the transplanted organ. Such a calculus may have been present but not noticed at the time of cadaveric renal retrieval. The position of the transplant kidney within the renal pelvis makes treatment of renal calculi relatively simple by percutaneous nephrolithotomy or extracorporeal shockwave lithotripsy.

4.4. *Gastrointestinal complications*

With improved immunosuppressive regimes, especially those with low dose steroid, the incidence of gastrointestinal complications such as duodenal ulcer with haemorrhage and the complications of diverticular disease have decreased considerably. With improved medical regimes for upper gastrointestinal disorder, operative intervention is now seldom required.

Most transplant surgeons are agreed that the retrieval of the kidney is probably the most important part of the operation but unfortunately this tends to be carried out by the most junior members of the transplant team. It is a pleasure to any surgeon to transplant an organ which has been carefully retrieved, even if there are vascular and excretory tract anomolies which have been carefully preserved and documented. The study of the vascular supply of the ureter and its preservation has contributed greatly to the reduced incidence of ureteric stenosis and necrosis. In the investigation of surgical complications and other causes of declining renal function, minimally invasive techniques are recommended. Hypertension due to stenosis of renal arteries should be treated as far as possible by anti-hypertensive drugs but the introduction of translumenal angioplasty has made surgical correction relatively simple and effective compared to open exploration and correction.

Unfortunately endo-urology has little to offer in the correction of excretory tract problems, especially ureteric stenosis due to its aetiology and nature.

Finally, there are three situations in which the transplant surgeon might be involved in an embarrassing position. Firstly, the donor cadaver should be treated with all due respect and left in a tidy anatomical condition, otherwise the wrath of the state pathologist expressed through the coroner may be incurred. Secondly, to avoid acrimonious communication from the receiving hospital, the surgeon retrieving the kidney should ensure that it is in optimal condition. Lastly, although tedious, after a retrieval procedure, the necessary forms should be completed with due accuracy to satisfy those concerned with their processing and subsequent implications.

Further reading

Donaldson, R. A., Jacobson, J. E., Pontin, A. R. Ureteric obstruction in renal allograft recipients. *South African Med. J.* 1977; 52: 1077–1082.

Donaldson, R. A., Jacobson, J. E., Pontin, A. R. Fluid collections associated with renal allografts. *South African Med. J.* 1978; 53: 51–53.

Henning, P. H., Bewick, M., Reidy, J. F. *et al.* Increased incidence of renal transplant arterial stenosis in children. *Nephrol. Dial. Transplant.* 1989; 4: 575–580.

Mehta, S. N. Kennedy, J. A., Loughridge, W. G. G. *et al.* Urological complications in 119 consecutive renal transplants. *Brit. J. Urol.* 1979; 51: 184–187.

CHAPTER 20

Early medical complications after renal transplantation

P. McNAMEE

1. Fluid balance

1.1. *Early post-operative management*

In the immediate post-operative period it is essential that monitoring of fluid balance begun in the operating room is continued. There is evidence that hypotension and hypovolaemia occurring in an ischaemic kidney may lead to more prolonged acute tubular necrosis. It is our policy to monitor central venous pressure (CVP), blood pressure and urinary output in the post-operative period to ensure optimum hydration and blood pressure.

A CVP catheter is inserted at the time of surgery and is maintained between 5 and 12 cm H_2O. Urinary output is measured hourly and fluid administered according to the CVP and the previous hour's output. The standard regime is to administer the previous hour's output +30 ml if the CVP lies within the normal range. If the CVP is below 5 cm H_2O the previous hour's output +50 ml (or sufficient to raise the CVP to within the normal range) is administered. If the CVP is greater than 12 cm H_2O then the previous hour's output is administered without supplement. If the patient has evidence of pulmonary oedema, fluid intake is decreased and if the graft is functioning a loop diuretic is administered.

The fluids administered are usually 0.9% saline and 5% dextrose in roughly equal proportions, although if the patient has diabetes or severe acidosis this regime may be altered accordingly.

Hourly measurement of the urinary output and appropriate replacement with intravenous fluids is continued for 24 hours post-operatively. At that time, if the patient has normal bowel sounds oral fluids may be administered. Urinary output is measured on a 12 hourly basis and fluids prescribed appropriately. Central venous pressure is monitored for a 24 hour period. Then unless there is concern about the patient's haemodynamic status, the central line is withdrawn.

Mary G. McGeown (ed.), Clinical Management of Renal Transplantation, 291–304.
© 1992 *Kluwer Academic Publishers, Dordrecht. Printed in the Netherlands.*

1.2. *Late post-operative management*

Following withdrawal of the central line, the patient's daily fluid requirements are assessed on clinical parameters i.e. daily output, blood pressure, jugular venous pressure, presence or absence of oedema and weight. The daily intake and output of fluids is recorded on a fluid balance chart. The patient is assessed on a daily basis with particular regard to blood pressure, presence of peripheral and pulmonary oedema and charted fluid balance. The patient is weighed regularly so that excessive weight gain is recognised early. Fluids are prescribed initially on a daily basis appropriate to the previous day's losses and the clinical state of hydration.

2. Electrolyte disturbances

Plasma electrolyte levels are reviewed one hour post-operatively and daily thereafter unless there is an indication for more frequent monitoring. Hyperkalaemia is the most frequent disturbance in the immediate post-operative period.

2.1. *Hyperkalaemia*

If hyperkalaemia is detected management depends on a number of factors:
1. the severity of hyperkalaemia
2. the state of renal function
3. the patient's volume status
The plasma potassium concentration is normally maintained between 3.5 and 5.0 mmol/l. If the concentration is greater than 6.5 mmol/l then action is necessary. There may be great variation in patient response to hyperkalaemia, due to whether factors such as acidaemia, pulmonary oedema, or hyperglycaemia are present, and whether digoxin is being given. It is therefore essential that in addition to the plasma potassium level, an ECG is carried out and muscle strength is tested.

ECG monitoring is commenced if the potassium concentration is greater than 6.5 mmol/l. If there is broadening of the QRS complex or significant tenting of the T waves then calcium gluconate is administered intravenously (10 ml, 10% solution). This will counter adverse membrane effects of hyperkalaemia although it will not remove or redistribute potassium.

The use of a cocktail of sodium bicarbonate, 50% dextrose and insulin administered intravenously leads to a shift of potassium from the extra- to the intra-cellular space and helps stabilise the membrane potential. The amount of intravenous fluids which can be given safely is related to the state of the patient's hydration. If there is evidence of pulmonary oedema and no sign of established renal function then urgent dialysis is necessary to remove excess potassium. If on the other hand the patient is euvolaemic and if renal function has been established conservative management is all that is necessary.

2.2. *Hyponatraemia*

Hyponatraemia occurs frequently in renal transplant patients as in most surgical patients. It is important to attempt to identify the factors responsible for the development of hyponatraemia since appropriate therapy depends upon correct diagnosis. Hyponatraemia may result from true total body sodium depletion, normal total body sodium with increased total body water or increased total body sodium with proportionately greater increase in total body water. Appropriate management of hyponatraemia hinges upon correct clinical assessment of the patient.

Since sodium is the principal determinant of extracellular volume, decreased total body sodium can be identified clinically by assessment of volume status. A patient who is truly sodium deficient will have a relatively contracted extracellular volume, characterised by hypotension (particularly postural hypotension) and an absence of peripheral oedema. The patient who has normal total body sodium but increased total body water leading to the development of hyponatraemia will have normal blood pressure without postural hypotension. There may or may not be mild oedema. The patient with increased total body sodium and even greater increase in total body water will have normal or high blood pressure and moderate to severe oedema.

If the patient is sodium deficient appropriate amounts of sodium chloride should be administered to return plasma sodium concentration to normal. This can be judged by:
1. normalisation of blood pressure
2. return of plasma sodium concentration to normal
3. when the patient has a functioning graft, increased urinary sodium excretion.

In the case of the patient with increased total body water but normal total body sodium, water intake should be restricted.

In the patient with increased total body sodium and increased total body water, restriction of sodium and water intake combined with loop diuretic therapy is appropriate, provided that the graft is functioning. If the graft is not functioning and the clinical situation demands it, dialysis therapy combined with ultra-filtration may be needed.

Hyponatraemia rarely develops in the early post-operative period unless inappropriate amounts of free water – from 5% dextrose – have been administered. Hyponatraemia developing later in the post-operative period is most often due to excessive water intake and decreased ability of the transplanted kidney to clear free water.

3. The diabetic transplant patient

The diabetic patient presents some special post-operative management problems.

3.1. *Fluid balance*

Diabetics are more likely to suffer from cardiovascular disease than non-diabetic patients. For this reason it is essential that care is exercised in the prescription of fluids to these patients.

3.2. *Hyponatraemia in the diabetic patient*

Hyponatraemia may occur in the diabetic patient as a consequence of hyperglycaemia. In the diabetic blood glucose should be estimated coincidently with plasma sodium level in order that the aetiology of hyponatraemia is accurately determined (see section 2.2.).

3.3. *Hyperkalaemia in the diabetic patient*

Insulin deficiency may lead to hyperkalaemia due to failure of trans-membrane potassium transportation. Particular attention must be paid to plasma glucose levels in order that trans-cellular potassium concentrations are regulated appropriately.

3.4. *Blood glucose regulation in the post-transplant diabetic patient*

The regulation of glucose and insulin administration to the diabetic transplant patient is similar to that of the diabetic patient undergoing any surgical procedure. Routine insulin is discontinued pre-operatively. An intravenous infusion of 5% dextrose and insulin is commenced and blood sugar concentration is checked by means of a glucometer four hourly or more frequently if clinical need demands it.

It must be appreciated that because of the effects of glucocorticoids and to a lesser extent cyclosporin (CYA), the post-operative insulin needs of the diabetic patient will be increased.

In the immediate post-operative period the diabetic patient's blood glucose is regulated by a sliding scale based upon frequent estimates of blood glucose concentration. As the patient returns to normal diet monitoring must be continued and increased insulin demands estimated. Requirements are particularly high during periods of anti-rejection therapy when four hourly blood glucose estimations are routine.

4. Graft non-function

Between 50 and 60% of patients undergoing renal transplantation in our unit have established renal function within 48 hours of transplantation. Early graft function has been associated with brief warm and total ischaemic time. However early graft function has not been shown to lead to better long term graft or patient survival. The best indicator of long term graft survival appears to be serum creatinine level one month after transplantation.

4.1. *Investigation of non-function*

In patients failing to show early graft function we perform a radioisotope renogram to verify the presence of blood flow to the graft. If isotope uptake is not seen, this has ominous implications for renal blood flow and renal arteriography is usually performed to determine whether the renal artery is patent.

Anuria may result either because of obstruction of the vesico-ureteric junction or because of detachment of the ureter from the bladder. We routinely perform an ultrasound scan of the graft if there is failure of early function, to look for evidence of free fluid indicative of a urinary leak, or pelvic dilatation found with obstruction. If there is evidence of a ureteric problem then early surgical consultation is sought. Ureteric re-implantation may be necessary.

The anuric post-transplant patient who has been shown by renography to have a viable graft presents particular management problems. It is essential that the patient's fluid, dietary and dialysis needs are assessed on a daily basis. Fluids are prescribed according to previous day's output and perceived clinical need. Dietary protein is restricted to 1 g/kg/day until renal function is established. Blood urea, creatinine and electrolyte levels are measured each day.

4.2. *Dialysis*

In the patient whose graft does not function within a few days of transplantation, despite strict control of fluid balance and diet, dialysis frequently is necessary to support the patient whilst awaiting the onset of graft function. Indications for dialysis are:
1. hyperkalaemia
2. pulmonary oedema
3. symptomatic uraemia

The mode of dialysis chosen for the individual patient is largely determined by the form of dialysis used pre-operatively. In the case of the patient maintained on peritoneal dialysis, it has been our policy to leave the dialysis catheter *in situ* at the time of surgery and to remove it later when function has been well established. If a patient previously maintained on peritoneal dialysis remains dialysis dependent after operation peritoneal dialysis is easily reinstituted.

Haemodialysis poses more problems in terms of cardiovascular instability than does peritoneal dialysis. If dialysis becomes necessary in a patient previously maintained on haemodialysis, it is embarked upon with some caution. It is essential that blood pressure is maintained in order that renal perfusion is not compromised as there is evidence that kidneys showing evidence of ATN are particularly vulnerable to vascular damage during the recovery period. An accurate clinical assessment of the patient's state of hydration is essential and the amount of fluid to be removed estimated. The blood pressure should be measured frequently during dialysis preferably with an automatic device such as Dynamap. If the blood pressure falls the rate of ultrafiltration should be reduced and if necessary measures taken to raise the blood pressure using intravenous colloid.

5. Graft rejection

Graft rejection remains a common complication. Acute rejection occurs in about 80% of transplant patients and is seen most frequently during the first month with a peak incidence between 7 and 14 days after surgery. Rejection must be recognised early and treated aggressively if good long term function is to be achieved. Increased immunosuppressive therapy should not be administered inappropriately. It is therefore important that an accurate diagnosis of rejection is made before treatment is commenced. A combination of clinical assessment, laboratory and radiological investigation helps the clinician arrive at a correct diagnosis.

5.1. *Clinical assessment*

Clinically the onset of acute rejection is characterised by:
1. deterioration in renal function
2. graft swelling
3, pyrexia
    If rejection is suspected it is important to assess the patient clinically. As described above we review the patient daily, noting fluid balance status and biochemistry. Graft function is demonstrated by increasing urinary output and improving blood biochemistry. The onset of rejection is characterised by a reversal of this trend i.e. decreasing urinary output and worsening renal function. It is however important that other factors which may cause similar changes are not overlooked. In this respect, detailed fluid balance charts are

essential if dehydration is to be detected. The creatinine clearance in the early post-transplant period is checked daily. If the urinary creatinine concentration is rising despite a fall in urine volume this may indicate improved renal concentrating ability which may account for decreased urine volume. Increased plasma urea level may also reflect dehydration or increased protein catabolic rate, rather than deteriorating renal function.

The graft should be examined daily. In the presence of rejection, inflammation within the graft may become manifest as swelling or increased pain due to compression of surrounding organs. On the other hand, urinary obstruction may lead to decreased output and graft swelling. An ultrasound scan of the kidney should be performed when rejection is suspected. This may show hydronephrosis or inflammation within the graft when it has an echo-dense appearance (Chapter 21).

Since acute rejection is an inflammatory process, it may be accompanied by pyrexia. However this may be due to infection. It is essential that infection (see below) is excluded before anti-rejection therapy is commenced.

5.2. Percutaneous renal biopsy

The definitive diagnosis of acute rejection may be made by means of a percutaneous renal biopsy. When there is sufficient clinical evidence of rejection, percutaneous renal biopsy is not performed routinely prior to initiation of the first anti-rejection course. If despite anti-rejection therapy, the patient shows no response to therapy, or deterioration in function occurs following return to baseline immunosuppression, then a percutaneous renal biopsy is performed (see chapter 17) prior to initiation of a further course of anti-rejection therapy.

5.3. Rejection and the non-functioning graft

When good graft function has been established and is followed by deterioration in function, rejection may be suspected. In the case of a graft which has not established function the diagnosis of rejection is much more difficult. Such grafts are frequently swollen and tender because of ATN and are echo-dense on ultrasound scan.

When non-functioning grafts are removed, even when a biopsy has shown ATN, acute rejection is almost always present. In such circumstances good clinical judgement is required. The development of pyrexia without evidence of infection may be the only clinical sign of acute rejection. Percutaneous renal biopsy distinguishes ATN from acute rejection. In many units, frequent fine needle aspiration is performed so that the onset of acute rejection may be recognised early. In other units, intra-renal pressure measurements have been used to distinguish between rejection and ATN.

5.4. *Anti-rejection therapy*

Anti-rejection therapy is described in chapter 15.

6. Infection after transplantation

The immunocompromised patient is at particular risk from infection. In the early period after transplant, when immunosuppression is frequently given at high dosage, the risk is greatest. Preventative measures are taken at this time and if infection occurs, it is important to recognise it rapidly and treat it appropriately.

Cardiovascular disease is the most frequent cause of death amongst long standing transplant patients, but infection is the most frequent cause of death in the early post-operative period. Attention to clinical assessment of the patient, protective barrier nursing and avoidance of over-immunosuppression will minimise the risks of infection.

6.1. *Prevention of infection*

Donors with evidence of systemic infection are not normally acceptable. It is essential that the potential recipient is assessed pre-operatively for signs or symptoms of infection. This is of particular relevance in the patient maintained on CAPD. If there is evidence of peritonitis or a recent history of peritonitis which may not have resolved completely, transplantation should be deferred. Overt evidence of other infection such as pneumonia or cellulitis also precludes transplantation.

Pre-operatively the patient is assessed for clinical evidence of infection. A mid-stream specimen of urine, throat and nasal swabs are sent for culture. Peritoneal dialysis is discontinued immediately pre-operatively. The last bag of fluid drained is sent for culture and 1 g of vancomycin is instilled into the peritoneal cavity prior to capping the line.

The Hb_sAg, HIV and CMV status of the donor and recipient are determined pre-operatively. Positive Hb_sAg or HIV serology are absolute contra-indications to transplantation. In many units it is policy not to transplant organs from CMV positive donors into CMV negative recipients because of the risk of overwhelming CMV infection particularly CMV pneumonitis. We still accept CMV positive grafts for CMV negative recipients. However we administer acyclovir prophylactically to sero-negative recipients receiving sero-positive grafts for a period of one month after transplantation. The standard dosage is 800 mg daily in a divided dose. Since introducing this regime two years ago, although we have seen patients sero-convert, there have been no serious CMV infections and no cases of CMV pneumonitis.

Following transplantation patients are nursed post-operatively in individual rooms and access to the rooms is limited to essential staff only. Staff who may be suffering from infections such as influenza or coryza do not see patients in the post-operative period.

6.2. Recognition of infection

Whilst it is possible that the immunosuppressed patient may develop any form of infection, clinical skill is of immense importance in its recognition. The site of infection and the most likely causative organisms will alter depending on when the transplant patient is assessed i.e. whether the patient is in the early or late post-operative period. The combination of clinical acumen and appropriate laboratory investigation allows the physician to embark early on rational treatment.

Early indicators of infection include development of pyrexia and rising white cell count. It is our practice to record the patient's temperature four times daily initially, and request a daily white cell count. If the temperature is greater than 38 °C blood cultures are sent and possible sources of infection are sought.

The daily assessment includes examination of the mouth and throat, searching for evidence of fungal infection of the buccal cavity or pharynx. Herpetic infection of the lips or hard palate may lead to pyrexia. The chest should be examined for clinical evidence of consolidation or atelectasis. The wound is examined. If the patient was previously maintained on CAPD, signs of peritonitis are sought. If suspected, fluid is drained from the peritoneal cavity and sent for gram stain and culture. If fluid cannot be easily obtained from the peritoneal cavity, 100 ml of normal saline are instilled, then withdrawn and examined as described above. If the abdomen is tender and there is clinical evidence of peritonitis, an ultrasound scan is helpful to exclude the formation of sub-phrenic abscess. The urine is examined daily and cultured. Interpretation of the significance of cultures obtained in a catheterised patient is always difficult. If there are signs or symptoms suggestive of urinary tract infection treatment is initiated with an appropriate narrow spectrum antibiotic while the urinary catheter remains in situ. Until the catheter has been withdrawn, it is not possible to eliminate infection. The use of broad spectrum antibiotic therapy in the treatment of urinary tract infection may lead to the development of multiply resistant organisms.

Indwelling intravenous lines are examined carefully. If there is any evidence of inflammation at the site of insertion, they are withdrawn and the tips of the lines sent for culture. In the febrile patient with a central line blood drawn from the line is sent for culture, then the line withdrawn and the tip sent for culture.

6.3. *Respiratory tract infection*

6.3.1. *Bacterial respiratory tract infection.* Immediately after operation, the source of infection is usually respiratory, particularly in patients who have previously smoked or have a past history of chest disease. Sputum is sent for culture and sensitivities of organisms determined. The expectoration of sputum may be encouraged by physiotherapy and inhalation of humidified hypertonic saline. Bronchodilators may also be used. Chest x-ray is performed and if the clinical situation appears to warrant it, blood gas analysis. Chest infections at this stage are hospital acquired. Such infections are treated with a third generation cephalosporin unless sensitivities of the organism cultured indicate an alternative antibiotic. If there is any evidence that aspiration has occurred metronidazole is added.

6.3.2. *Opportunistic respiratory tract infection.* The principal opportunistic respiratory tract infections which affect the transplant population are:
1. cytomegalovirus infection
2. pneumocystis pneumonia
3. mycoplasma pneumonia

Opportunistic respiratory tract infections are more likely to occur in the later post-operative period particularly if increased immunosuppression has been given for the treatment of rejection. The most frequently occurring opportunistic infection is CMV infection. However the incidence of CMV pneumonitis has fallen significantly since the introduction of prophylaxis as described above.

6.3.2.1. *Cytomegalovirus infection.* Onset of CMV infection is characterised by the onset of fever occurring three to six weeks after transplantation. The fever is usually high ($>39\,°C$) and swinging in character. It is accompanied by granulocytopaenia. Atypical lymphocytes may be found but are not diagnostic of CMV infection. CMV retinitis has been reported but is rare. Diagnosis may be made by virus culture or may be based upon the finding of a rising anti-CMV-antibody titre. Virus culture is difficult and the anti-CMV-antibody titre may not be detected until after the illness has largely resolved. The diagnosis therefore is largely clinical, but is greatly assisted by knowing the CMV status of the donor and recipient pre-operatively.

CMV infection may follow a relatively benign course characterised by swinging pyrexia and leucopaenia which persists for seven to 14 days and then resolves. On the other hand it may be extremely serious with associated hepatitis and pneumonitis. In patients with symptoms clinically suggestive of CMV infection immunosuppressive therapy is reduced immediately. Azathioprine is withdrawn if the white cell count falls below $4.0 \times 10^{3-}$, prednisolone and cyclosporin therapy reduced while there is evidence of active infection. Evidence of pulmonary infiltrates is sought from chest x-ray and blood gas analysis performed. The transaminase level is checked. The presence of pulmonary infiltrates and development of hypoxaemia are ominous. If there is doubt as to the aetiology of the infection, broncho-alveolar lavage and trans-bronchial biopsy are performed to exclude pneumocystis carinii infection and to determine if viral inclusion bodies are present.

If there is evidence of CMV pneumonitis, gancyclovir and anti-CMV immunoglobulin are administered. If hypoxaemia develops, there is urgent consultation with the intensive care unit. Ventilatory support in the form of either continuous positive airways pressure (CPAP) or ventilation is needed.

6.3.2.2. *Pneumocystis carinii pneumonia*. Pneumocystis pneumonia rarely occurs in the early period. Onset is usually delayed until after discharge from hospital. The mode of presentation is with cough and increasing dyspnoea, associated with fever. On chest x-ray pulmonary infiltrates are seen and hypoxaemia is found on blood gas analysis. The picture is similar to that of both CMV pneumonitis and mycoplasma pneumonia.

The febrile transplant patient presenting with the above symptoms and signs is admitted and intensively investigated. We seek urgent advice from the respiratory specialists. Broncho-alveolar lavage is performed and the pneumocystis organism sought. Trans-bronchial biopsy is performed in search of both the pneumocystis organism and also viral inclusion bodies found in CMV pneumonitis. Anti-mycoplasma antibodies and cold agglutinins are sought.

If pneumocystis is found or if there is a strong clinical suspicion that pneumocystis may be present the patient is treated with co-trimoxazole in high dosage, appropriate to the level of renal function.

6.3.2.3. *Mycoplasma pneumonia*. This opportunistic infection also usually presents late in the post-operative period. The mode of presentation is similar to that of CMV and pneumocystis. The diagnostic procedures are as described above and therapy is with erythromycin.

6.3.2.4. *Urinary tract infection*. A daily urine culture is routine in the immediate post-operative period. Positive urine cultures are frequent while the urinary catheter remains *in situ*. Treatment is not initiated unless there is clinical evidence suggesting significant urinary tract infection. The catheter is removed on the fifth post-operative day. Following removal of the catheter the urine usually becomes sterile. If there is clinical evidence of infection, this is treated with an appropriate antibiotic.

6.4. *Peritonitis*

Peritonitis occurs not uncommonly in the transplant patient previously maintained on peritoneal dialysis. If at the time of transplantation there is evidence of tunnel infection of if there is a recent history of successfully treated peritonitis the dialysis catheter is removed at the time of surgery. A specimen of peritoneal fluid, and the catheter tip, are sent for culture.

Peritonitis is recognised by the usual features of abdominal pain, guarding and rebound. As described above, in a patient who still has a catheter *in situ*, peritoneal fluid is withdrawn and sent for gram stain and culture. If there is clinical evidence of peritonitis, treatment is commenced with intravenous vancomycin and gentamicin. The most commonly isolated organisms are gram positive cocci, which are usually vancomycin sensitive. When the organism and its sensitivity has been determined, the appropriate antibiotic is continued for a period of ten days. When gentamicin and vancomycin are used, serum levels should be checked regularly.

If there is very severe pain or poor response to intravenous antibiotic therapy, the drugs should be administered intraperitoneally. The catheter should be withdrawn if there is a slow response to treatment or if fungus is isolated from the peritoneal fluid.

6.5. *Fungal infection*

Immunosuppressed transplant patients are at increased risk of the development of fungal infections particularly mucocutaneous candidiasis. Although this may cause discomfort, it is rarely life-threatening.

6.5.1. *Mucocutaneous fungal infection.* During the daily physical examination the mouth is examined for signs of oral candida. Patients particularly at risk are those with poor dental hygiene, those using dental prostheses and those recently treated with high dose steroids for rejection. Good oral hygiene is encouraged. Oral candidiasis is treated with oral nystatin or amphotericin mouth wash.

Patients with a history of oral candida infection may develop oesophageal involvement. This is characterised by the development of severe dysphagia and has characteristic appearances on both barium swallow and oesophagoscopy. Treatment is with oral nystatin or amphotericin.

6.5.2. *Systemic fungal infection.* Systemic fungal infection rarely occurs after transplantation. When it does occur it is characterised by fever and a rapidly deteriorating clinical condition. Infection usually results from contamination of indwelling intravenous lines by mucocutaneous fungi. Diagnosis is made by the finding of fungi on blood culture or the characteristic appearance on CT scan of the liver. Systemic fungal infection is associated with considerable mortality and must be treated with great urgency.

In proven or suspected systemic fungal infection, it is essential to remove contaminated indwelling lines and reduce immunosuppressive therapy. An appropriate anti-fungal agent is begun at once. In the past amphotericin was used as the principal anti-fungal agent, combined with flucytosine. More recently we have used fluconazole which is not nephrotoxic and unlike keto-conazole does not significantly interact with cyclosporin.

6.5.3. *Other viral infections.* Herpes simplex occurs commonly in the transplant patient, most frequently as a result of recurrence of previously acquired infection. The sites involved are the lips, hard palate and labia. Genital herpes has rarely occurred here but has been reported to be a severe problem in some units.

Oral herpes is usually treated symptomatically by application of acyclovir cream. If the infection seems clinically severe oral or intravenous acyclovir should be administered. Genital herpes is treated with systemic acyclovir.

6.5.4. *Hepatitis C.* It has been recognised increasingly that hepatitis C may be transmitted by both blood products and solid organ transplants. We are now able to screen potential donors or recipients for the presence of hepatitis C. Hepatitis may be recognised by elevation of transaminases. At present there is no effective means of treatment.

6.5.5. *Varicella zoster.* Varicella infection is rarely a problem in the early period. Patients previously exposed to the varicella virus may report a history of having had chicken pox. If there is no such history, anti-varicella antibodies may be detected in the serum. If serology is negative the patient should be informed that he is at risk should he be in contact with an individual suffering from chicken pox. Close contact should be avoided and the patient is given gamma globulin. If clinical infection occurs, systemic acyclovir therapy should be administered.

Herpes zoster infections after transplantation are treated with systemic acyclovir in order to reduce both the severity of symptoms and the incidence of post-herpetic neuralgia.

Further reading

Balfour, H. H. Jr, Chace, B. A., Stapleton, J. T. *et al.* A randomized placebo-controlled trial of oral acyclovin for the prevention of cytomegalovirus disease in recipients of renal allografts. *New Engl. J. Med.* 1989; 320: 1381–1387.

Halloram, P., Aprile, M. Factors influencing early renal function in cadaver kidney transplants. *Translantation* 1988; 45: 122–127.

Myers, B. D., Moran, S. M. Hemodynamically mediated acute renal failure. *New Engl. J. Med.* 1986; 314: 97–105.

Pereira, B. J. G., Milford, E. L., Kirkman, R. L. *et al*. Transmission of hepatitus C virus by organ transplantation. *New Engl. J. Med.* 1991; 325: 454–460.

Rose, B. D. *Clinical physiology of acid-base and electrolyte disorders*. 3rd ed. 1989, London, McGraw-Hill.

CHAPTER 21

Diagnostic imaging of the post-transplant kidney

A. LARKIN

Detailed radiological imaging of the newly transplanted kidney is usually required in one of three clinical settings.

Firstly, the kidney which has failed to demonstrate any significant function and in which the clinical course is felt to be atypical for the short lived acute tubular necrosis (ATN) which is not infrequently encountered. At this stage the main considerations are to differentiate between vascular occlusion, unusually severe prolonged ATN, or more rarely hyperacute rejection.

Secondly, the kidney which has exhibited some initial function but this gradually or abruptly ceases. In addition to the complications already mentioned, CYA toxicity, ureteric obstruction or rejection are further possibilities.

Thirdly, the situation where graft function is maintained but clinical assessment of the graft points to a developing local complication, such as an increasing swelling adjacent to the kidney suggesting a perinephric collection of fluid.

In a few centres radiological imaging, including isotope renography and ultrasound are routinely employed to follow the course of the newly transplanted kidney. The hope is that serial observations will enable complications to be identified and dealt with before they manifest themselves clinically or even biochemically, and allow the effectiveness of any therapeutic measures to be more closely monitored. Recent studies suggest that this approach may be of value with isotope studies where a baseline scan is useful against which to assess developing trends. The case for routine ultrasound scanning seems less well established.

Using radiological techniques the so called 'surgical complications' such as ureteric obstruction, perinephric fluid collections and renal vascular thrombosis can be reliably identified and distinguished from the potential 'medical complications' such as rejection, prolonged ATN or CYA toxicity. It is a more difficult task to separate these 'medical complications' from each other, particularly as in some cases the deterioration in function is due to several coincidental processes acting together. Despite these limitations

Mary G. McGeown (ed.), Clinical Management of Renal Transplantation, 305–327.
© 1992 *Kluwer Academic Publishers, Dordrecht. Printed in the Netherlands.*

Table 48. Methods of imaging the transplanted kidney

1. Ultrasound
2. Doppler ultrasound
3. Radionuclide studies
4. Angiography
5. Antegrade pyelography
6. Intra-venous urography
7. Computerized axial tomography
8. Magnetic resonance imaging

radiological imaging offers a worthwhile and often crucial adjunct to the clinical assessment.

There are several imaging options widely available for the assessment of the transplanted kidney (Table 48). I will consider each of these in turn.

1. Ultrasound

Ultrasound scanning (US) represents a major advance for the assessment of the recently transplanted kidney. It has largely replaced some earlier modalities such as intravenous urography (IVU) and with the evolution of more sophisticated scanning techniques promises to be of even greater benefit in the years ahead.

As ultrasound is independent of renal function and does not employ nephrotoxic contrast agents it is particularly appropriate in the situation of a 'failing graft'. It allows inspection of both the internal morphology of the kidney and the perinephric region where graft threatening complications can sometimes develop. Being non-invasive it is usually well tolerated even by the most distressed patients and as ultrasound machines are portable it is possible for those in strict barrier nursing to be examined safely by the bed side. An absence of ionizing radiation with its attendant long term risks is a further advantage when dealing with the younger age group and those requiring repeated studies, especially as some of the alternative modalities such as CT scanning or angiography require relatively high radiation doses.

One major disadvantage with US is that appearances are often nonspecific. Other factors such as overlying tenderness, changes over serial scans, and the patient's biochemistry require consideration. Ultrasound scanning therefore relies very heavily on an experienced operator familiar with the wide spectrum of normal appearances and capable of appropriately interpreting abnormal appearances within their clinical setting.

1.1. *Theory of ultrasound*

Ultrasound uses sound energy, at a frequency many times above the audible range, produced by a transducer mounted within a housing, referred to as the probe.

As sound waves pass through the patient, some sound energy is absorbed, some is scattered and a small but useful proportion is reflected at the interface between adjacent organs and also from the parenchyma within organs. By producing a short burst of sound and then falling silent, the transducer can also be used to detect these faint returning echoes. If an approximation of the speed of travel through a particular tissue is made it is possible by measuring the time between the transmission of the sound pulse and return of the echo to pin-point the depth of the reflecting interface. The strength of these returning echoes can be applied to a 'gray scale' and displayed on a video monitor, the brighter dots representing the more intense echoes. By mounting multiple small separate transducers side by side along the face of a probe and then producing short bursts of sound in sequence from each it is possible to obtain a composite picture of the underlying structures. Using this linear array arrangement and by generating new images rapidly, events can be displayed as they occur, arteries pulsing, valves shutting, etc. This is aptly called real time scanning.

An alternative approach is to mechanically nod the transducer within the probe assembly and in this way sweep the ultrasound beam across the region of interest. With this design the probe has a much smaller rather bulbous scanning head. This is useful when there is limited access for scanning. The image it produces is sector shaped with the probe head and skin surface being towards the apex. As a result, views of superficial structures are rather restricted.

Probes generate sound energy at a unique frequency dependant upon their construction characteristics. Higher frequency sound waves produce images with better resolution but penetrate poorly through the soft tissues. Fortunately, the superficial location of the graft permits the use of these relatively higher frequency probes.

1.2. *Distal acoustic enhancement*

Sound waves are exponentially attenuated as they pass through soft tissue and the resultant echo received from the deeper interfaces is correspondingly reduced in strength. In an attempt to compensate for this the longer the delay in receiving a returning signal, the more that signal is electronically boosted. However liquid structures with few interfaces are good transonic media and do not attenuate the sound energy to any appreciable extent, while the speed of transmission of sound through them remains approximately the same as for soft tissue. Thus the echoes returning from

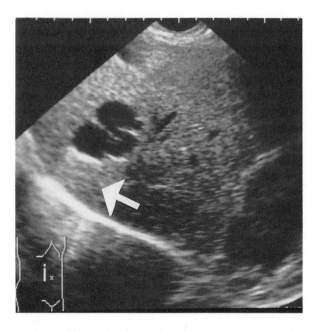

Figure 57. The ultrasonic phenomenon of distal acoustic enhancement is, clearly demonstrated in this case of hepatic cysts. There is increased brightness (arrow) in the hepatic parenchyma immediately beneath these fluid filled structures.

immediately deep to a fluid filled structure are much stronger than those adjacent echoes returning from a similar depth in soft tissue (Figure 57). Yet both have taken the same time to return and are amplified by a similar proportion. This results in increased brightness in the soft tissue immediately beneath a fluid filled structure and is known as distal acoustic enhancement (DAE). This is a useful phenomenon as both simple fluid collections which have no internal echoes, and more complex fluid collections which may well have low level echoes floating within them will both exhibit DAE betraying their fluid consistency. It should be appreciated, however that on occasions solid lesions may also be echo free as the paucity of returning echoes only indicates a very uniform internal structure, i.e. echo free does not always imply fluid filled.

1.3. *Acoustic shadowing*

Calcified lesions reflect all of the incident sound energy and consequently a clear cut echo-free acoustic shadow is cast beyond the brightly reflective lesion. While some non-calcified structures, such as bowel gas or fat can also produce this acoustic shadowing, it is generally not as marked, persistent or well defined.

1.4. *Technique*

Unlike native kidneys the transplant is superficially sited allowing direct acoustic access and does not undergo any respiratory movement. The images obtained are usually of excellent quality.

During scanning the patient is placed in a supine position. It is particularly important to achieve good acoustic coupling between the probe and the patient's skin using ultrasound jelly. This can be difficult in the patient with recent transplant where the wound is still fresh. In order to minimise the risk of wound infection sterile ultrasound jelly should be used or it may be feasible to scan through the dressing if a thin transparent covering has been used.

A full bladder is not required for assessment of the graft itself but does provide an excellent fluid filled acoustic window through which to view the deeper perinephric structures. It has the added advantage of displacing any obscuring loops of air filled bowel out of the pelvis. Unfortunately this full bladder technique is not without risk in the immediate post operative period as overdistension may result in leakage at the vesico-ureteric anastomosis, and consequently it is not routinely used.

1.5. *Normal ultrasonic appearances*

The sonographic appearance of a transplanted kidney, initially at least, is similar to that of a normal native kidney. The renal cortex is composed of medium level echoes, while the renal pyramids in comparison usually appear slightly hypoechoic. Small echogenic foci frequently seen at the corticomedullary junction represent the arcuate arteries. The centre of the kidney is intensely echogenic and within this the collecting system, fat and vessels are hidden.

Very soon following transplantation the appearance of the kidney alters. Most importantly its volume increases by around 20% after 2 weeks and approaching 30% after 3 weeks. Slight splitting of the central bright echoes is common and this does not reflect hydronephrosis or suggest obstruction. This changing and variable appearance of the normal graft partly explains the difficulty in assessing for developing complications. It is only when appearances become sufficiently unusual that problems are suspected.

1.6. *Sonographic features of acute rejection*

The prompt diagnosis of acute rejection is of critical importance as early treatment significantly improves graft survival. Although there has been considerable debate concerning which sonographic features reliably reflect

310

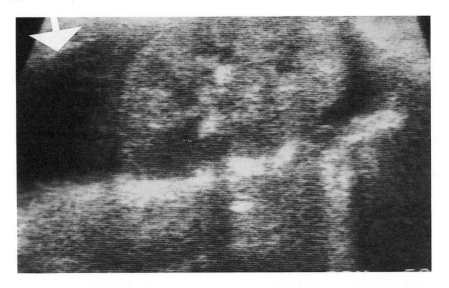

Figure 58. The renal cortex exhibits a haphazard pattern of echo poor and echo bright regions due to haemorrhage and infarction. There is a large associated perirenal fluid collection (arrow). Appearances were very suggestive of an acutely rejecting kidney. This was subsequently confirmed by percutaneous biopsy.

developing acute rejection some of those which are generally accepted include:-

1. an increase in volume of the graft outside the normal range.
2. enlarged and abnormally echo-poor pyramids which result in a more distinct corticomedullary boundary.
3. alternating echo-poor and echo-bright regions within the cortex due to haemorrhage or infarction.
4. associated perirenal fluid collections.

Despite most of these sonographic changes being rather subjective, when combined with appropriately abnormal radionuclide and Doppler studies, they may point strongly towards acute rejection and may obviate the need for renal biopsy.

1.7. *Sonographic features of acute tubular necrosis*

Ultrasound scanning has proved of little value in detecting ATN. Obvious changes in the acoustic pattern of the graft are usually absent and radionuclide studies are needed.

1.8. *Sonographic features of perirenal fluid collections*

The detection of perirenal fluid collections, along with the exclusion of unsuspected ureteral obstruction is the primary role of US, as either of these processes can clinically mimic the rejection syndrome. It is not uncommon to find a thin rim of fluid around a freshly transplanted kidney and this should not cause any undue concern. More discrete larger collections consisting of urine, blood, pus or lymph in the perirenal region may however jeopardize graft survival. When they attain a sufficient size they may cause compression of adjacent structures, such as the ureter with resultant hydronephrosis. Alternatively, if they become infected there is a serious risk of sepsis spreading to involve the graft directly as well as the likelihood of the patient becoming systemically toxic. Often the most straightforward approach to determine the composition of these perirenal collections is to aspirate to dryness under ultrasonic guidance using a fine guage needle. The risks of this type of intervention are negligible and it serves both a diagnostic and sometimes a therapeutic role.

There may however be sonographic clues as to the nature of the fluid and the clinical context may be of help.

1.8.1. *Lymphocoeles*.

Lymphocoeles are due either to lymph leaking from the patient's own lymphatics divided during surgery or from fluid oozing from the graft lymphatics. They occur in association with approximately 20% of grafts. Although they have a variable appearance, the majority show fine septa within an echolucent region which usually has a fairly well defined border.

1.8.2. *Urinomas*.

Urinomas occur in up to 5% of patients, and are usually caused by leakage from the vesico-ureteric anastomosis. Again they are echo free and well defined. Supplementary imaging with IVU or radionuclide studies is useful to confirm the diagnosis.

1.8.3. *Haematoma*.

Haematoma may be as a direct result of surgery or related to biopsy or even to fulminant rejection. Sonographic appearances alter as the haematoma matures. It is echo-poor initially, but as clotting progresses it may eventually become quite echogenic.

1.8.4. *Abscess*.

An abscess is usually less well defined and may have echoes within it representing debris. There may be overlying tenderness, although immunosuppression with steroids may dampen any inflammatory response masking this useful sign.

1.9. *Sonographic appearances of ureteric obstruction*

Ureteric obstruction in the post transplant situation is a relatively common surgical complication occurring in up to 7% of patients. When a declining urinary output is combined with deteriorating function and obstruction is suspected, ultrasound should be the initial investigation as it is quick, sensitive and non-invasive. It relies upon the sonographic demonstration of hydronephrosis where there is splaying of the normally compact renal sinus echoes by echo free spaces. In florid cases, the calyces and infundibula become readily visible and can be demonstrated in continuity (Figure 59). Unfortunately the spectrum of appearances of hydronephrosis can be very wide ranging from mild splitting of the bright central echogenic complex to the obvious ballooning of the pelvicalyceal system seen with gross hydronephrosis. It is tempting to assume that the presence of hydronephrosis invariably equates with obstruction and in turn that the degree of hydronephrosis reflects the severity of this obstruction. This however is not always the case as the degree of dilatation of the collecting system is dependent upon several factors including urinary output, compliance of the collecting system, as well as the degree of outflow obstruction. In circumstances

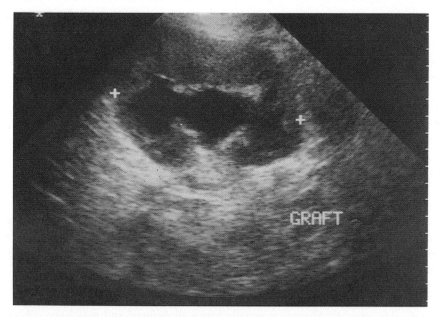

Figure 59. A recently transplanted kidney had shown progressive decline in urinary output. An ultrasound demonstrates that the normal bright central echo pattern has been replaced by echo free distended calyces which can be seen to be in continuity with the renal pelvis. This case of hydronephrosis was due to a progressive stricture at the vesico-ureteric anastomosis.

where there is poor urinary output due to intrinsic renal failure and coincidental severe ureteric stenosis any resultant hydronephrosis may be very unimpressive.

It is important to realise that a mild degree of splitting of the central echogenic complex is not uncommon in the recent graft and although it may reflect fullness of the collecting system it does not necessarily indicate obstruction. The presence of a full bladder can cause a degree of functional obstruction which will resolve once the patient has micturated. This is not a significant problem in the post transplant patient who is having catheter drainage. A brisk diuresis may also produce some pelvicalyceal fullness but this does not usually lead to confusion with an obstructed system which is associated with a falling urinary output.

If there is increasing calyceal dilatation developing over a series of scans this certainly suggests obstruction. Intrinsic ureteric conditions such as oedema or stricture must be considered along with obstructing lesions within the ureter such as clot or calculus.

2. Doppler ultrasound

During recent years this development has gained prominence in renal imaging as it allows evaluation of blood flow within arteries in a non-invasive fashion.

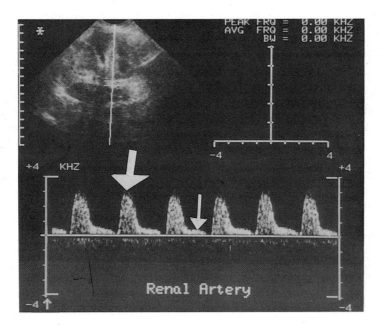

Figure 60a. Doppler ultrasound of a recently transplanted kidney with declining function. The distribution of blood cell velocity within the renal artery is displayed in histogram form. Although there is a good systolic flow as shown by the peak (large arrow) there is relatively poor diastolic flow represented by the flat plateau (small arrow).

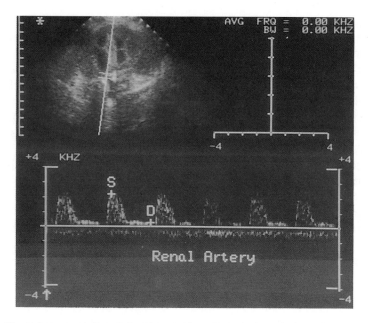

Figure 60b. Follow-up studies of the kidney shown in Fig. 60a shows a trend of diminishing diastolic flow. This combined with typical morphological changes within the graft suggests acute rejection. Following antirejection therapy graft function recovered.

It depends upon the principle that when the ultrasonic beam is reflected from a moving object, the frequency of the returning wave will be altered by a phenomenon known as the Doppler shift. As flowing red cells reflect sound waves it is possible to measure a Doppler shift which is directly related to the velocity of flow. This frequency change is fortuitously in the audible range and can be presented as an audible signal. A visual representation of the returning echoes in the form of a histogram however, gives more information as it essentially is a display showing the distribution of blood cell velocity and hence indicates the direction of flow and reveals the presence of any turbulent flow (Figure 60a).

Recent advances have allowed this Doppler analysis to be applied to all of the frame in a real time image, the resultant image depicting blood flow towards the transducer a red colour and away from it flow a blue colour. This colour Doppler imaging allows even small patent vessels to be readily identified and these can then be further scrutinized by conventional Doppler techniques to reveal the velocity and pattern of flow within them.

The Doppler ultrasound technique stimulated much excitement as initially it was felt it would be feasible to reliably distinguish acute rejection from ATN or CYA toxicity.

The rationale was that the normal Doppler signal has antegrade flow throughout the cardiac cycle, but as resistance in the renal vascular bed increases, the diastolic flow diminishes and possibly reverses. This change in pattern of flow can be easily monitored with Doppler sonography and a quantitative parimeter, the resistive index derived. As acute rejection usually involves a combination of a cellular type reaction with resultant swelling of the interstitium, combined with an endovasculitis, it seemed highly likely that this should be reflected by an increase in the vascular resistance within the graft. While early work was very promising, further studies raised serious doubts about the validity of this approach. In some cases of rejection for instance, the process is almost entirely confined to a cellular type response with no vascular component. Hence the vascular resistance is unaltered and these cases will not be detected. Others have pointed out that the dynamics of vascular resistance were a more complex physiological hotch-potch depending upon such diverse factors as cardiac output, perinephric collections and presence of fistula. Any or all of these factors could so distort the results obtained as to reduce their validity. At present the consensus seems to be that Doppler ultrasound may serve as a useful technique for predicting rejection when considered along with the morphological changes already discussed. Indeed some centres have constructed scoring systems combining both these Doppler and morphological criteria in an attempt to assess the likelihood of rejection. In addition it is felt that serial studies with a constantly rising resistive index are probably of more significance than a single isolated measurement.

However Doppler ultrasound is of indisputable value in assessment of the patency of the renal vessels. Occlusion of the renal artery is readily identified. Early stenosis of the renal artery may also be detected by the presence of turbulent flow. Less reliably, renal vein thrombosis can be detected and is usually associated with a high vascular resistance within the graft. Venography may have a complementary role in demonstrating the iliac vein thrombosis which is so commonly associated with this condition.

3. Radionuclide studies

Radionuclide studies are used primarily to quantify renal perfusion or function in an non-invasive manner. There is a wide selection of suitable radiopharmaceutical agents available. Methodology and the interpretation of results differs from one centre to the next. Despite these disparities certain generalizations are broadly accepted. A base line study is essential, followed by serial scans each of which is performed under a strict protocol to ensure that the differences between successive scans are genuine and do not simply reflect some subtle alteration in technique. In this way developing trends can be revealed and it is these, rather than any single study which are the strongest pointers to possible complications.

The amount of radiation associated with these studies is several orders less than that involved in most radiological imaging and therefore x-ray film cannot be used as it is not sufficiently sensitive. A large diameter rounded disc of a fluorescent substance, usually sodium iodide, is used to detect incident radiation. This sodium iodine crystal responds to incoming radiation by emitting a corresponding photon of light. An array of photomultiplier tubes immediately behind the sodium iodide disc registers these flashes of light and a micro-processor will pin-point the position of the event on an X Y axis by noting the relative intensities of current in each different photomultiplier tube. This whole assembly is mounted in a rather unwieldy housing referred to as a gamma camera, as it is mainly gamma rays which are imaged.

By scanning a fixed area for a period of time and aggregating all the scintillations an image reflecting the distribution of radio-isotope is produced. This information can be stored in digital form and it is possible to analyse an image for any short span of time and hence produce a snap shot or alternatively a dynamic image showing the changing distribution of isotope with time. By indicating a region of special interest within the image, usually the graft, it is possible to produce a graphical representation of change in radio-activity against time within this small demarcated area. In serial studies it is the comparison of these time activity curves which proves most useful in identifying trends.

Among the radiopharmaceuticals available those most commonly used include:

3.1. *Technetium diethylenetriamine penta-acetic acid*

Diethylenetriamine penta-acetic acid (DTPA) is a soluble molecule with a molecular weight of 500 which is eliminated only by glomerular filtration, i.e. there is no tubular secretion. Only a small percentage is protein-bound (3–5%) and as the bulk of the agent is freely filtered it can be used to assess glomerular filtration rate. DTPA does not possess radio-activity but can be tagged to an active isotope such as technetium[99]. This agent is particularly suitable as it has a relatively short half life (approximately 6 hours) and during its decay it emits only gamma rays, hence there is a lower radiation dose to the patient as compared to other radionuclides. A further advantage is that the construction characteristics of the gamma camera favour the energies of the gamma photons released by the decaying technetium.

3.2. *Iodine[131] hippuran*

Iodine[131] hippuran is eliminated by a combination of tubular secretion (80%) and glomerular filtration (20%). As a result this agent is eliminated from the body up to 5 times faster than technetium[99] DTPA. This property tends to reduce the background count and may make any abnormalities in the scan more obvious.

Disadvantages of this agent include the high radiation dose absorbed in obstruction of renal failure and the relative insensitivity of current gamma cameras at detecting the energy spectrum of the radiation emitted by this agent.

3.3. Technetium^{99} – mercapto acetyl triglycine

This agent (MAG 3) is eliminated by a combination of tubular secretion and filtration. Its short biological half life and technetium^{99} label are responsible for its low radiation dose and its excellent imaging properties.

3.4. Renogram

The renogram is the term applied to the time activity curve obtained by analysing the pattern of radio-activity over the graft. Conventionally it is divided into 3 phases:

Phase 1. The vascular phase

Phase 2. Tubular transit
This phase is up-sloping and represents continuing accumulation of isotope in the kidney due to recirculation. It also reflects transport of isotope down the tubules. The peak occurs when the isotope reaches the collecting system and passes into the ureter and out of the region of interest.

Phase 3
This phase which follows the peak is down-sloping and is due to loss of isotope into the collecting system.

3.5. Graft perfusion

Any of the agents already mentioned can be used to assess graft perfusion. The presence of a normal rapid first phase on the renogram confirms that the kidney is vascularised, excluding renal artery occlusion. By relatively straightforward analysis of the renogram curves it is feasible to produce perfusion indices and differentiate between normal perfusion and impaired perfusion. In the past this could be used to discriminate between ATN with normal perfusion and acute rejection which was usually associated with impaired and falling perfusion. With the use of CYA which causes vaso-constriction, the discrimination is less clear.

318

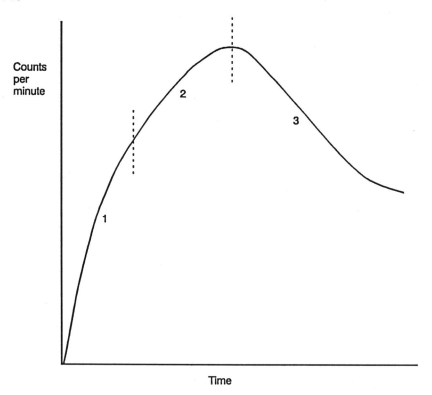

Figure 61. Normal renogram. Mag 3 or I^{131} hippuran.

3.6. *Graft function*

Graft function is best assessed by an agent which is actively secreted such as I^{131} orthoiodohippurate. As renal tubular function becomes compromised the second phase becomes increasingly less steep so that the transit time is no longer discernible and the entire curve becomes flattened. This may be coupled with relatively good perfusion as in ATN or with reduced perfusion as in acute rejection.

In an early obstructed graft there will be a normal first phase but the second phase will show no definable peak or excretory phase. If the obstruction is unrelieved there will be a progressive deterioration in renal function.

3.7. *Rejection*

Rather than assessing different aspects of graft function using radiopharmaceuticals and drawing conclusions from these, an alternative approach is to use labelled agents which preferentially accumulate within a rejecting graft.

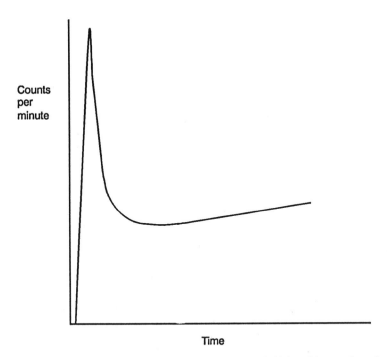

Figure 62. D.T.P.A. renogram of a kidney with ATN. The initial rapid upstroke reflects good perfusion but characteristically there is little extraction of D.T.P.A. as shown by the low flat plateau.

Various agents including gallium[67], I[125] fibrinogen, Tc-sulphur[99m] colloid and In[111]-labelled white cells have been tried.

4. Angiography

In the early years of renal transplantation angiography had a prominent role in the detection of complications. This has gradually declined as non-invasive methods such as Doppler ultrasound and isotopic studies have become more reliable.

As with the other imaging modalities advancing technology has had a considerable impact on the practice of angiography. Significant developments include the advent of non-ionic contrast media which not only are inherently less toxic but also do not induce the excruciating pain previously experienced when ionic contrast was injected directly into the arterial tree. Catheters used in angiography have also steadily reduced in calibre with a consequent reduction in post-procedural haematomas. The manner in which the angiographic images are recorded has also changed considerably since the arrival of digital subtraction imaging. This system relies upon registering incident radiation electronically in digital form, producing an image on the video

320

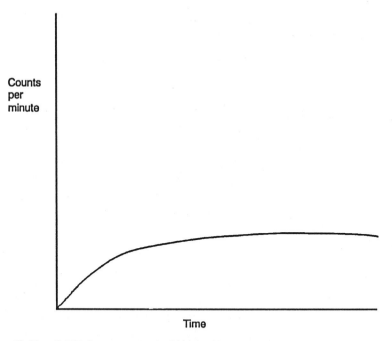

Figure 63. Tc – D.T.P.A. renogram of a kidney with severe rejection. There is slow and poor uptake of isotope with little excretory function.

monitor composed of innumerable small dots, the density of each relating to a specific numerical value on 'a gray scale'. If a 'mask' of this image is generated by reversing the digital values of each dot, and this is electronically superimposed on the initial image, the numbers will cancel and the screen will become blank. However if the detectors continue to register incident radiation and this mask is continuously subtracted in real time from all subsequent images only changes within the scene, such as contrast injected into the arterial tree will be shown. In this manner unwanted background, such as bone and soft tissues will be eliminated leaving the contrast filled vessels displayed in isolation.

As the image is a digital representation it can be processed and amplified electronically. Consequently the system is many times more sensitive than normal film and the amount of contrast required to produce images of diagnostic quality is greatly reduced. The images so produced are stored on a video tape and can be rerun and rapidly inspected.

In addition it is possible to manipulate the digital images to obtain optimum filling of vessels of interest. The flexibility of this imaging system is much greater than conventional systems as the x-ray tube can be tilted or angled easily to display the renal artery to best advantage. Motion artefacts are troublesome in the upper abdomen, but are less of a problem within the pelvis. Although a digital system has a restricted field of view it can easily encompass the region of interest in these situations.

4.1. *Technique*

Puncture of the contralateral femoral artery is usually preferred as this avoids both the transplant and the site of recent surgery which may be tender and make post-procedural compression less efficient. A small gauge (4 or 5 French gauge) non-selective straight or pigtail catheter is usually sufficient and once positioned with its tip at the aortic bifurcation, contrast can be injected and appropriate views obtained.

4.2. *Appearance of angiogram*

In a normal transplant the arteries appear smooth in outline and the cortical vessels are well filled. Contrast is rapidly washed out of the arterial system and a dense nephrogram soon appears. Contrast may then be identified within the renal veins and finally it appears within the collecting system.

There is a wide spectrum of abnormal appearances, some of which can be loosely related to specific pathological processes. In acute rejection for instance, the kidney is enlarged and the associated vasculitis may produce vessel stenosis or obliteration with a prolonged arterial washout time. The resultant nephrogram is usually faint and there may be simultaneous filling of arteries and veins indicating some degree of arterio-venous shunting. Acute tubular necrosis usually produces much less dramatic changes. Indeed the arteries themselves usually appear entirely normal with the only finding of significance being delay and reduction in excretion of contrast.

Renal artery occlusion may occasionally occur abruptly in a hitherto normally functioning kidney. In these instances selective catheterization of the renal artery and streptokinase infusion has been advocated for graft salvage.

A markedly prolonged arterial washout time on arteriography is suggestive of renal vein thrombosis. In association with arterial occlusion it suggests that the vein has thrombosed due to advanced rejection. Venography may be required to confirm the diagnosis. This is performed safely by injecting contrast into a small vein on the foot and obtaining spot views, of the iliac system in particular, as contrast reaches it. Graft vein thrombosis frequently extends to involve the iliac system where it may be outlined as a filling defect within the vein. Collateral vessels suggest the occlusion has been present for some time. Unfortunately it is usually impossible to assess the upper extent of the thrombus as very little contrast will pass beyond and it will then be necessary to demonstrate patency of the inferior vena cava using venous access from the contralateral side.

Thrombus confined to the graft vein can be satisfactorily demonstrated with venography only by selectively catheterising the vein via an ipsilateral transfemoral approach and gently injecting a small volume of contrast. As there is the risk of dislodging thrombus and provoking a pulmonary embolus, when this is thought to be present other non-invasive techniques such as Doppler ultrasound or radionuclide studies are to be preferred.

5. Antegrade pyelography

Antegrade pyelography is an interventional radiological tool which may be required in very particular circumstances. The failing graft which shows ultrasonic evidence suggestive of hydronephrosis and in which it proves technically impossible to perform a retrograde study is one such situation. Using this technique it is possible to confirm that the pelvicalyceal system and ureter are dilated and to identify the site of any obstruction within the ureter. There is a natural reluctance to embark upon this investigation, as there is the theoretical risk of introducing infection into an obstructed collecting system in a patient who is already immunocompromised, with possibly catastrophic results. The trauma to the transplant is reduced by the use of small gauge needles and ultrasound scanning to direct the procedure. Once the renal pelvis is entered the system is decompressed by aspiration of some urine which is reserved for both bacteriology and biochemistry. Contrast medium is then instilled slowly and spot films are obtained under direct screening.

The significance of any ureteric strictures encountered can be confirmed by a 'Whitaker' perfusion test which is performed by passing a guide wire through the needle and introducing a catheter into the dilated pelvis. Fluid is then infused via this catheter at a rate of 10 ml per minute and the pressure recorded and compared to the bladder pressure monitored through a transurethral catheter. A pressure gradient of less than 10 mm Hg is within the normal range, while readings of greater than 20 mm Hg suggest significant obstruction at some point between the two catheters.

A final consideration is that antegrade pyelography permits direct access to the collecting system allowing removal of calculi or dilatation of ureteric strictures without the need of general anaesthesia.

6. Intravenous urography

The role of IVU has reduced dramatically during the last few years and many would argue it no longer has a place in transplant evaluation. This decline in popularity is partly due to the availability of alternative imaging modalities, particularly those which are independent of renal function and because of the potential nephrotoxic effect of the contrast agents used further compromising the kidney's already deteriorating function. In this respect the older conventional ionic contrast agents were particularly hazardous and in general were not well tolerated by the post-transplant patient. In addition to the allergic type reactions the injection of up to 200 ml of an intravenous fluid with an osmolality ranging from 1200–2000 m osmol/kg H_2O could pose particular problems for patients in a precarious state of fluid balance with the risk of provoking acute pulmonary oedema.

New non-ionic contrast agents which have been developed over the last 10 years have reduced all of these problems somewhat. Their non-ionic composition has resulted in an intrinsic reduction of over 50% of osmolality and as they are also associated with fewer allergic side-effects, ill patients tolerate them better. Several studies also suggest these newer agents have less direct nephrotoxicity as compared to their ionic forerunners and their universal adoption as IVU contrast agents seems inevitable, in spite of their relative expense. Certainly in the post-transplant assessment they are the agents of choice.

Formerly the IVU was employed to detect urological complications, such as anastomotic leaks or ureteric obstruction. However, alternative approaches such as radionuclide imaging, ultrasound and direct antegrade studies are now more commonly used in these situations. It is only rarely therefore where these modalities are thought to be unsuitable or prove equivocal that the IVU still has a contribution to make.

6.1. Urographic appearances of obstruction

When urinary output is poor and renal function declining it will usually be necessary to increase the volume of contrast injected significantly by a factor of up to 3 or 4 times the standard dose. If there is severe obstruction there will be delay in the appearance of the nephrogram and once this has appeared it tends to become increasingly dense. Delayed films may be required to demonstrate contrast filling into the dilated collecting system down to the level of obstruction. Associated back pressure changes, such as dilatation of the ureter and blunting of the normally sharp calyceal fornices are usually present. Obstruction to the ureter can be due to a variety of causes including ureteric strictures which usually occur at the vesico-ureteric anastomosis, clot, or rarely calculi lodged within the ureter. When there is slight dilatation of the collecting system administration of an intravenous diuretic may help distinguish ectasia from significant obstruction. If the diuretic promotes clearance of contrast from the renal pelvis and ureter, the fullness of the collecting system is unlikely to be related to obstruction.

6.2. *Urographic appearances of leakage*

Although radionuclide studies are inherently more sensitive in demonstrating actively accumulating urinomas, they lack the resolution to localise the site of extravasation, whereas this can usually be identified fairly accurately with IVU by obtaining early films.

7. Computerized axial tomography (CT)

By employing a rotating x-ray tube and a battery of detectors mounted in a gantry sufficient information can be gathered to allow a computer to reconstruct a thin cross sectional image of the region being scanned. In the upper abdomen and chest the quality of the image generated is dependent on the patient's ability to control their breathing. These respiratory movement artefacts are not a problem when imaging the transplant within the pelvis. However the presence of very dense material such as a hip prosthesis within the scan plane can produce strong streaking artefacts which seriously degrade the image. When viewed on the monitor it is possible to manipulate the raw data to change the contrast between different tissues. Estimates of distance, area and volume are easily and accurately obtained and it is also feasible to measure an exact density for any tissue of interest.

Although the vast majority of peri-transplant collections are readily demonstrated by ultrasound and can be simply aspirated if desired, there are exceptional occasions, particularly if the collections are deep seated, or ultrasound views are suboptimal when CT scanning offers significant advantages in demonstrating its size and exact relationships. This allows even small perirenal collections which are close to critical structures to be safely aspirated under CT guidance. Without resorting to aspiration, CT can often give useful clues about the nature of the fluid. The density of lymphocoeles and urinomas for instance, is usually similar to that of water. In contrast, fresh haemorrhage has a relatively high density which declines as the haematoma ages and becomes more serous. The presence of small bubbles of gas within a high density collection suggests abscess formation.

The administration of intravenous contrast causes a fairly rapid increase in the density of circulating blood and in turn those structures which are richly perfused will also display a significant but less dramatic increase in their density. This so-called enhancement effect can be used to confirm graft perfusion. Some recent studies have even suggested that by measuring the changing density of the renal cortex over several rapidly repeated scans it is possible to obtain a quantitative assessment of glomerular filtration. In practice however, radionuclide evaluation supported by Doppler ultrasound and in difficult cases, arteriography is the preferred method for assessing graft perfusion.

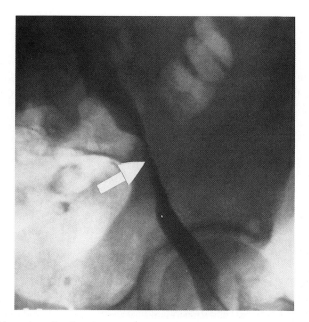

Figure 64a. This patient developed marked ipsilateral leg oedema within a few days of transplantation. A venogram carried out by a direct femoral route to exclude venous thrombosis instead demonstrated extrinsic compression on the medial aspect of the external iliac vein (arrow). An ultrasound scan subsequently showed this to be due to a deep-seated perirenal collection of fluid.

Most graft complications are investigated adequately without resorting to CT scanning, but in certain exceptional cases it may prove invaluable.

8. Magnetic resonance imaging

The theory underlying MRI has been well described elsewhere. When nuclei of certain atoms are placed in a strong magnetic field they can absorb and emit radio-frequency energy. By analysing the radio-frequencies which are absorbed and emitted conclusions can be drawn regarding the chemical environment of the nuclei under observation. It is also possible to generate a two dimensional image of any scan plane desired. Initially it was hoped that by yielding information concerning the chemical make-up of tissues it would be possible to draw firm conclusions about the potential disease processes at work. Some early studies had suggested that acute rejection and CYA nephrotoxicity could be reliably distinguished but other work has cast doubt on the value of MRI in these situations. At present it seems to offer few advantages over more generally available imaging techniques, and its limited availability and high cost ensure that it will remain essentially a research tool in graft assessment for some time to come.

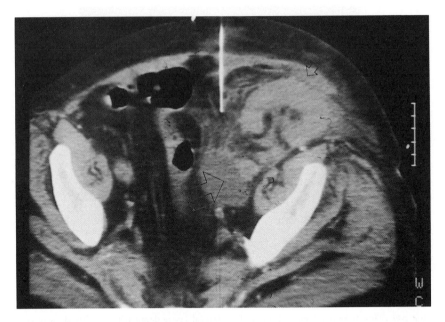

Figure 64b. A CT scan confirmed the presence of a low density rounded collection (large arrow) deep and medial to the graft (small arrow), seen sited superficially within the left iliac fossa. Under CT guidance a fine guage needle has been inserted and advanced towards this collection.

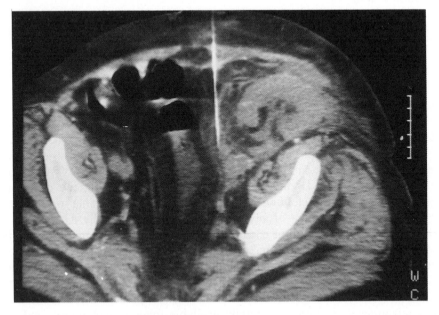

Figure 64c. A repeat CT scan some minutes later shows the needle in position after aspirating 25 ml of clear fluid. Following drainage of the urinoma the patient's leg oedema disappeared within a few days.

Further reading

Dubbins, P. A. Doppler ultrasound in renal disease. *Current Imaging* 1989; 1: 32–38.

Dubovsky, E. V., Rossel, C. D. Radionuclide evaluation of renal transplants. Seminars in Nuclear Medicine 1988; 18: 181–198.

Genkins, M., Sanfillippo, F., Carroll, B. Duplex Doppler sonography of renal transplants. *A.J.R.* 1989; 152: 535–539.

Hall, J. T., Kim, E. E., Pjura, G. A. Correlation of radionuclide and ultrasound studies with biopsy findings for diagnosis of renal transplant rejection. *Urology* 1988; 32: 172–179.

Kittredge, R., Brensilver, J., Pierce, J. Computed tomography in renal transplant problems. *Radiology* 1978; 127: 165–169.

CHAPTER 22

Management after discharge from hospital

W. NELSON

1. Review visits

1.1. *Purpose*

Follow up after discharge from hospital aims to achieve the optimum short and long term health of the patient by maintaining the benefits of good graft renal function with the minimum of complications. Frequent review during the initial months after transplantation makes possible early detection and treatment of rejection, the major cause of graft loss. It also affords the opportunity to check the patient's compliance with and tolerance of potentially toxic therapy. As progress is monitored the necessary adjustments can be made to immunosuppression and other treatment.

1.2. *Review arrangements*

Prior to discharge and at each subsequent visit medical staff inform the patients of the time of their next visit. This is recorded in the medical notes. When unexpected early review is necessary there is in addition direct communication between medical or nursing and secretarial staff. In addition to booking outpatient appointments the transplant secretary also tries to ensure the patient's attendance by sending reminders to those attending infrequently and assisting with transport bookings where appropriate. The value to patients and staff of dedicated and efficient individuals in this position is immense.

In their pre-discharge briefing patients have been instructed in the detail of an accurate 24 hour urine collection, which they are asked to bring with them to each outpatient visit. Those taking cyclosporin A (CYA) are also informed of the need to withhold their morning dose until after blood is taken, allowing assay of trough blood levels of the drug.

Mary G. McGeown (ed.), Clinical Management of Renal Transplantation, 329–347.
© 1992 *Kluwer Academic Publishers, Dordrecht. Printed in the Netherlands.*

1.3. *Frequency of review*

It is the universal experience of all transplant units that the greatest graft loss occurs in the initial months after transplantation. For this reason following their discharge from hospital, usually at two to three weeks post-transplantation, it is Belfast policy to review patients twice weekly for the first three months. Following this, review is at weekly intervals to six months and two weekly intervals to nine months after transplant. If renal function remains stable review is extended by two weeks at three monthly intervals until visits are every six months in long term patients. Some may consider less frequent review adequate.

It is made clear to all patients that they may expect to be recalled after review if there is any question about deterioration in renal function or other reason for concern. While this will frequently involve no more than a check of chemistry, the importance of the early detection and, usually successful, treatment of rejection is also underlined. In the initial weeks after discharge from hospital patients are likely to be recalled to the transplant unit and asked to await results in case admission for further assessment is necessary. Later, with minor changes, an earlier outpatient review may suffice.

Following an episode of rejection, or other intervention more frequent review is usual until a stable situation is again achieved. Early review may also be arranged in spite of stable graft function, to monitor the effect of change in treatment. Most commonly this will be a planned reduction of immunosuppression, such as steroid, though an increase in dose or change of immunosuppressive or other drug may similarly call for earlier review.

1.4. *Patient assessment*

At each clinic visit the patient's height and weight are recorded. In children these are entered at regular intervals on standard growth charts. A midstream sample of urine is provided for culture and dip-stick urinalysis. Blood is taken for a series of routine investigations including estimation of creatinine clearance using the 24 hour urine collection, which also allows measurement of urinary protein excretion.

The patient is then seen by the physician who reviews his/her progress and assesses any current problems. This is facilitated by a flow chart on which are recorded creatinine and creatinine clearance, 24 hour urine protein excretion, urea and electrolytes, haemoglobin and white cell count, urine culture result, blood pressure and drug therapy at each visit. Additional spaces allow recording of CYA blood level, bone profile, blood glucose and glycosylated haemoglobin where appropriate. The flow chart allows any result to be seen in the context of previous and subsequent results as well as any change in treatment. This can usually be noted in a brief glance while enquiring about the patient's welfare.

1.4.1. *History*. In a busy outpatient clinic with between 40 and 80 patients to be seen it is not practical to take a full medical history. As many patients are well known to staff it is often unnecessary to review background history summarised in correspondence in the records. However, a number of points are worthy of note:

1.4.1.1. Specific complaints are recorded with the results of relevant enquiry. A patient's view of his own progress and general well-being is frequently worth obtaining as it may lead to the discussion of problems which would not otherwise be volunteered.

1.4.1.2. Patients who have recently been discharged from hospital after transplantation are asked about their wound and any discomfort or swelling in relation to it.

1.4.1.3. At each visit drug treatment must be fully reviewed including names, dosage, timing and frequency of administration. A card containing this information is given to each patient at discharge from hospital and should be checked and updated at each visit. A sample of each individual tablet or capsule can be taped on each line aiding identification as well as confirmation of formulation. Where comprehension is limited or in doubt suitable supervision must be arranged. Memory aids, such as pill dispensers are also occasionally of value.

Tolerance of therapy should be checked particularly, allowing opportunity for concerns about side effects of immunosuppression to be discussed. Planned dose reductions or options for change can be outlined. If there is doubt about compliance with treatment after such discussion the risks of non-compliance must be made clear.

1.5. *Systems review*

Again comprehensive review is not practical in this situation but frequently patients are known to have or to be at risk of problems affecting one or more systems and these can be the target of specific enquiry.

1.5.1. *Urinary tract*. All renal transplant recipients have had surgical intervention to their urinary tracts with urethral catheterisation and might be regarded as at risk of urethral or ureteric stricture formation or infection. In fact urinary symptoms are relatively uncommon in those without a background of urological disease. Dysuria, urgency and frequency of micturition with suprapubic discomfort may point to lower urinary infection, while loin pain, fever and malaise may indicate involvement of native kidneys and pyelonephritis. However, as the transplanted kidney is denervated localising symptoms may be absent. Poor urine stream may point to urethral stricture, bladder outflow obstruction or primary bladder dysfunction (which will usually be known). Polyuria may reflect tubular disease in relation to resolving ischaemic injury, rejection or other cause of interstitial reaction. It may also signal an osmotic diuresis reflecting inadequate glycaemic control. Visible haematuria may accompany symptomatic infection but if asymptomatic requires full investigation in its own right.

1.5.2. *Cardiovascular system.* After infectious disease the major cause of long-term morbidity and mortality is cardiovascular disease. Symptoms reflecting ischaemic heart disease, hypertension, left ventricular and congestive cardiac failure, peripheral and cerebro-vascular disease commonly call for enquiry. These include chest pain, exercise tolerance and other factors inducing dyspnoea, headache, palpitation, dizziness, visual symptoms, claudication on walking, cold peripheries and focal weakness.

1.5.3. *Respiratory system.* While symptoms most frequently reflect previous chronic chest disease of bronchitic, asthmatic or emphysematous type the chest is an important site of infectious disease in the previously healthy patient on immunosuppression. Infection is commonly with the usual bacterial and viral respiratory pathogens though infection with pneumocystis, aspergillus, candida, CMV, varicella and acid-fast bacilli should be borne in mind, particularly in patients who are unwell with respiratory symptoms following increase in immunosuppression to treat rejection. Breathlessness unexplained by cardiovascular disease or anaemia may be the only symptom pointing to the chest in such a patient in whom further investigation may be required urgently. Other important symptoms include cough, sputum production, wheeze, haemoptysis, pleuritic pain and exercise limitation.

1.5.4. *Gastro-intestinal tract.* Oral discomfort may relate to aphthous ulceration or candidiasis. If severe there may be associated oesophageal involvement with dysphagia making swallowing difficult. It is more commonly seen with increased immunosuppression especially if accompanied by broad spectrum antibiotic therapy. Poor oral hygiene may also contribute and is more easy to treat. Gum hypertrophy in relation to CYA is the commonest long term oral complaint contributing to poor oral hygine and aggravated by it.

Dyspepsia is common. Timing in relation to various precipitating and easing factors, as well as its nature and location may point to the cause. While nausea may be associated with dyspepsia as in cholelithiasis it may also herald the onset of significant uraemia in chronic graft failure. More acute abdominal pain may reflect perforation of an ulcer or diverticulum, pancreatitis, cholecystitis, or appendicitis.

Changes in appetite and weight should also be noted. An increase in both usually accompanies improved general health and renal function following successful transplantation. However, freedom from the dietary restrictions of renal failure, especially when accompanied by steroid treatment and any inherited tendency to obesity, result in the all too common picture of excessive weight gain. Loss of appetite and weight, on the other hand, should prompt further detailed enquiry especially if associated with alteration in bowel habit, tenesmus, rectal bleeding or non-specific dyspepsia.

1.5.5. *Nervous system.* Aside from cerebrovascular and pre-existing neurological disease symptoms are uncommon. Peripheral neuropathy in relation to diabetes or prior uraemic neuropathy may result in peripheral sensory impairment or less commonly pain or weakness such as a foot drop. Symptomatic autonomic neuropathy may also occur when diabetes or amyloidosis have caused the initial renal disease. Acute infective neurological problems are dealt with elsewhere.

1.5.6. *Skin.* Changes in the skin are common. Hirsutes in relation to CYA is perhaps the most obvious and greatly concerns females and children. The skin may also become more coarse in texture. In contrast, steroid produces thinning of the skin with resulting bruising. Skin tumours are the most common variety of neoplasm induced by immunosuppression as well as being the most amenable to treatment. Our patients have generally been informed of this and will usually point out any doubtful lesion. Fungal rashes and viral warts are also common reasons for dermatology referral.

1.5.7. *Social history.* It is worthwhile checking on rehabilitation in the spheres of domestic, occupational and leisure activities. Habits which are potentially hazardous to health such as smoking and excessive alcohol consumption should be monitored.

1.6. *Physical examination*

The extent and nature of the examination are guided by the knowledge of recent problems, past history and complaints. Where these and the patient's appearance point to good health, recording of the blood pressure may be sufficient though often further examination is required along the following lines:

1.6.1. *General appearance.* The patient's habitus may point to steroid treatment though often this is indistinguishable from simple obesity. The skin changes noted previously may also correlate with the therapy. Complexion is also noted and mucous membranes observed for pallor or plethora and the presence of peripheral or central cyanosis. However, simple observation of the way a patient walks frequently gives clues to the way he or she feels.

1.6.2. *Cardiovascular system.* As most patients will have been hypertensive or have required hypotensive therapy at some time, recording of blood pressure at each visit is mandatory. A check should be made for peripheral oedema. Corroborating information is obtained from examination of the radial pulse, neck veins, praecordium with auscultation to assess heart sounds, murmurs and triple rhythm, and lung fields for evidence of pulmonary congestion. Symptoms may point to the need for assessment of neck and lower limb pulses. The presence of a bruit over a large vessel may relate to a stenotic area but its radiation and associated findings are important. For example, a bruit at the base of the neck is frequently heard with a good elbow fistula but might instead radiate from a calcified aortic valve or be associated with a history of vertebro-basilar insufficiency.

Sites of previous vascular intervention should be observed. While many fistulas continue to function well without ill effect, some will thrombose producing a local thrombophlebitis. Peripheral ischaemia is more likely to occur beyond a fistula or graft and may be aggravated by venous hypertension. Prosthetic grafts are also a potential source of sepsis.

1.6.3. *Respiratory system*. The chest has been mentioned as part of the cardiac assessment but is an important source of pathology in its own right. The presence of chronic chest disease or any pointer to recent primary infection requires more detailed examination. This may indicate localising signs of infection, fluid accumulation or consolidation, or more generalised bronchial secretions or airway obstruction requiring further investigation.

1.6.4. *Abdomen*. Examination of the transplanted kidney is usual at initial review and on any subsequent occasion when there is doubt about graft renal function. The health of the operation scar is noted with any visible or palpable swelling of the graft or adjacent structures. Any local tenderness or bladder distension is also recorded. The presence and nature of a graft bruit is compared with previous documentation of this. While a soft bruit is unremarkable, an increase in pitch with the onset of hypertension may point to the need to exclude a graft artery stenosis.

Further abdominal examination may reveal local signs of inflammation in relation to peptic ulcer, cholelithiasis, diverticular disease or rarely appendicitis or pancreatitis when there is a history of abdominal pain. In such situations admission for further investigation is usual. Enlargement of liver, spleen or native kidneys is sought, with any local tenderness.

Recently transplanted patients may still have their peritoneal dialysis catheters in place. The exit sites should be examined and when graft function is stable arrangements made for their removal to eliminate a potential source of peritonitis.

Evaluation of lower urinary symptoms may require examination of the urethral meatus and vagina for evidence of urethritis or vaginitis. Rectal examination may be necessary to assess prostatic symptoms or any rectal bleeding or change in bowel habit. Testicular swelling on the side of the graft is not uncommon and usually transilluminates indicating a hydrocoele occasionally requiring surgical correction.

1.6.5. *Head*. Changes in facial features such as rounding and hirsutism may be immediately apparent. Herpetic ulceration of the lips can be easily seen. Observations of the state of mouth, teeth and gums may also reveal effects of therapy such as gum hypertrophy and the need for advice about improved oral hygiene and dental care.

Any visual complaint warrants examination of the eyes, indeed there is a good case for regular screening. Immunosuppression increases the severity of infective disease particularly those of viral aetiology such as herpetic keratitis and CMV retinitis. Digital tonometry should be performed and if any doubt exists as to the cause of visual deterioration formal checking of intra-occular pressure should be arranged in view of the relation between steroid therapy and glaucoma. A more common late steroid complication is cataract formation which may obscure views of the retina. Background hypertensive retinal changes are not uncommon and indicate the extent of the problem. Diabetic patients should have regular checks for evidence of proliferative retinopathy requiring referral for photocoagulation.

Hearing loss has been associated with immunosuppression though at transplant review it is usually only possible to exclude obvious conduction defects and referral for fuller ENT assessment is indicated.

1.6.6. *Other systems*. When skeletal, joint and neurological complications are seen at transplant review full orthopaedic or neurological assessment will usually involve relevant referral or admission.

1.7. *Advice*

The patient should be informed of his or her progress. This will usually be encouraging and allay any anxiety. Where a problem has been detected the plan for investigating and managing it should be outlined.

A review of drug therapy including discussion of its tolerance and any options or plans for change is essential. The patient should understand the reason for taking each prescribed drug and the potential consequences of failure in compliance.

Advice and encouragement may be needed regarding resumption of normal activities. Some may need advice about adjustments in lifestyle including increased exercise, stopping smoking and a healthy diet to maintain correct weight and nutritional balance. The dietitian plays an important role in the long term health of our patients.

The next review visit is arranged and if there is a possibility of earlier recall the patient should be warned of this. When patients are moving to a different region or country it is important that they understand clearly details of the unit and individual who has agreed to take over their care and are given a sufficient supply of medication to allow time to find a new general practitioner.

1.8. *Records*

It is Belfast policy to keep current transplant outpatient charts in the unit office to allow rapid easy access to information.

In addition to the usual patient identity and contact information they contain four main sections:

1.8.1. *Letter file*. Copies of all discharge summaries, outpatient clinic letters, out-going referrals and in-coming replies dating from the transplant.

1.8.2. *Flow charts*. A single column entry for each clinic visit contains the information previously listed. When printed laboratory results are returned the doctor who reviewed the patient enters the relevant results on the flow sheet. Though laborious this ensures that no result needing action is overlooked. The original report can then be destroyed. The flow chart allows a summary of the patient's progress to be contained in compact form, showing clearly the timing of changes in therapy and effects of these. In children height and weight growth charts are added to this section.

1.8.3. *Clinical notes*. Urinalysis results, height and weight are recorded by the nursing staff at each visit. Notes are made of any problems or findings at medical examination.

1.8.4. *Reports*. Results not filed on the flow sheet are stored.

1.9. *Communication with general practitioners*

Any need for change in treatment apparent at outpatient review is communicated by a hand written note to the family doctor given to the patient. When results are returned a letter is dictated to the family doctor outlining any recent problems, investigations and plans for management. After the first few months if the patient is well and no changes needed progress reports are sent out less frequently. The long term patient who is stable on baseline immunosuppression has a report sent covering each visit at six month intervals. Where a patient is also being followed in the long term by another specialty it is helpful to forward copies of letters there. When a patient moves domicile it is essential to ensure that a detailed summary is sent in advance to those taking over their follow up. It is also important to provide a summary for those travelling abroad.

1.10. *Supervision*

Although up to six members of medical staff may assist at any clinic, a single senior and junior member of staff are clearly designated as responsible for dealing with problems. Thus any doctor seeing a patient may, for example, suspect from the drift of previous results that leucopaenia is likely in a patient on azathioprine or from symptoms that a urinary infection is present. He or she will usually check the relevant result personally at the earliest opportunity, but if not will convey the need to do so to the physician responsible for the clinic at that time. If subsequent investigation, admission or change of drugs is necessary they will contact the patient.

Deterioration in graft function may not be suspected from chart review or clinical assessment. For this reason the supervising team check the results of each patient's renal function on the clinic day. Linkage between unit and laboratory computers greatly facilitates this. Cyclosporin blood results are reviewed on the same day allowing prompt action to increase inadequate doses and to reduce toxic doses. The commonest explanation of an apparently toxic trough level is that the patient has taken the morning dose of CYA before the blood sample was withdrawn giving a peak rather than a trough level. Caution in interpretation is therefore needed.

An unexplained deterioration in renal function indicates need for checking the result, re-assessment of the patient and further investigation. The urgency with which this is carried out is influenced by the extent of the change and how recently the patient has been transplanted.

2. Investigations

2.1. *Routine monitoring*

The following investigations are performed routinely on all patients at each visit:

2.1.1. *Serum creatinine*. This is the most reliable and consistent simple indicator of short term change in renal function. Although a reflection of muscle mass and therefore influenced by growth or wasting its levels in patients with stable renal function are remarkably consistent between visits. It is our experience that a rise of 10% is usually significant and warrants further attention.

2.1.2. *Creatinine clearance*. Although less consistent than serum creatinine estimation and subject to all the inaccuracies of 24 hour urine collection this produces a more meaningful and linear measure of renal function showing reduction earlier than the serum creatinine.

2.1.3. *24 hour urine protein*. Accurate monitoring of urine protein loss is an additional advantage of regular urine collection. While it may assist in the short term differentiation between, for example, urinary obstruction and rejection, it is also useful in long term monitoring of possible chronic rejection or recurrent glomerulonephritis.

2.1.4. *Serum urea*. While not a reliable indicator of the level of renal function the serum urea is a useful pointer to nitrogen balance and catabolism. Elevated levels in patients with poor renal function also herald impending uraemic complications which frequently occur at lower levels of serum creatinine in steroid treated transplant recipients than in other patients with chronic renal failure.

2.1.5. *Electrolyte block*. Knowledge of the electrolyte balance is important in patients who may have renal impairment or tubular disease in relation to drugs, rejection, obstruction or infection. The connection between the electrolyte block and the physiological effects of various drugs should be remembered. These include diuretics, angiotensin converting enzyme inhibitors, CYA and steroids.

2.1.6. *Full blood picture*

2.1.6.1. *Haemoglobin*. This usually rises to normal levels with the return of normal renal function. Failure to do so prompts a search for blood loss, deficiency of haematinics, haemolysis or bone marrow failure. Macrocytosis is usual in patients on azathioprine and in most is not associated with adverse effects. In a few mild anaemia may reflect marrow sensitivity to azathioprine though marked hypoplastic anaemia is rare and when it occurs is reversible on temporary withdrawal of azathioprine.

2.1.6.2. *White cell count*. Leucocytosis may be an early marker of bacterial infection, in which clinical signs may be masked by immunosuppression. However steroids, particularly in high doses, also produce a polymorph leucocytosis with relative lymphopaenia due to sequestration of the latter. Thus in a patient on steroid with a falling white cell count a higher level may point to more marked bone marrow suppression than anticipated. This has led us to take the relatively high white cell count of 4.0 e9/1 as the cut off point below which azathioprine is withheld. Leucopaenia most commonly reflects azathioprine excess or CMV infection. Despite the effect of steroid it may still be possible to detect a relative lymphocytosis in the latter. Occasionally the presence of virus inclusion bodies may help confirm the diagnosis.

2.1.6.3. *Platelet count*. This is occasionally reduced along with red and white cell series by the various causes of marrow hypoplasia. High levels when not reflecting splenectomy may point to increased risk of thrombosis.

2.1.7. *Cyclosporin blood level.* Adjusting CYA dose to achieve and maintain blood levels within the therapeutic range is probably the single most important factor in minimising toxicity. We use a specific radio-immunoassay for measuring whole blood CYA aiming to maintain a level between 100 and 200 µg/l. In the early months after transplantation and while tailing off other immunosuppressive agents, if monotherapy is planned, the upper figure is targeted, while in the stable long term patient the lower figure is the aim.

2.1.8. *Urine culture.* As urinary infection is not uncommon in the transplant population and pyelonephritis in a denervated graft can be clinically silent, midstream urine is cultured on each visit. The urine is transported in a container with boric acid as preservative so that microscopy can be carried out later in those samples with positive cultures. A colony count of 10^6 or greater is regarded as significant. Significant culture of a single organism associated with the presence of pus cells on microscopy is regarded as an indication for antibiotic therapy. Repeated infection is an indication for further investigation.

2.2. *Specific investigation*

While the preceding investigations are carried out routinely on all patients additional investigation needs to be carried out regularly in certain patient groups.

2.2.1. *Hyperparathyroidism.* Adequate control of secondary hyperparathyroidism in the dialysis patient can be difficult. With improved phosphate clearance and vitamin D metabolism by the functioning transplant hyperparathyroidism generally improves. However, a few patients may develop tertiary hyperparathyroidism with hypercalcaemia and bone disease despite successful transplantation. Any patient whose serum calcium has tended to be high especially if there is elevation of alkaline phosphatase or radiological evidence of renal osteodystrophy should have these parameters checked regularly to confirm their return to normal. Failure to do so, or further elevation, signals the need to consider parathyroidectomy.

Patients who have required parathyroidectomy while on dialysis may need long term vitamin D supplement. In this group the serum calcium must be followed carefully after transplant as dose reduction may be necessary,

2.2.2. *Diabetes mellitus.* The diabetic transplant patient requires particularly close attention. In addition to the management of their all too common vascular disease (peripheral, coronary and cerebral), hypertension, retinopathy and neuropathy, regular review provides an opportunity to optimise their glycaemic control. This is usually done in co-operation with a metabolic physician who suggests the most appropriate insulin regime, or oral agent. The majority of patients perform home glucose monitoring and can provide a record for checking their progress. This can be validated against random blood glucose and glycosylated haemoglobin estimations and any necessary adjustment in insulin dose made.

The insulin resistant effects of both steroid and CYA can make diabetic control difficult particularly if antirejection therapy is needed. Increased doses of insulin are usually required and patients previously controlled on diet may require oral hypoglycaemic agents or the introduction of insulin. Overt diabetes may develop for the first time in the non-diabetic following exposure to these drugs. Glycosuria will be detected on routine urinalysis and polyuria will be noted from the urine volume. This may not appear for some time after transplantation and continued vigilance is important.

2.2.3. *Hyperlipidaemia*. Patients at risk from hyperlipidaemia, most commonly elevation of cholesterol, may previously have been detected and commenced diet or drug therapy. Following transplantation drug therapy and increased appetite can potentiate the lipid disturbance and continued monitoring and advice are needed. Although it is not currently our policy there is a strong argument for more widespread screening of the transplant population for hyperlipidaemia in view of their premature morbidity and mortality from vascular disease.

2.2.4. *Recurrent renal disease*. Certain diseases causing failure of native kidneys may recur in the transplanted organ. Where serological markers exist it may be reasonable to follow these at intervals. Certainly they should be checked when considering possible causes for deterioration of graft renal function. In only a few will specific treatment beyond current immunosuppression be of value. Serological markers include:

2.2.4.1. *Anti-glomerular basement membrane (AGBM) antibody*. It is advisable to wait for at least 6 months after AGBM antibody titres have fallen to baseline levels before proceeding to transplantation to avoid early appearance of disease in the graft. Although late relapse is rare we have seen it after 3 years in a patient with stable graft function on baseline immunosuppression. In this case the introduction of plasma exchange and cyclophosphamide halted the process and restored modest renal function.

2.2.4.2. *Anti-neutrophil cytoplasmic antibody (ANCA)*. When renal failure is due to ANCA positive vasculitis or crescentic glomerulonephritis, as in Wegener's granulomatosis or microscopic polyarteritis, it is usual not to proceed to transplantation until the ANCA titre is low or negative. Although the antibody is probably not directly implicated in disease pathogenesis, titres tend to parallel its activity. Patients should be checked at intervals since the ANCA positive diseases tend to follow more of a relapsing and remitting long term course than does anti-GBM disease.

2.2.4.3. Anti-nuclear antibody (ANA). Despite the on-going nature of systemic lupus erythaematosis recurrent lupus nephritis in the graft appears to be uncommon. DNA antibody levels may be useful in following the course of the disease.

2.2.4.4. C3 complement. As well as in lupus nephritis a reduced C3 complement level is seen in membrano-proliferative glomerulonephritis of dense deposit type. This frequently recurs in the transplanted kidney. Complement level may not reflect disease activity and no intervention has been of demonstrable value.

2.2.4.5. Immunoglobulin A (IgA). The serum IgA level may be elevated in up to 50% of cases of IgA glomerulonephritis. While IgA deposits may be found in subsequent graft biopsies it is often clinically silent.

2.2.4.6. Other conditions. Regular monitoring may be important in a variety of medical conditions. Any patient with a history of hepatitis should have liver function tests followed. Thyroid function tests are usually used to guide maintenance thyroid replacement.

Drug levels in peripheral blood are useful in the regulation of treatment with anticonvulsants, digoxin, theophyllines and less commonly in outpatient practice, some parenteral antibiotics.

Patients maintained on oral anticoagulation will require adjustment of the courmarin dose to achieve a target range of prothrombin time or International Normalized Ratio (INR).

The further investigation and management of common problems such as deterioration in graft function, hypertension, urinary and other infection is outlined in detail in chapters 15, 16, 17 and 18.

3. Drug treatment

3.1. Comprehension

It is important that all patients have a full understanding of the drugs they are taking at any time. This involves an explanation of the purpose for which each drug is given, along with its timing, frequency and dose. Where a drug may be available in different tablet sizes, strengths and formulations both the patient and the doctor asked to prescribe the treatment must understand the prescription in detail. Prior to initial discharge from hospital all of these details are reviewed with the patient and a card recording the information is supplied. This should accompany the patient on each visit to the family doctor or hospital so that current treatment can be confirmed and any change recorded.

3.2. *Compliance*

Medical and nursing staff must be continually alert to situations where deficiencies of memory or intellect may result in poor compliance. If necessary a family member or friend should be asked to supervise drug taking. They should be fully instructed in the treatment and receive details of subsequent changes.

The possible consequences of poor compliance with treatment must be made clear. Freedom from dialysis and the effect of renal failure is sufficient to ensure compliance in the vast majority. Intentional non-compliance is probably most frequently encountered in the adolescent or young adult who finds drug side effects unpleasant, particularly in relation to changes of body image. The patients should be informed in advance of possible drug effects and encouraged to discuss difficulties as they arise so that these can be reduced as far as possible.

3.3. *Supply of drugs*

Difficulty with the supply of drugs is not a common problem in our experience. However, it is important that on leaving hospital an adequate supply is provided to allow for any delay in obtaining drugs. Adequacy of supply can be underestimated when holidays, moves or other travels occur. We advise our patients that they should contact us directly if in doubt about drugs supplied to them or if supply is a problem. Reassurance is generally all that is required and problems are easily dealt with. Correcting the few genuine errors is worth any inconvenience involved.

3.4. *Effect of renal function*

While many transplant recipients have normal renal function as measured by the usual parameters, some will have significant impairment of renal function. For many drugs and their metabolites excretion occurs largely by the kidney and dosage adjustment is necessary in the presence of impaired renal function. Nephrotoxic drugs should be avoided if at all possible.

3.5. *Effect on renal function*

The healthiest possible transplanted kidney will be functioning with less than 50% of the normal nephron mass and might be regarded as in a state of mild hyperfiltration. In many there will have been further loss from ischaemic damage or rejection. Glomerular haemodynamics are frequently further compromised by CYA though measured renal function appears very satisfactory. Thus drugs with potential for detrimental effect on renal function should only be used with the greatest caution in renal transplant patients. Common examples of such drugs are the non-steroidal anti-inflammatory agents (NSAIDs) and angiotensin converting enzyme inhibitors (ACE inhibitors).

3.6. *Immunosuppressive agents*

The therapeutic regimens for the use of these drugs has been fully described in chapter 15.

3.7. *Other drugs*

The use of certain groups of drugs commonly used in the renal transplant population will be briefly considered. A comprehensive review is not possible and most drugs not mentioned are used as in normal clinical practice.

3.7.1. *Cardiovascular system*

3.7.1.1. *Diuretics*. These are widely used in the control of hypertension, congestive heart failure and oedema or fluid retention in relation to steroid and vasodilator therapy. Patients on steroid therapy are more prone to hypokalaemia requiring potassium supplement especially if taking cardiac glycosides or at risk of arrhythmia on the basis of ischaemic heart disease.

3.7.1.2. *Beta-blockers*. These agents are used in the treatment of hypertension as well as the control of angina and, less frequently, arrhythmias. They may be used on their own or as an addition to vasodilators which may produce a reflex tachycardia. Beta blockers may precipitate left ventricular defeat and should be used with care when left ventricular function is known to be compromised. Their use may also aggravate poor peripheral circulation and bronchospasm as well as masking symptoms of hypoglycaemia in the diabetic. Atenolol, one of the most frequently prescribed and best tolerated of this group, is water soluble and excreted by the kidneys. In the presence of renal impairment the dose may need reduction to avoid profound bradycardia.

3.7.1.3. *Calcium-channel blockers*. This family of drugs are also used in the treatment of hypertension, angina and arrhythmias with different members having a more pronounced effect in each area. Nifedipine, particularly in the sustained release formation, is a widely prescribed and effective hypotensive agent. Flushing and oedema occasionally limit its use (cautious use is necessary in those with poor cardiac reserve). Unlike other members of the group it does not appear to interact with CYA and may have a protective effect against CYA nephrotoxicity.

3.7.1.4. *Other vasodilators*. Nitrates are primarily used as anti-anginal agents. Since the advent of nifedipine and other newer hypotensive drugs the use of hydralazine has declined. Despite vasodilator side effects and an occasional lupus reaction it is an effective hypotensive agent. Alpha-adrenoreceptor blocking drugs also have vasodilator properties and are useful hypotensive agents. Prazosin and more recently, in once daily form with less dramatic postural effect, doxazosin are the usually prescribed members of this group. Diazoxide and minoxidil are potent hypotensive drugs which are not used frequently because of side effects.

3.7.1.5. *Angiotensin converting enzyme (ACE) inhibitors*. These drugs are useful hypotensive agents and help the failing left ventricle. Their effect is most obvious in high renin states where particular caution must be exercised. When the patient with heart failure on diuretic is treated hypotension may occur adding to any existing pre-renal uraemia. If hypertension reflects renal ischaemia its control with an ACE inhibitor is likely to result in substantial deterioration of renal function. This is especially relevant to a single functioning kidney such as a transplant, and in situations where glomerular perfusion may already be compromised by other drugs such as non-steroidal anti-inflammatory agents or possibly CYA. In less critical situations, however, they are often well tolerated and free of the side effects of other hypotensive drugs.

Patients being treated with an ACE inhibitor should have their renal function carefully monitored. In the presence of impaired renal function, even if this is not deteriorating, hyperkalaemia may occur, when this treatment should be withdrawn.

3.7.1.6. *Centrally acting hypotensive agents*. Methyldopa remains an effective hypotensive drug without the adverse effects on renal or cardiac function seen with many other drugs. In view of its reputation for causing lethargy, postural hypotension and impotence it is often better tolerated than expected. Clonidine is often well tolerated but used infrequently because of the need for complete certainty about compliance to avoid the dangers of rebound hypertension.

Lipid lowering agents. These should be considered only after appropriate modification of diet and lifestyle have failed to improve a dangerously abnormal lipid profile. Debate continues regarding the indications for intervention with expensive long term treatment when resulting improvement in mortality has not been clearly demonstrated. In the renal population the incidence of side effects with the clofibrate group is high, including deterioration in renal function and myositis-like symptoms. In contrast simvastatin appears to be well tolerated though liver function must be regularly checked.

3.7.2. *Gastrointestinal system*

Ulcer healing drugs are extensively prescribed for the renal transplant population. This may reflect the characteristics of a group which has moved from the situation of increased gastric acid output of chronic renal failure to drug treatment rendering them more prone to dyspepsia and ulcer complications. Treatment is therefore more likely to be necessary in the early months after transplantation. We routinely use ranitidine prophylactically in patients with a history of ulcer related disease when they receive high dose steroid for treatment of rejection. Treatment should not be continued longer than is strictly needed. Cimetidine is used less often because of its capacity to bind to microsomal cytochrome P450 resulting in increased levels of CYA, warfarin, phenytoin and theophylline. We have not encountered complications with the use of raniditine.

Smoking should of course be discontinued and antacids may be used if necessary. When resistant disease is encountered there may be benefit from increasing the dose of ranitidine or introducing omeprazole, a proton pump inhibitor.

3.7.3. *Infections*

Increased risk of infection is a major side effect of immunosuppression. This subject is also dealt with in chapters 15 and 20. Some points relevant to outpatient follow up are considered here.

3.7.3.1. *Bacterial infection.* This is managed as in other clinical situations. Care must be taken when using potentially nephrotoxic antibiotics where dose reduction is needed on account of impaired renal function. Drugs in these categories include aminoglycosides, cephlosporins, tetracyclines, trimethoprim and the 4-quinolones.

The most frequently encountered interaction between antibiotic and immunosuppressive agents is elevation of CYA levels when erythromycin is given.

The use of broad spectrum antibiotics is more likely to result in overgrowth of resistant bacteria or fungi in patients taking immunosuppression.

Prophylactic antibiotic treatment is seldom used. However because of the risk of bacteraemia with major dental procedures a short course of ampicillin or (for those not on CYA) erythromycin should be given commencing on the day of dental treatment. Anti-tuberculous therapy is used prophylactically for the first 6 months after transplantation in those who have previously required this treatment.

3.7.3.2. *Viral infection.* Acyclovir is active against the herpes viruses, though it should be started at the onset of the infection. It is used in the systemic treatment of varicella-zoster and the systemic and topical treatment of herpes simplex infections of the skin, mucous membranes and eyes. We give it prophlactically for the first 6 weeks to patients who are sero-negative to the cytomegalovirus (CMV) receiving a kidney from a CMV positive donor. Gancyclovir is reserved for life threatening CMV infection.

3.7.3.3. *Fungal infection.* The risk of fungal infection increases with the level of immunosuppression though cutaneous and mucosal involvement may occur on low levels of maintenance treatment. Oral candidiasis is the commonest problem seen. In addition to oral hygiene measures and modifying any contributing therapy it generally clears with oral nystatin, amphotericin or miconazole. For more severe infection with pharyngeal or oesophageal involvement oral fluconazole may be required. Dose adjustment of the latter is necessary with renal impairment.

Vaginal candidiasis is treated with nightly insertion of vaginal pessaries for 2 to 4 weeks. Any superficial involvement is treated with cream which must also be used by the partner. In addition to the previously mentioned contributing factors hyperglycaemia and oral contraception may predispose to infection and should be modified. The imidazole group of drugs appear equally effective in shorter courses of between 3 and 14 days.

Cutaneous fungal infection should be confirmed by examination of scrapings and an appropriate antifungal agent applied topically. Tinea infection of the nail or scalp may require systemic treatment with either griseofulvin or itraconazole.

3.7.3.4. *Protozoal infection.* Pneumocystis infection is dealt with in chapter 18. This has been rare in Belfast and prophylactic treatment is not used, but co-trimoxazole is used in many centres.

3.7.4. *Endocrine system*

3.7.4.1. *Drugs used in diabetes.* The range of insulins and oral hypoglycaemic agents are used as usual. The antagonistic effects of steroid, CYA and diuretics should be remembered when treatment changes are made. Additional treatment and advice may be needed to cope with the increased appetite of the transplant patient. Close liaison with diabetic services as well as patient understanding and monitoring of their own blood glucose levels produces the best results.

3.7.4.2. *Growth hormone.* Where children fail in catch up growth there is evidence that supplements of growth hormone will be useful if given before fusion of epiphyses. Steroid therapy contributes to growth retardation and this should be maintained at the lowest possible dose, preferably using an alternate day treatment regimen. The use of CYA may allow steroid withdrawal and for this reason is used routinely in children.

3.7.4.3. *Oral contraceptive agents.* Because of the increased incidence of hypertension and risk of thrombotic events we discourage the use of these agents advising alternative forms of contraception where possible.

3.7.5. *Musculo-skeletal and joint disease*

Rheumatoid arthritis, lupus and other connective tissue disease usually become quiescent on immunosuppressive therapy. Degenerative disease, sometimes contributed to by treatment, trauma or gout more commonly cause problems. The hazards of treatment with non-steroidal anti-inflammatory drugs have already been mentioned. There is the risk of adverse effects on renal function. Furthermore gastric upset is more likely in this group of patients. It is best to try to control symptoms with simple analgesia and any possible local measures. Where the risk of a non-steroidal drug is felt to be justified renal function must be closely monitored. Limited evidence suggests that sulindac may carry less risk to renal function and this agent is often used.

3.7.6. *Central nervous system*

The interactions of many anticonvulsants with other drugs, particularly immunosuppressive agents have been previously considered. An anticonvulsant less likely to cause hepatic microsomal enzyme induction such as sodium valproate should be chosen. Other groups of drugs are used as in usual clinical practice.

CHAPTER 23

Rehabilitation after renal transplantation

J. H. BROWN

Successful renal transplantation will return to essentially normal health the patient whose sole problem was chronic renal failure. This implies that a definite improvement in quality of life is experienced. The restoration of adequate energy levels and increased subjective well-being, should permit a return to the activities undertaken prior to the onset of renal failure. This transition requires considerable psychological adjustment by the patient, who may need help and support to achieve rehabilitation. The misinformed attitudes of some of the people who surround the patient may hamper the rehabilitation process.

Some studies have shown that there is no difference in the mortality of patients with end-stage renal failure between those who are maintained by dialysis and those who receive cadaver donor grafts. Therefore, the improvement in quality of life attained by successful transplantation needs to be greater than just removing the need to perform dialysis several times per week to justify the risks of the procedure.

1. Psychological and psychiatric problems

A considerable number of patients on regular dialysis suffer from multiple psychological and psychiatric problems related to their disease and there is a wide variation in the ability of patients to cope with these problems. Depression and anxiety are common, patients expressing fear of death if treatment should fail is also commonly reported.

Additional stresses are caused by the frequent decline in socio-economic status, the constraints imposed by the need regularly to allow time for dialysis, the limitations on travel and the rigid controls on diet and fluid consumption. Patients are often less well off financially, and have a changed role within the family. Some patients are unable to accept the fact that they have been selected for chronic ill-health. They deny their illness and ignore the necessary rigours of its treatment, so that a non-compliant rebellious individual emerges. Fortunately the majority of dialysis patients cope well

Mary G. McGeown (ed.), Clinical Management of Renal Transplantation, 349–356.
© 1992 *Kluwer Academic Publishers, Dordrecht. Printed in the Netherlands.*

with their changed circumstances as they realise that acceptance of illness may mean the difference between survival and death, rehabilitation and non-rehabilitation. The combination of family support and the promise of much better times ahead, following a successful transplant, can be crucial factors in enabling the individual to come to terms with renal failure and dialysis.

Renal transplantation creates its own psychological and psychiatric problems. Some patients have excessively high expectations of transplantation which, if they are not achieved, may be followed by depression. Pre-transplantation counselling is important to ensure that the prospective recipient obtains a realistic perspective of the effects of transplantation, both good and bad. The possibility of graft failure needs to be discussed. Early post-transplant complications and an extended hospital stay can be associated with depression. Those patients so affected will often be surrounded by others with similar problems and so may obtain a distorted view of the results of transplantation rather than see that the vast majority have a successful outcome. Successful transplantation results in increased independence which in itself may cause new anxieties, as once more the patient's role within the family is changed and further psychological adjustments are required. There is often initial euphoria or a "honeymoon period" after grafting, particularly with a trouble free initial course, which may be ended abruptly by a major complication and subsequent psychological stress. An occasional patient may develop difficulties with his/her sexual identity if they learn that the donor of their graft was of the opposite sex.

Side effects of drug therapy can cause alteration of body image post-transplantation. Steroid therapy may cause the well recognised Cushingoid habitus with truncal obesity, hirsutism and characteristic moonface. Adoption of low dose regimens or alternate day administration may lessen these effects. Cyclosporin-induced hirsutism and coarsening of features can be particularly distressing, especially in young females. Fortunately these post-transplantation psychological and psychiatric problems are significant in only a minority of patients. The vast majority readily manage the necessary psychological adjustments, but some patients do need assistance to enable them to rehabilitate satisfactorily.

1.1. *Preparation in hospital*

An important part of the inpatient care of the allograft recipient is the psychological preparation of the patient for the changes that will occur on his/her discharge from hospital. Counselling by the nursing staff on matters such as immunosuppressive therapy, signs of rejection, avoidance of infection are all straightforward, but there is an important role for the nurse in preparing the patient for the greater degree of independence that he/she will have post-transplantation. An important part of counselling is discussion of the possibility of graft failure and its management. Some patients, particularly if they have been on dialysis for a long time may have become very dependent on the hospital and its staff. These individuals need to be helped to loosen these links and adopt a greater degree of independence. The involvement of marital partners and other family members often improves the post-discharge rehabilitation. The unit social worker and the unit dietician are important contributors to the preparation for discharge from hospital. The majority of patients will gain weight post-transplantation and steroid related obesity can be a cause of long term morbidity making early dietary advice necessary. If a patient support group exists, participation in the activities of the group both pre-and post-transplantation can be of great benefit to the individual patient.

2. Employment

The ability to return to useful employment is often taken as a yardstick of the success of any given therapy. Several studies have shown that between 70% and 90% of successfully transplanted patients return to fulltime employment (including fulltime housework and study). This is generally achieved within one year of grafting. Studies have often reported that the number of patients fit for work considerably exceeds the number employed, particularly in regions of high unemployment. The perception by the general population, and in particular employers, of the state of health of individuals who have had a successful renal transplant is such that transplant recipients are often regarded as less suitable candidates for employment than is actually the case. Another reason for a larger than expected difference between the number suitable for employment and the number in work, may be seen amongst the lower socio-economic groups. If the difference in financial terms between taking a poorly-paid job, with low job satisfaction, and continuing to receive state benefits is small, a number of patients may settle for the status quo and use the time to enjoy their increased level of activity. A considerable number of individuals, who were involved in very physically demanding occupations before they developed renal failure, are unable to resume their former job and the return to employment is to a less strenuous post.

Several studies have compared the employment status of patients on dialysis with that of patients who have undergone renal transplantation and have found that the employment rate was higher in the transplant group. Evans *et al.* studied 859 patients attending several different centres in the U.S.A. – 74% of the transplanted patients were in fulltime employment compared with 44% of the dialysis patients. Subdivision by mode of dialysis revealed a considerable variation in the number employed in each group – 59% of home haemodialysis patients were working compared to 25% of the CAPD treated patients.

The results of this and similar surveys must be interpreted with caution. The two groups were not matched and therefore may not have the same age distribution or incidence of co-existent medical problems, factors that affect the potential for employment regardless of the presence of renal failure. These studies are also flawed as they do not evaluate how successful transplantation has affected factors such as type of job, job satisfaction, career progress, financial reward and performance ability. Despite these reservations it is clear, from both the literature and personal clinical experience, that successful transplantation both increases the number of patients capable of fulltime work and the number in gainful employment, and also improves their performance at work.

3. Exercise/recreation

Unless impeded by coexistent cardio-respiratory or musculoskeletal disabilities the recipient of a successful renal allograft will be able to increase his/her level of physical activity. They will once again be able to participate in sports on both a recreational and a competitive basis. Positive encouragement to participate in regular exercise is advised especially for children and young adults. However, contact sports should be avoided because of the risk of trauma to the transplanted kidney which is less well protected than the native kidney.

Events like "Transplant Olympics" provide an excellent vehicle for patients to participate in competitive and recreational sporting activities with fellow transplant recipients. This can provide an often much-needed psychological morale boost as well as providing excellent publicity about the success of transplantation and maintaining the public awareness of the continuing need for organ donation.

Some individuals, who have received a transplant, have had some outstanding achievements in the world of sport. An Olympic athlete returned to successful competition after transplantation, a group of recipients formed the crew of a boat that completed the Fastnet Ocean Yacht race, and another group swam the English Channel in relay. These are just some examples of the degree of rehabilitation possible after successful renal transplantation.

4. Renal transplantation in children

One of the most important consequences of successful paediatric renal transplantation is the effect on growth and physical development. All children with chronic renal failure are growth retarded in terms of height and in terms of bone age, with the majority being below the third centile. Growth retardation can cause psychological problems both within the family, particularly when the younger siblings outgrow the affected child, and within the peer group. Studies have shown that growth velocity increases post-transplantation although catch-up growth is not always achieved. The final growth deficit is often most pronounced when transplantation occurs at an older age, when chronic renal failure has been present for many years.

Steroid therapy hinders growth in a dose dependant manner by causing premature closure of the epiphyseal plate. Changing to alternate day administration considerably lessens the growth retarding effect. However, care is necessary in selecting both the timing and the rate of change from every day to alternate day steroid therapy as rejection episodes may occur during this conversion. Many paediatric nephrologists favour a CYA monotherapy immunosuppressive regime to avoid the growth retarding effect of steroids. Thirty percent of patients on CYA monotherapy will require the addition of steroids to treat and to prevent rejection.

The recent development of recombinant human growth hormone has provided an additional therapeutic measure to maximise the growth potential after transplantation of children with chronic renal failure. One of the biggest obstacles preventing the return to normal physical activity post-transplantation is deforming renal osteodystrophy. Therefore it is important to gain early control of calcium and phosphate levels during the pre-transplantation period.

In addition to retardation of physical growth approximately one third of paediatric recipients may suffer impairment of sexual development with either delayed puberty or incomplete sexual development. Manipulation of the steroid therapeutic regime may lead to improvement but androgenic supplements may be necessary. Assessment of bone age radiologically is an important part of the management of these children. Adolescents with pubertal delay require sympathetic counselling as there is often a considerable degree of associated anxiety and peer group ridicule about both pubertal delay and short stature.

The child with chronic renal failure is frequently absent from school as a result of hospitalisation, dialysis and general ill-health and, unless home tuition is arranged, often falls back educationally. Considerable improvement occurs post-transplantation with 95% of children returning to fulltime schooling. This has the dual benefit of improving education and enhancing social development by reintegration with the peer group. Returning to fulltime education improves the child's chances of gaining employment in later life.

Following transplantation readjustments within the family are often necessary. If the graft was from a living-related donor, usually a parent, a stronger relationship may develop between the child and the donor, and the link with the other parent weakened. Supportive counselling may be required to avoid unnecessary conflict within the home. The child with a transplant often benefits from meeting other children who have been successfully transplanted and events such as "Transplant Olympics"/"Transplant Games" provide an excellent opportunity for this to take place.

5. Comparison of dialysis and transplantation

Both modalities of treatment can satisfactorily support the patient with end-stage renal failure. Several studies have been performed to compare the relative merits of each form of renal replacement therapy. Simmons *et al.* assessed 766 patients who had been on renal replacement therapy for one year. One hundred and seventy-five patients had been transplanted and the majority of the remainder were treated by CAPD. The transplanted group had significantly better scores for physical well-being, emotional well-being and health satisfaction. Evans *et al.* in another large multi-centre study (859 patients) also reported a better quality of life amongst those patients who had been transplanted, with a significantly increased level of physical activity and rate of employment. There have been several smaller studies most of which have drawn the same conclusions, although one or two reported no differences between the two forms of therapy. The result of these smaller studies must be interpreted with caution as patients were not randomised to a treatment modality which will influence outcome, as will a relatively low transplant centre success rate.

The long term complications of grafting may adversely affect the rehabilitation of transplanted patients. Steroid-induced avascular necrosis of the hips causes considerable pain and immobility, thus removing a lot of the benefits of increased activity and ability to work. Cardiovascular disease, symptomatically represented by angina and intermittent claudication, will also reduce activity levels and in some cases can be extremely incapacitating. There is evidence to suggest that the development of cardiovascular disease is accelerated post-transplantation. Steroid therapy may cause posterior polar cataract formation leading to visual loss, another major disability. The high level of cardiovascular disease and the increased incidence of malignancy amongst the transplanted population result in a higher mortality rate. Premature death may lead to considerable social and financial hardships for the surviving family members.

5.1. *Cost of renal replacement therapy*

Comparison of the costs of the various methods of renal replacement therapy has been made and also of the survival rates following each treatment. If the initial high cost of the first year post-transplantation is spread over the subsequent years, the cost of transplantation is significantly cheaper. This differential has become smaller with the almost universal change from aza-thioprine and prednisolone to cyclosporin. In the USA the 1984 annual cost estimates for transplantation was $15000 and for dialysis, $25000. A study in Canada, which averaged costs over a seven year period, calculated an annual difference of $6600 between the two forms of treatment. In the UK the average cost of transplantation after the first year has been estimated (1991) at £3000 per annum (for drugs and hospital reviews) compared with £13–18,000 per annum for dialysis. In less well developed countries without an end-stage renal failure programme, costs cannot be compared, as often the only available treatment is a living related donor graft, frequently performed in another country. If transplantation is successful the benefits cannot be measured in financial terms.

5.2. *Patient survival after renal transplantation*

Initially survival rates after transplantation were worse than those now being achieved. This was mainly due to the relatively large number of deaths from sepsis, partly the consequence of the large doses of immunosuppressive drugs, especially steroids, that were used. Early comparative studies found no difference in survival between patients treated by dialysis and those treated by transplantation, although patients receiving living related donor grafts had a better survival rate. However the improvements in surgical technique and better use of immunosuppressive agents, particularly the use of low-dose or steroid-avoiding regimes, have improved patient survival after transplantation and more recent studies demonstrate that successful transplantation is better than longterm dialysis.

6. Quality of life studies

There have been many studies documenting rates of survival of both patients and grafts following transplantation and others detailing the incidence and prevalence of medical and surgical complications. However there are relatively few studies that have scientifically assessed the improvement in quality of life. The majority of these have been cross-sectional in nature and have compared two groups of patients, one having undergone transplantation, the other remaining on dialysis. In these studies the patients were not randomised to a mode of treatment nor were attempts made to evaluate the changes in quality of life that transplantation induced in individual patients. There are, however, studies at present being undertaken in the United Kingdom to assess longitudinally the effect of transplantation on quality of life.

Various questionnaires have been designed to assess health status and quality of life. These examine variables such as physical well-being, emotional well-being, happiness scores, mood profiles, anxiety and depression levels and social well-being. Examples of questionnaires that are frequently employed include the Nottingham Health Profile, the Sickness Impact Profile, the Campbell Index of Well-being, the Rosenberg Happiness Scale, the Bradburn Happiness items and the Psychological Adjustment to Illness Scale. The results of studies can be significantly influenced by the degree of counselling before transplantation provided for patients and the subsequent expectations that they have for successful transplantation. The quality of life studies that have been performed have generally involved small numbers of patients apart from the two sizable studies by Simmons and by Evans, commented upon earlier.

A parameter that is receiving an increasing amount of attention in quality of life studies is quality adjusted life years (QALYs). This mathematically derived parameter has been designed for use in the setting of imperfect health to assess the quality of life attained by a treatment intervention, rather than the enhanced survival. QALYs have a role in the allocation of funding by ranking different projects in the order of benefit to patients. Treatment decisions are now being influenced by the cost per QALY of alternative forms of therapy. Usually transplantation is considerably cheaper per QALY than hospital haemodialysis. This difference will only remain if patient selection is appropriate. As financial stringencies and budgeting play an increasingly important role in the running of healthcare systems the relative cost of QALYs is likely to influence the availability and practice of transplantation in the future.

7. Conclusion

The published literature generally indicates that successful rehabilitation following transplantation is important in achieving an enhanced quality of life. The management of the transplant recipient must include measures designed to achieve successful rehabilitation and provision for adequate counselling. It is highly likely that quality of life, cost effectiveness, and QALY assessment will play an increasingly important role in the practice of transplantation in the years to come.

Further reading

Evans, R. W., Manninen, D. L., Garrison, L. P. Jr. *et al.* The quality of life of patients with end-stage renal disease. *N. Engl. J. Med.* 1985; 312: 553–559.

Evans, R. W. Quality of life assessment and the treatment of end-stage renal disease. *Transplant Reviews* 1990; 4: 28–51.

Keown, P. A., Stiller, C. M. Dialysis or transplant: An integrated approach to end-stage disease management. *Kid. Int.* 1988; 33: S145–S149.

Simmons, R. G., Abress, L. Quality of life issues for end-stage renal disease patients. *Am. J. Kid. Dis.* 1990; 15: 201–208.

Simmons, R. G., Abress, L., Anderson, C. R. Quality of life after kidney transplantation. A prospective, randomized comparison of cyclosporine and conventional immunosuppressive therapy. *Transplantation* 1988; 45: 415–421.

CHAPTER 24

Reproduction after renal transplantation

J. H. BROWN

The presence of chronic renal failure markedly reduces fertility in women of childbearing age. It has been reported that only 1 in 200 women on dialysis become pregnant, with a minority progressing successfully to term. Amenorrhoea is common in uraemia, which causes disruption of the usual menstrual and ovulatory pattern. Some women have irregular anovulatory vaginal bleeding. Hormonal studies have revealed the presence of hypothalamic suppression and hypogonadatrophic hypogonadism. Regular dialysis results in only slight improvement of this situation. Functional sexual disorders are also common in chronic renal failure with most patients suffering from diminished libido.

A normal menstrual pattern will return between one and 12 months posttransplantation, most women achieving a normal cycle after four to six months. In 1958 the first documented successful pregnancy in a transplant recipient occurred, the mother having received a kidney from her identical twin. No immunosuppressive therapy was used in this case. However it illustrated the potential improvement in fertility following transplantation, and there have now been over 2000 recorded cases of pregnancy in women with renal allografts.

Chronic renal failure also has a deleterious effect on the sexual and reproductive function of the male patient. Approximately 50% will experience diminished libido or impotence or both. Hypogonadism is present causing both decreased spermatogenesis and decreased testosterone production. These factors combine to produce the subfertility state of the male with chronic renal failure that is little altered by dialysis. Successful transplantation greatly improves both libido and fertility, but it is important that the surgeon preserves the spermatic cord at operation (chapters 13, 19).

1. The kidney in pregnancy

During pregnancy anatomical and physiological changes take place in the normal kidney. Both kidneys increase in size (bi-polar diameter) and weight

Mary G. McGeown (ed.), Clinical Management of Renal Transplantation, 357–368.
© 1992 *Kluwer Academic Publishers, Dordrecht – Printed in the Netherlands.*

due to a combination of an increase in glomerular size and an increase in renal water content. More striking are the changes that occur in the collecting system. Dilatation of the calyces, pelves, and ureters is seen and is accompanied by hypertrophy of the ureteric smooth muscle and hyperplasia of the connective tissue. This causes stasis of urine and is one of the reasons for an increase in urinary infection in pregnancy.

Characteristic alterations also take place in glomerular filtration rate (GFR) and effective renal plasma flow (ERPF). Both increase early in the first trimester reaching a maximum by 9–11 weeks of gestation. The rise in GFR may be as much as 40–50% above non-pregnancy levels and that of ERPF 50–90% greater than non-pregnant levels. In the third trimester, particularly following the 36th week of gestation, both GFR and ERPF fall by about 15–20% and return to normal by the end of the third month postpartum. Tubular function alters during pregnancy with changes in acid-base balance and increased amounts of glucose, amino acids, and uric acid are excreted in the urine – it is not uncommon for pregnant women to be dipstick positive for glucose. Total body water is increased but blood pressure falls because of a relatively greater reduction in peripheral vascular resistance.

Similar anatomical and physiological changes occur throughout the pregnancy of a woman with renal transplant. The alterations in GFR and the changes in urinary protein excretion have been well documented and have been shown to be more pronounced with better pre-conception renal function. The increase in protein excretion is much greater in the transplanted female and can lead to diagnostic confusion. The dilatation of the collecting system and the short transplant ureter both increase the risk of acute pyelonephritis during pregnancy.

The effect of pregnancy on parenchymal renal disease is unclear and depends on the level of renal function. Certain conditions such as disseminated lupus appear more sensitive to changes of pregnancy. The physiological changes of the gravid state, particularly the greater degree of proteinuria make the interpretation of possible disease progression difficult.

2. Maternal complications

2.1. Hypertension

Hypertension is the commonest maternal ante-natal complication, occurring in 27–30% of patients. This is four times the incidence of pregnancy induced hypertension in non-transplanted pregnant females. A considerable proportion of the transplant population are hypertensive before pregnancy, and these women often require additional treatment or hospital admission to control their blood pressure during the pregnancy, particularly during the third trimester. Our own experience is similar to that reported in the literature with 26% of patients being hypertensive. However the true incidence of pre-eclampsia is uncertain as the diagnosis is difficult in the transplanted patient. Renal disease, and the transplant itself, may cause proteinuria, hypertension, oedema and deteriorating renal function. The best method of confirming the diagnosis is renal biopsy: this investigation however is infrequently carried out.

The treatment of hypertension in the pregnant transplant recipient is no different from that in any other pregnant female. Angiotensin-converting enzyme inhibitors should be avoided as animal studies have shown that these drugs decrease placental blood flow.

2.2. Graft dysfunction and acute rejection

The renal allograft undergoes the same changes in GFR during pregnancy as does the normal kidney, with a decline observed in the third trimester. In 15% of patients this decline in GFR persists post-partum and is the beginning of a steady progression to graft failure. It is not possible to predict which patients will be so affected, but if the serum creatinine before pregnancy is greater than 180 μmol/l the chances are significantly increased that graft dysfunction will progress following pregnancy. Thirty to forty percent of transplant recipients develop proteinuria during pregnancy. This reaches a maximum during the third trimester and disappears by the twelfth week post-partum. As glomerular hyperfiltration is thought to be implicated in the progression of a variety of renal diseases, there is speculation that the natural hyperfiltration of pregnancy is implicated in the progressive decline in GFR that is seen in 15% of patients after pregnancy. There has been however no convincing evidence to support this hypothesis.

Acute rejection episodes are seen in approximately 9% of patients during the course of pregnancy, which is similar to the incidence in non-pregnant transplanted individuals over the same period. This is somewhat unexpected as pregnancy is regarded as an immunologically privileged state and it might be anticipated that the frequency of rejection episodes would fall. There have been reports of a reduction in the requirements for immunosuppressive drugs during pregnancy, and in a very few cases even successful total withdrawal of immunosuppression. However it is not recommended that any alteration be made to immunosuppressive therapy during pregnancy. Clinically, acute rejection in pregnancy resembles acute rejection occurring in the non-pregnant state, with pyrexia, a swollen tender kidney, fall in urine output and rise in serum creatinine. It is advisable to confirm the diagnosis histologically as other conditions such as acute pyelonephritis (common in pregnancy), recurrent glomerulopathy, pre-eclampsia and cyclosporin (CYA) nephrotoxicity, may cause similar clinical pictures. The potential adverse effects of additional immunosuppressive therapy on the foetus require a firm diagnosis to be made before treatment is instituted.

2.3. *Infections during pregnancy*

All types of infection – bacterial, viral and fungal – are more likely to occur in pregnancy and are commoner in the immunosuppressed transplanted patient. These infections have varying potential to injure the foetus. Bacterial urinary infection is the commonest infection in pregnancy. Usually this is of low severity and responds promptly to antibiotic treatment with no adverse effect on the foetus. Of more importance however, are the potentially terato-genic viral infections such as cytomegalovirus (CMV), herpes virus and hepa-titis B, all of which are more prevalent in the transplant population. CMV infection has the most foetal damaging potential and can result in an acute illness at birth with jaundice and hepatosplenomegaly, microcephaly, growth and mental retardation, ocular and auditory defects and congenital heart disease.

2.4. *Parathyroid dysfunction*

After successful renal transplantation up to 20% of women develop tertiary hyperparathyroidism requiring parathyroidectomy. As calcium is actively transported across the placenta, especially during the third trimester when 80% of foetal skeletal calcification occurs, maternal hypercalcaemia can result in suppression of the foetal parathyroid glands. Consequently neonatal hypocalcaemia may occur and is a potential cause of seizures and brain damage. Conversely, if parathyroidectomy is performed and maternal hypo-calcaemia ensues, maternal convulsions and foetal parathyroid dysfunction become potential problems. It is therefore important to monitor carefully calcium and phosphate levels during pregnancy and prescribe calcium and vitamin D supplements as appropriate.

3. Foetal complications

At least 50–60% of the infants are born alive and healthy and have no neonatal problems. There have been reports of higher success rates with 70–80% of infants born without neonatal complications. This has been the case in our own series. However, there are certain foetal problems that occur more frequently in these high risk pregnancies.

3.1. *Prematurity*

Prematurity is a frequent occurrence with between 30–60% of deliveries taking place before 37 weeks of gestation. The high incidence of prematurity is multifactorial in aetiology. Impaired renal function, urinary tract infection and pyelonephritis, intrauterine infection, and pregnancy induced hypertension, all may contribute to the early onset of labour. However the commonest reason for delivery occurring before the 37th week of gestation is premature rupture of the membranes, which occurs in 20–40% of pregnancies. It is believed that the higher rate of infection that exists in the immunosuppressed patient is partly to blame, although it has also been postulated that steroid therapy weakens the amniotic membrane by altering the composition of the connective tissue.

The average maturity at delivery is 34–35 weeks gestation, a figure repeated in our own series, which had a prematurity rate of 55% mainly due to premature rupture of the membranes.

3.2. Growth retardation

After transplantation between 15 and 20% of pregnancies are associated with infants who are born small for gestational age – birth weight below the 10th centile – a rate greater than that of the non-transplant population. Hypertension, which has a high prevalence in transplanted individuals, contributes significantly to intrauterine growth retardation, mainly by its effect on the placenta. Chronic renal impairment is another of the factors involved in the aetiology of this problem. Concern has been recently expressed that CYA has an adverse effect on intrauterine growth. Pickrell et al reported in 1988 a series of cases of growth retarded infants born to women taking CYA, in which there was no other obvious cause for the growth retardation. However there have been no other subsequent reports, and information provided by the manufacturers does not show evidence to implicate CYA as a cause of intrauterine growth retardation.

3.3. Congenital abnormalities

A review of the current literature suggests that congenital abnormalities do not occur any more frequently among the children of transplanted women than in the rest of the population. The overall incidence of congenital abnormalities appears to be less than 3%. This is reassuring considering the teratogenic potential of the various drugs that these women are obliged to take. As one would expect, there are a considerable number of case reports of different malformations occurring in infants born to women taking immunosuppressive drugs but very little definite evidence of a causal relationship between drug and malformation.

3.3.1. *Azathioprine.* Azathioprine has been shown to be teratogenic in animals but only at much higher concentrations (6 mg/kg/day) than are used in clinical transplantation. Transient gaps and breaks in lymphocyte chromosomes may be caused by azathioprine but these usually disappear 5–32 weeks after transplantation. However germ cell and other tissues have not been studied, and more permanent chromosome damage may occur in these tissues. We have performed lymphocyte chromosomal analysis on children born to parents who had been transplanted and were taking azathioprine. Chromosomal abnormalities were detected in less than 10% of the children tested with a mean rate of cell damage of 3.3%. The foetus may be protected from damage by azathioprine because at the time of organogenesis it does not possess the enzyme inosinate pyrophosphorylase which converts azathioprine to thioinosinic acid, the metabolite that is active on dividing cells.

3.3.2. *Prednisolone*. While animal studies have suggested that prednisolone causes intrauterine growth retardation, and abnormalities such as cleft lip and cleft palate, human experience of steroids used therapeutically in pregnancy has not revealed the same problems. The active metabolite of prednisolone does not appear to cross the placental barrier in large quantities, measured levels in the foetal circulation being one tenth of those in the maternal blood. Maternal side effects of steroid therapy – hypertension, hyperglycaemia and increased susceptibility to infection – may themselves predispose to foetal problems.

3.3.3. *Cyclosporin*. The experience of CYA in pregnancy is limited to reports of small groups of patients, usually less than 10. Most of the information available is from data collected by the manufacturer. They have information on 166 pregnancies in 157 patients. Cyclosporin crosses the placental barrier achieving foetal blood levels similar to those in the maternal circulation. There is therefore a potential for neonatal nephrotoxicity; however Sandoz report only one infant having significant renal dysfunction at birth and requiring dialysis. It would seem prudent to minimise the dose of CYA prescribed to the expectant mother.

The data provided by the manufacturer reveal that 50% of live births were of low birth weight (below 2500 g) with 22% below the tenth centile. Seventy-five per cent of the infants were healthy at birth.

Sandoz have documented 6 cases where the infant was born with a congenital malformation. There is no evidence to date that CYA is teratogenic in animals. *In vitro* studies of chromosomal function have shown the potential of CYA to induce mutagenic changes. Cyclosporin has been shown to impair spermatogenesis and sperm maturation in rats.

4. Obstetrical aspects

4.1. *Abortion*

In many series the loss in the first trimester exceeds 40%. This high early foetal loss can be attributed partly to the large number of therapeutic abortions that take place. Some 22–28% of pregnancies are electively ended in the first trimester. The indications for therapeutic abortion include significant hypertension or renal impairment prior to conception, worsening hypertension or renal function during pregnancy, uncertainty about the maternal risk of a continuing pregnancy, the possibility of hereditary renal disease, uncertainty about the longterm maternal prognosis and the subsequent loss of parental care, and the various psychosocial problems that accompany an unplanned pregnancy. This latter indication is probably the most common as women, who have become used to the subfertile state of uraemia, often do not realise that they have returned to a fertile state and therefore do not take adequate contraceptive measures. Spontaneous abortion occurs in 13–16% of pregnancies, a rate similar to that of the normal pregnant population.

4.2. *Ectopic pregnancy*

Transplanted patients are at greater risk of ectopic pregnancy. The incidence of ectopic pregnancy in the reported series ranges from 0.2–0.5%. In this group of patients pelvic adhesions are more common, either as a result of previous surgery or CAPD related peritonitis, and predispose to ectopic pregnancy. This diagnosis can be difficult to make because irregular bleeding and amenorrhoea may accompany both deteriorating renal function and extrauterine pregnancy. A misdiagnosis is the more likely because pelvic symptomatology is often attributed to the transplanted kidney with less consideration given to the possibility of symptoms arising from other pelvic organs.

4.3. *Delivery*

Vaginal delivery is preferable and caesarian section should be reserved for purely obstetrical indications, and if possible performed electively. However the reported caesarian section rate is approximately 25% – higher than would be expected. This probably reflects a high degree of clinical caution, although pelvic abnormalities are more common – renal osteodystrophy and avascular necrosis of the hip – and provide an additional indication for caesarian section. In our series 8 out of 23 (35%) pregnancies were delivered by caesarian section though all had accepted obstetrical indications.

The renal allograft is located in the false pelvis and therefore in normal circumstances does not interfere with vaginal delivery. Neither does vaginal delivery cause damage to the transplanted kidney. Because of the immunocompromised state of the mother, rigorous aseptic technique is important to prevent maternal sepsis and prophylactic antibiotics should be administered when instrumentation is required. During the period of induction and delivery, when oral intake may be curtailed it is advisable to administer immunosuppressive drugs intravenously. The additional stress of labour necessitates increasing the dose of steroid given to those women on longterm prednisolone therapy. Our practice is to administer 100 mg hydrocortisone intravenously at the onset of labour and again at the end of delivery.

5. Pre-pregnancy counselling

Ideally pregnancies after transplantation should be planned to take place when the prospective mother is in good health with stable renal function and conditions are optimum for achieving a successful outcome. The reduced life expectancy of the transplant recipient necessitates that consideration should be given to the social setting into which the child will be born, as the possibility exists that the mother will not survive to bring up the child. (Ten percent of mothers with allografts die within 7 years of childbirth). Survival following transplantation is maximum amongst those patients who have normal renal function at two years. We therefore would recommend that pregnancy should be postponed for at least two years following transplantation, at which stage immunosuppressive therapy will have been reduced to baseline. There is some evidence to suggest that this is associated with enhanced birthweight.

When counselling potential mothers certain additional guidelines are recommended that should maximise the chances of an uncomplicated, successful pregnancy:
- normotensive
- no evidence of rejection
- minimal/absent proteinuria
- serum creatinine less than 180 μmol/l (preferably less than 130 μmol/l)
- stature compatible with good obstetrical outcome
- azathioprine less than 2 mg/kg, CYA less than 5 mg/kg, prednisolone 10 mg/day or less

6. Antenatal care

The confinements of women with renal allografts should be regarded as high risk pregnancies and should be managed as such in a specialist referral centre. The team approach is best with obstetrician, nephrologist, and in the latter stages, paediatrician, all involved and where appropriate a diabetic physician. It is generally recommended that after early referral the patient should be seen at least every two weeks until the thirty-second week of gestation, and then weekly until term. As well as clinical assessment it is important to monitor closely mother, maternal renal function, and foetal progress. Each visit should include measurement of blood pressure, urinary protein, biochemical markers of renal function, haematological parameters, CYA level, if taking this drug, and urine culture. At least once each trimester calcium and phosphate levels should be assessed, and maternal blood checked for evidence of infection with cytomegalovirus and herpes simplex virus, the presence of hepatitis B antigens and antibodies, and also for the presence of circulating antibodies that may cause haemolytic disease of the newborn (these women often have had multiple blood transfusions).

The full array of modern foetal assessment techniques should be available and be used appropriately. Regular ultrasound scans and other non-invasive tests should be carried out. Other investigations should be undertaken where obstetrically indicated. Monitoring of urinary oestriol is not useful in transplanted patients as levels are usually low, both as a result of adrenal suppression by steroid therapy and the presence of an abnormal excretory pattern by the transplanted kidney. If oral steroids are part of the immunosuppressive regime an oral glucose tolerance test should be performed during the pregnancy.

Pregnant allograft recipients may need a considerable amount of counselling both before and during the pregnancy. They will have considerably more concerns and questions than non-transplanted women. Is pregnancy advisable? Will the pregnancy be complicated? Will it do any harm to my kidney? Will it produce a healthy child? Such women often need more emotional and psychological support than other pregnant women and facilities to meet this need should be available during the pregnancy and puerperium. This may best be achieved by having a specified midwife/obstetric nurse involved with the patient throughout her confinement.

7. Contraception

This is an important matter and recipients need counselling before discharge from hospital and preferably before transplantation. The high incidence of therapeutic abortions for unwanted pregnancies suggests that this area of management requires improving.

Barrier methods of contraception, e.g. diaphragm or sheath, have the least risk to the patient but are not the most efficient. However we would recommend these as the preferred methods. The oral contraceptive pill is the most efficient method but possesses the accompanying risks of increased thromboembolic disease and aggravation of hypertension. These complications may be reduced by the use of the low-dose combined oestrogen/progesterone pill or the progesterone only preparation. Oral contraceptives should be restricted to those women who are normotensive, non-smokers and have no other medical condition likely to be aggravated by the treatment. For those women where the risk of non-compliance is high and the risks of pregnancy (medical and social) are great, depot preparations of progesterone may be considered.

Intra-uterine contraceptive devices (IUCD) are generally not recommended. They are associated with menstrual irregularities which may obscure the signs and symptoms of abnormalities of early pregnancy. Immunosuppressed women are more at risk of IUCD-associated pelvic infections and there is also some evidence that the IUCD is less effective in the immunosuppressed individual as a result of alterations in the leucocyte response. Where appropriate, sterilisation should be considered early.

Following transplantation an annual cervical smear should be performed as the risk of cervical neoplasia is thirteen times greater in immunosuppressed women.

8. Breast feeding

Breast feeding has many advantages, both to the mother by accelerating involution of the uterus and by decreasing ovulation and therefore the risk of an immediate second pregnancy, and to the infant from enhanced nutrition and the transfer of immunoglobulins and immunocompetent cells. Prednisolone, CYA, and to a lesser extent azathioprine and its metabolites, are excreted in breast milk. The amount of steroid excreted is less than required to have a therapeutic effect and as the infant has been exposed to azathioprine or CYA throughout the gestation it could be argued that breast feeding is not contraindicated. However there is no definitive evidence to support this assumption and most centres recommend that breast feeding should be avoided.

9. Reproduction and the male recipient

Successful transplantation also improves male fertility. A considerable number of the partners of male recipients conceive in the months following transplantation. Little has been written about these children but there does not appear to be any increase in the number of congenital abnormalities. Our own studies have shown a very low incidence of chromosomal abnormalities in children whose fathers have received a renal transplant. Ten children were studied, one was a Trisomy 21 but the other nine were normal, with a mean chromosome damage rate of 1.4% cells (within the normal range). Penn et al. reported only two congenital abnormalities in their series of 60 babies.

Often such pregnancies are unexpected/unplanned with resultant social and family upsets, particularly if the other siblings have grown up. Because of the increased mortality of transplant recipients there is the possibility of the premature death of a parent with its subsequent social problems. It is therefore important to counsel male recipients (as well as female recipients)

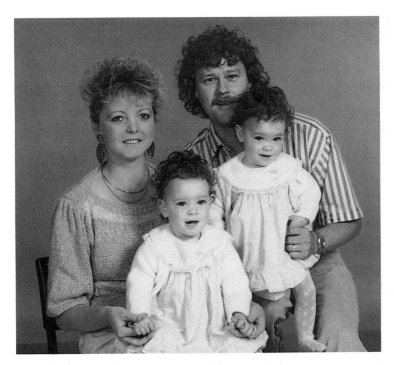

Figure 65. A 31 year-old transplant recipient with her identical twin daughters, aged 1 year.

about improved fertility after transplantation and the need to take appropriate contraceptive measures.

Conclusion

The improvement in fertility that occurs following successful renal transplantation allows the young woman with chronic renal failure to greatly enhance her life by becoming a mother. This is strikingly illustrated in Figure 65 which shows a 31 year-old woman, transplanted 3 years previously, with her two identical twin daughters, aged 1 year. The fulfilment of the desire for a child should not be denied if not strongly contraindicated on medical grounds.

If the guidelines for successful outcome are followed and the appropriate specialist medical attention received from an early stage, and ideally before conception, the success rate for pregnancy following transplantation is high. The close co-operation between all disciplines involved is one of the keys to success. There are no doubt inherent risks for both mother and foetus and every effort must be made to minimise these. The importance of supportive and compassionate counselling cannot be over-emphasized. Future research should be directed at understanding the pathophysiology of the problems

368

specific to this group of patients, especially hypertension, pre-eclampsia and graft dysfunction, and how best these can be managed.

Further reading

Brown, J. H., Maxwell, A. P., McGeown, M. G. *Outcome of pregnancy following renal transplantation: the Belfast experience. Irish J. Med. Sci.* 1991; 160: 255–256.

Davison, J. M. Pregnancy in renal allograft recipients: prognosis and management. *Clin. Obstet. Gynecol.* 1987; 1: 1027–1045.

Gaudier, F. L., Santiago-Delpin, E., Rivera, J., Gonzales, Z. Pregnancy after renal transplantation. *Surg. Gyn. Obstet.* 1988; 167: 533–543.

Hou, S. Pregnancy in organ transplant recipients. *Med. Clin. North. Am.* 1989; 73: 667–683.

McGeown, M. G., Houston, J. K. Chronic renal disease. *Clin. Obstet. Gynecol.* 1982; 9: 101–113.

Penn, I, Makowski, E. L. Harris, P. Parenthood following renal transplantation. *Kid. Int.* 1980; 18: 221–233.

CHAPTER 25

Results of renal transplantation

MARY G. McGEOWN

Comparisons made between the results of different centres, combined with careful descriptions of the methods of treatment should make it possible to decide on the best form of treatment. However it is very difficult to ensure that the comparisons between different centres are valid. Many factors need to be considered when deciding whether groups of patients are comparable. These include those which may affect the life expectancy of the patient, irrespective of the presence of the graft (i.e. those that would be present if the patient continued on dialysis and did not have a renal transplant) and those which primarily affect the survival of the graft (Table 49). Some of

Table 49. Factors which affect patient and graft survival

Factor	Patient survival	Graft survival
Source of kidney (live or cadaver)	−	+
Age	+	−
Severe cardiac disease	+	±
Severe hypertension	+	±
Insulin dependant diabetes mellitus	+	±
Systemic infection (tuberculosis)	+	−
Disseminated collagen disease	+	±
Severe pulmonary disease	+	−
Severe malnutrition	+	−
Severe obesity	+	−
Amyloidosis	+	+
Severe psychiatric disturbance	±	+
Oxalosis, cystinosis, Fabry's disease	±	+
Urinary diversion required	±	±
Type of glomerulonephritis	−	+
High level cytotoxic antibodies	−	+
Blood transfusion	−	+
High antigen mis-match	−	+
Repeat transplantation	−	+
Immunosuppression	+	+
Length of time on dialysis	+	−
"Centre effect"	+	+

Mary G. McGeown (ed.), Clinical Management of Renal Transplantation, 369–377.
© 1992 *Kluwer Academic Publishers, Dordrecht. Printed in the Netherlands.*

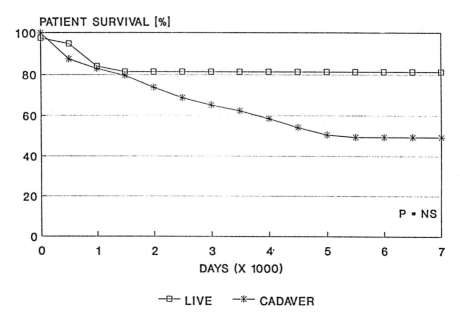

Figure 66. Acturial patient survival after live and cadaveric transplantation.

course may affect both life expectancy and graft survival, one more than the other, or the effect may be indirect – a patient with a severe psychiatric disturbance may fail to take the necessary immunosuppressive drugs.

Multifactorial analysis should make possible valid comparisons between results from different centres, but since the number of factors to be taken into account is large, a very large number of patients in each group is needed. Many centres, including our own, have performed more than 500 renal transplants, and some more than 1000, but even these numbers when sub-divided into groups for the numerous factors involved, are not sufficient for satisfactory multifactorial analysis. Several studies combine results from many centres to give large numbers of patients, but this approach simply multiplies the differences.

The results from the Belfast centre can perhaps provide some pointers to factors of importance for the survival of patients and grafts. The methods used here, already discussed in detail in the earlier chapters, changed rela-tively little from 1968 until the end of 1988.

Kidneys taken from live related donors have usually been associated with higher graft and patient survival rates than those from cadavers. The source of the kidney has therefore an important bearing on the result. As already stated, the Belfast centre has used mainly cadaveric donors throughout and the results of cadaveric and live donation are shown as separate lines in Figures 66 and 67.

For primary cadaveric (417) and primary live (38) donations the results

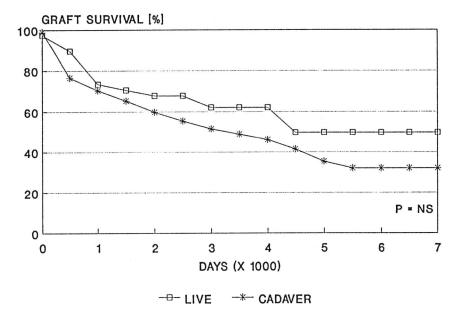

Figure 67. Actuarial graft survival after live and cadaveric transplantation.

of patient and graft survival do not differ significantly up to 7000 days (19 years). However the number of live donations is small.

During the first half of the period under review the age of the recipients at time of transplantation was 15 to 50 years, later 7 to 56, and finally patients were accepted at any age provided they were considered fit to undergo surgery. The age of the recipient did not affect significantly the results of transplantation of our patients, but as the numbers of older patients receiving transplants increases more may be expected to suffer from severe cardiac and peripheral vascular disease.

During the first five years of our programme patients were excluded if they had a previous history of myocardial infarction, cerebrovascular accident, severe disease in other organs, or insulin dependant diabetes mellitus. Gradually these conditions for exclusion were abandoned as transplants succeeded in patients marginally unfit in one or other system. Patients with severe hypertension had been accepted from the beginning. About 80% of patients with end-stage renal failure have hypertension and to exclude hypertensive patients would exclude the great majority of those needing transplantation. After transplants succeeded (for long periods) in two patients who had been turned down for coronary bypass operation because of the severity of their coronary disease, patients were accepted for transplantation irrespective of their cardiac condition. Indeed several had coronary bypass operations in preparation for successful transplants. Longer experience has shown that transplantation should not be offered to all patients with cardiac problems. Intractable heart failure despite good dialysis is a contra-indication to transplantation. Severe rare cardiac malformations also contra-indicate transplantation.

From 1978 onwards occasional patients with insulin dependant diabetes mellitus were accepted for dialysis and transplantation. As older non-insulin dependant diabetic patients are accepted more can be expected to have intractable cardiovascular problems. Patients were treated who had disseminated collagen disease, primary amyloidosis, bronchiectasis (in a patient whose renal disease was later found to be due to amyloid), severe malnutrition or severe obesity (one patient weighed 110 kg), urinary diversion, or moderately severe psychiatric disturbance. The psychiatric patients proved very difficult to treat by dialysis, three lapsed from treatment and one had a transplant but died within a short time of discharge after failing to take the immunosuppressive drugs and refusing to attend hospital.

During the early part of the transplantation programme in Belfast, either good bladder function or an ileal conduit was regarded as essential, and if a conduit had not been fashioned already one was prepared before the patient was put on the recipient list. More recently we have found that careful assessment of bladder function quite often shows that the patient's own bladder can be used. Other patients can be taught to carry out self-catheterisation safely. None of the patients had active tuberculosis or known infection at the time of transplantation, although several were known to have had tuberculosis in the past.

The significance of the type of disease in those patients who originally had some type of glomerulonephritis has been fully discussed in Chapter 18.

Immunological details of the patients including the degree of tissue match obtained, number of recipients highly sensitized, and the effect of match grade and sensitization on graft and patient survival have been described already in Chapter 9 (Figures 22 to 27). The concept of beneficial matching has been discussed. Patients with zero mismatch had a significantly higher graft survival than those with five or six antigens mismatched. There was a significant improvement in graft survival with fewer mismatches at the HLA-A locus but not at the -DR locus (however only 45 recipients received a kidney with two HLA-DR mismatches). No difference was associated with increasing number of mismatches at the -B locus. Long before the introduction of HLA-DR matching Belfast had reported a one year cadaveric graft survival rate of 82%.

In this analysis only "broad" antigens have been considered. Over the last 10 years an increasing number of "antigen splits" have been recognised, although many laboratories cannot type for these because of lack of suitable sera. Opelz has found in an analysis of a very large number of first cadaver grafts that when splits are used there is a much better correlation between matching and graft survival. Using splits he finds a difference of over 30% between zero and six antigen matches.

Long term graft survival is much reduced in highly sensitized patients. High current panel reactive antibody (PRA) level is associated with 44%

reduction in graft survival at 10 years, and similarly elevated historic PRA with 30% reduction (Chapter 9, Figures 26 and 27).

There is another important reason which is often over-looked when searching for a good tissue match for the first graft. High sensitization, especially in male patients, often results from a previous failed graft. It is therefore important to avoid giving grafts carrying mismatched antigens. It is particularly important to avoid mismatched common antigens, which will make it very difficult to find a second or subsequent graft, should the first one be rejected.

Opelz and Terasaki reported in 1973 that pretransplant blood transfusion had a beneficial effect on renal allograft survival, and the improvement was later shown to be between 10 and 20%. More recent studies have questioned the benefit of transfusion in patients given CYA and it has been suggested that the transfusion benefit is present only when the immunosuppression is azathioprine and prednisolone. The less obvious improvement associated with blood transfusion in recent times may be attributed at least in part to the improvement in early graft survival seen generally. However, Opelz's on-going study (1992) suggests that blood transfusion is still beneficial.

While blood transfusion may lead to cytotoxic antibody formation this is not usually significant in patients not previously sensitized by pregnancy or a previous failed graft. Unnecessary transfusions should be avoided in such patients. In general transfused patients do not have to wait longer for kidneys than non-transfused ones.

All except six of our patients received pretransplant transfusions.

The very important effect of immunosuppressive drugs on both patient and graft survival has been discussed in Chapter 15. The patients shown in Figures 63 and 64 (Chapter 25) were transplanted between 1968 and 31 December 1988. All received azathioprine and low dose steroid following the regime described in Chapter 15. From the beginning of 1989 onwards CYA began to be introduced for individual patients and it was some time before a clear-cut policy for its use was evolved. The end of 1988 was chosen as the end-point of the report as there had been no significant changes in immunosuppressive therapy throughout the entire period.

The length of time on dialysis prior to transplantation has some bearing on the results of the latter. The nutritional state may become poor in patients on CAPD who have repeated bouts of peritonitis. Longer term haemodialysis may necessitate repeated blood transfusions and a greater hazard of a high degree of sensitization, though this problem should be reduced by the more general use of erythropoetin for treatment of anaemia in patients with chronic renal failure.

Dialysis amyloidosis, associated with very high B_2 microglobulin levels, seldom develops before five years on dialysis but after that is increasingly common in patients treated by haemodialysis, less so in those on CAPD. The commonest symptoms are joint pains, particularly affecting shoulders, due to deposition of amyloid in joint capsules, synovium, articular cartilage,

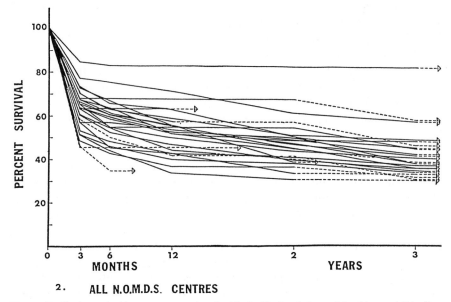

PERCENT SURVIVAL

MONTHS   YEARS

2.   ALL N.O.M.D.S. CENTRES

Figure 68. Graft survival in centres associated with the National Organ Matching and Distribution Centre, 1976. Each line represents one centre. Interrupted lines indicate fewer than 10 grafts per annum over this period.

bone and tendons, but the most disabling problem is a severe form of carpal tunnel syndrome. There is some evidence of resorption of amyloid after transplantation, but it is best avoided by early transplantation.

The last factor listed in Table 49 is the so-called "centre effect". By this is meant the innumerable small differences in the management of renal transplantation found when the details of practice of one centre are compared with that of another. This was the subject of two surveys arranged by the British Transplantation Society and carried out, with an interval of five years between them by the three "wise men". The "wise men" were senior, highly respected members, two of whom have been Presidents of the Society. They visited eight centres (those represented by the four top and bottom lines shown in Figure 68 which shows cadaveric transplants only; it is noteworthy that the top line represents the results of Belfast). Exhaustive enquiries were made into all aspects of transplantation, including the factors listed in Table 49. In the first study 50 consecutive first cadaveric grafts were scrutinized, and in the second 100 consecutive cadaveric grafts immediately prior to the date of the study. In the second study second and subsequent grafts, and live donations were also scrutinized. By the time of the second study the difference in cadaveric graft survival at one year between the best and worst centres had narrowed (54–81%), but the "centre effect" was still important. Patient survival was not different between the two studies. At the time of the second study, Belfast was the one centre using azathioprine and low dose steroid as the only immunosuppression, yet still remained amongst the centres with the best results. One commentator on the study remarked on the rather disappointing effect of CYA as the main immunosuppressive therapy. It was noted that the use of CYA seemed to have helped most the centres with the poorest results at the time of the first study. They concluded that the "centre effect" had a greater influence on the results than any other individual factor.

Belfast results

The good survival rate of patients and grafts during the first year after transplantation (the one year cumulative survival rate for the first 100 grafts was 82%) contributed greatly to the long term survival shown in Figures 66 and 67.

The remarkably low early death rate from infection (two patients died before eight months) was probably due to both the low dose of steroid from the beginning and stringent criteria for its use in the treatment of rejection, and the precautions taken to protect the patients from hospital-borne infection.

Although seven patients died from infection, five deaths occurred after eight months. This figure included two with subacute bacterial endocarditis (one following surgery for aortic stenosis); four due to pulmonary infection, and one from sepsis following removal of a Thomas shunt removed more than three years previously.

Cardiovascular disease was the commonest cause of death following transplantation, causing 49% (24 of 51) of deaths which occurred before 10 years. More effort needs to be made to encourage patients with chronic renal failure to stop smoking and to modify their dietary habits.

The increased incidence of neoplasia in patients receiving immunosuppression is well recognised. In this series there were five deaths from malignant neoplasms (including one patient from acute monoblastic leukaemia) within 10 years and four deaths later (2 at 11 and 2 at 12.5 years after transplantation). Skin neoplasia, of squamous and basal cell type, has occurred in at least 10 transplant recipients, some of whom have had multiple lesions. None have died but the number with skin neoplasms increases with time, in spite of warnings to avoid as much as possible exposure to sunlight, and to use sun-screen cream when exposed.

Acute rejection was a surprisingly infrequent cause of graft failure, accounting for 19 graft losses. However slow decline in graft function led to the loss of six further grafts before 10 years after surgery. When histology was available, sclerosed glomeruli and interstitial fibrosis with tubular loss dominated the picture, sometimes with vascular thickening. These lesions were probably the end result of earlier acute rejection, but two patients had not received anti-rejection therapy as there had been at no time clinical suspicion of rejection. One lost three grafts in this way, each of which had functioned for from three to five years.

The rehabilitation of the patients, including the fertility of females of child-bearing age and excellent fertility of the males after transplantation has been described in Chapters 23 and 24.

Avascular necrosis of the head of femur (or other joint surfaces) is a very disabling complication of transplantation. Fortunately only two patients have developed it, though in one young woman it occurred in both hips. She was given the usual increased dose of oral steroid once only for an early severe episode of rejection after which excellent graft function returned. The low incidence of avascular necrosis is probably related to the sparing use of steroid.

Conclusion

Azathioprine combined with low dose steroid without other imunosuppression has given good long term graft and patient survival in our hands. Any method of immunosuppression must be judged by the incidence of serious side effects it produces as well as its efficacy in preventing rejection. The incidence of side effects we have encountered while not negligible is relatively modest. The combination of these two drugs seems to give adequate immunosuppression for the majority of recipients, and is relatively easy to prescribe. The results of CYA, with or without steroid for maintenance therapy have not been shown so far to be better in the longer term than the combination of azathioprine and low dose steroid. Cyclosporin is a more difficult drug in use, because of its nephrotoxicity and interaction with many other drugs which may be necessary for these patients. It has unpleasant side effects, including hirsutism, gum hypertrophy (in which squamous cell carcinomatous change recurring after removal and metastasizing has just been reported), and coarsening of the features, which are difficult to accept for those who develop them.

It is my personal opinion that the initial treatment for most patients receiving their first graft should be azathioprine combined with low dose steroid. Cyclosporin should be considered for patients noted to have leucopoenia when on dialysis, in whom the white cell count remains low during the first few days after transplantation, or who do not tolerate the usual doses of azathioprine we have used at later stages; and for the patient who has rejected more than one previous graft. The addition of CYA may be helpful when a rejection episode has proved to be steroid resistant. However a short course of ALG or OKT3 may be more effective than CYA in this situation. The future may give us new drugs more suited to our patients' needs.

The Holy Grail we seek is a safe, non-toxic totally effective immunosuppressive drug. This has not yet been found. The shortage of donor kidneys is a continuing problem for all transplant centres, to which we must all address ourselves. There are still some hospitals who never contribute donors yet continue to refer patients who need renal replacement therapy.

Further reading

Briggs, J. D. Renal transplantation. *Quart. J. Med.* 1989; 267: 589–597.

Cook, D. J. Long-term survival of kidney allograft. In Terasaki, P. ed. *Clinical Transplants.* Los Angeles; UCLA Tissue Typing Laboratory 1987: 277–285.

McGeown, M. G., Douglas, J. F., Brown, W. A. *et al.* Advantages of low dose steroid from the day after renal transplantation. *Transplantation* 1980; 29: 287–289.

McGeown, M. G., Doherty, C. C., Douglas, J. F. *et al.* Ten year results of renal transplantation using only azathioprine and low dose prednisolone as immunosuppression. In Terasaki, P. ed. *Clinical Transplants.* Los Angeles; UCLA Tissue Typing Laboratory, 1989: 191–199.

Middleton, D., Gillespie, E. L., Doherty, C. C. *et al.* The influence of HLA-A, -B and -DR matching on graft survival in primary cadaveric renal transplantation in Belfast. *Transplantation* 1985; 39: 608–610.

Opelz, G. Comparison of immunosuppressive protocols in renal transplantation: a multicenter view. *Transplantation Proc.* 1988; 20, Suppl. 8: 31–36.

Index

380

Developments in Nephrology

1. J.S. Cheigh, K.H. Stenzel and A.L. Rubin (eds.): *Manual of Clinical Nephrology of the Rogosin Kidney Center*. 1981   ISBN 90-247-2397-3
2. K.D. Nolph (ed.): *Peritoneal Dialysis*. 1981 ed.: out of print
   3rd revised and enlarged ed. 1988 (not in this series)   ISBN 0-89838-406-0
3. A.B. Gruskin and M.E. Norman (eds.): *Pediatric Nephrology*. 1981
                                                                 ISBN 90-247-2514-3
4. O. Schück: *Examination of the Kidney Function*. 1981   ISBN 0-89838-565-2
5. J. Strauss (ed.): *Hypertension, Fluid-electrolytes and Tubulopathies in Pediatric Nephrology*. 1982   ISBN 90-247-2633-6
6. J. Strauss (ed.): *Neonatal Kidney and Fluid-electrolytes*. 1983   ISBN 0-89838-575-X
7. J. Strauss (ed.): *Acute Renal Disorders and Renal Emergencies*. 1984
                                                                 ISBN 0-89838-663-2
8. L.J.A. Didio and P.M. Motta (eds.): *Basic, Clinical, and Surgical Nephrology*. 1985
                                                                 ISBN 0-89838-698-5
9. E.A. Friedman and C.M. Peterson (eds.): *Diabetic Nephropathy*. Strategy for Therapy.
   1985   ISBN 0-89838-735-3
10. R. Dzúrik, B. Lichardus and W. Guder: *Kidney Metabolism and Function*. 1985
                                                                 ISBN 0-89838-749-3
11. J. Strauss (ed.): *Homeostasis, Nephrotoxicy, and Renal Anomalies in the Newborn*.
    1986   ISBN 0-89838-766-3
12. D.G. Oreopoulos (ed.): *Geriatric Nephrology*. 1986   ISBN 0-89838-781-7
13. E.P. Paganini (ed.): *Acute Continuous Renal Replacement Therapy*. 1986
                                                                 ISBN 0-89838-793-0
14. J.S. Cheigh, K.H. Stenzel and A.L. Rubin (eds.): *Hypertension in Kidney Disease*. 1986
                                                                 ISBN 0-89838-797-3
15. N. Deane, R.J. Wineman and G.A. Benis (eds.): *Guide to Reprocessing of Hemodialyzers*. 1986   ISBN 0-89838-798-1
16. C. Ponticelli, L. Minetti and G. D'Amico (eds.): *Antiglobulins, Cryoglobulins and Glomerulonephritis*. 1986   ISBN 0-89838-810-4
17. J. Strauss (ed.) with the assistence of L. Strauss: *Persistent Renalgenitourinary Disorders*. 1987   ISBN 0-89838-845-7
18. V.E. Andreucci and A. Dal Canton (eds.): *Diuretics*. Basic, Pharmacological, and Clinical Aspects. 1987   ISBN 0-89838-885-6
19. P.H. Bach and E.H. Lock (eds.): *Nephrotoxicity in the Experimental and Clinical Situation*, Part 1. 1987   ISBN 0-89838-997-1
20. P.H. Bach and E.H. Lock (eds.): *Nephrotoxicity in the Experimental and Clinical Situation*, Part 2. 1987   ISBN 0-89838-980-2
21. S.M. Gore and B.A. Bradley (eds.): *Renal Transplantation*. Sense and Sensitization.
    1988   ISBN 0-89838-370-6
22. L. Minetti, G. D'Amico and C. Ponticelli: *The Kidney in Plasma Cell Dyscrasias*. 1988
                                                                 ISBN 0-89838-385-4
23. A.S. Lindblad, J.W. Novak and K.D. Nolph (eds.): *Continuous Ambulatory Peritoneal Dialysis in the USA*. Final Report of the National CAPD Registry 1981–1988. 1989
                                                                 ISBN 0-7923-0179-X

Developments in Nephrology

Kluwer Academic Publishers – Dordrecht / Boston / London